P9-DIG-206

Physicians'
Cancer Chemotherapy
Drug Manual
2010

Other Jones and Bartlett Oncology Titles

Breast Cancer Treatment by Focused Microwave Thermotherapy, Fenn

Cancer in Children, Carroll/Finlay *NEW*

Dx/Rx: Breast Cancer, Lake

Dx/Rx: Cervical Cancer, Dizon/Robinson

Dx/Rx: Colorectal Cancer, Holen/Chung

Dx/Rx: Genitourinary Oncology, Galsky

Dx/Rx: Leukemia, Burke

Dx/Rx: Lung Cancer, Azzoli

Dx/Rx: Lymphoma, Persky

Dx/Rx: Palliative Cancer Care, Malhotra/Moryl

Dx/Rx: Prostate Cancer, Kampel

Dx/Rx: Upper Gastrointestinal Malignancies: Cancers of the Stomach and Esophagus, Shah, also Series Editor

Glioblastoma Multiforme, Markert, et al.

Gynecologic Tumor Board: Clinical Cases in Diagnosis and Mgmt of Cancer of the Female Reproductive System, Dizon/Abu-Rustum

Handbook of Breast Cancer Risk-Assessment, Vogel/Bevers

Handbook of Cancer Emergencies, Marinella *NEW*

Handbook of Cancer Risk Assessment and Prevention, Colditz/Stein

Handbook of Radiation Oncology: Basic Principles and Clinical Protocols, Haffty/Wilson

Hospital for Sick Kids, Handbook of Supportive Care in Pediatric Oncology, Abla *NEW*

How Cancer Works, Sompayrac

Management of Nausea and Vomiting in Cancer and Cancer Treatment, Hesketh

Medical and Psychosocial Care of the Cancer Survivor, Miller *NEW*

Molecular Oncology of Breast Cancer, Ross/Hortobagyi

Molecular Oncology of Prostate Cancer, Ross/Foster

Pancreatic Cancer, Von Hoff/Evans/Hruban

Pediatric Stem Cell Transplantation, Metha

Pocket Guide to Cancer Chemotherapy Protocols, 6e, Chu

Pocket Guide to Hematologic Cancer Chemotherapy Protocols, Chu *NEW*

Pocket Guide to Targeted Therapies in Cancer, Chu *NEW*

The Johns Hopkins Breast Cancer Handbook for Health Care Professionals, Shockney/Tsangaris

For a complete list of our oncology titles see *www.jbpub.com/oncology*

Physicians' Cancer Chemotherapy Drug Manual 2010

Edward Chu, MD

Deputy Director, Yale Cancer Center
Chief, Section of Medical Oncology
Professor of Medicine and Pharmacology
Yale University School of Medicine
New Haven, CT

Vincent T. DeVita, Jr., MD

Amy and Joseph Perella Professor of Medicine
Professor of Epidemiology and Public Health
Yale University School of Medicine
New Haven, CT

JONES AND BARTLETT PUBLISHERS

Sudbury, Massachusetts

BOSTON   TORONTO   LONDON   SINGAPORE

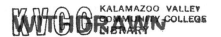

World Headquarters

Jones and Bartlett Publishers	Jones and Bartlett Publishers	Jones and Bartlett Publishers
40 Tall Pine Drive	Canada	International
Sudbury, MA 01776	6339 Ormindale Way	Barb House, Barb Mews
978-443-5000	Mississauga, Ontario L5V 1J2	London W6 7PA
info@jbpub.com	Canada	United Kingdom
www.jbpub.com		

Jones and Bartlett's books and products are available through most bookstores and online booksellers. To contact Jones and Bartlett Publishers directly, call 800-832-0034, fax 978-443-8000, or visit our website, www.jbpub.com.

Substantial discounts on bulk quantities of Jones and Bartlett's publications are available to corporations, professional associations, and other qualified organizations. For details and specific discount information, contact the special sales department at Jones and Bartlett via the above contact information or send an email to specialsales@jbpub.com.

The authors, editor, and publisher have made every effort to provide accurate information. However, they are not responsible for errors, omissions, or for any outcomes related to the use of the contents of this book and take no responsibility for the use of the products and procedures described. Treatments and side effects described in this book may not be applicable to all people; likewise, some people may require a dose or experience a side effect that is not described herein. Drugs and medical devices are discussed that may have limited availability controlled by the Food and Drug Administration (FDA) for use only in a research study or clinical trial. Research, clinical practice, and government regulations often change the accepted standard in this field. When consideration is being given to use of any drug in the clinical setting, the healthcare provider or reader is responsible for determining FDA status of the drug, reading the package insert, and reviewing prescribing information for the most up-to-date recommendations on dose, precautions, and contraindications, and determining the appropriate usage for the product. This is especially important in the case of drugs that are new or seldom used.

Production Credits
Chief Executive Officer: Clayton Jones
Chief Operating Officer: Don W. Jones, Jr.
President, Higher Education and Professional Publishing: Robert W. Holland, Jr.
V.P., Design and Production: Anne Spencer
V.P., Manufacturing and Inventory Control: Therese Connell
V.P., Sales and Marketing: William J. Kane
Executive Publisher: Christopher Davis
Editor: Kathy Richardson
Production Director: Amy Rose
Production Editor: Dan Stone
Director of Special Markets: Eileen Ward
Interactive Technology Manager: Dawn Mahon Priest
Cover Image: © MedicalRF.com/agefotostock
Cover Design: Kristin E. Parker
Printing and Binding: Malloy, Inc.
Cover Printing: Malloy, Inc.

6048

Printed in the United States of America
13 12 11 10 09   10 9 8 7 6 5 4 3 2 1

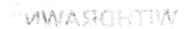

Table of Contents

Editors

Edward Chu, MD
Deputy Director, Yale Cancer Center
Chief, Section of Medical Oncology
Professor of Medicine and Pharmacology
Yale University School of Medicine
New Haven, CT

Vincent T. DeVita, Jr., MD
Amy and Joseph Perella Professor of Medicine
Professor of Epidemiology and Public Health
Yale University School of Medicine
New Haven, CT

Contributing Authors

M. Sitki Copur, MD
Associate Professor of Medicine
University of Nebraska
Director, Saint Francis
    Cancer Center
Grand Island, NE

Hari Deshpande, MD
Assistant Professor of Medicine
Yale Cancer Center
Yale University School of Medicine
New Haven, CT

Laurie J. Harrold, MD
Nora F. Pfriem Cancer Center
Bridgeport Hospital
Oncology Associates
Trumbull, CT

Arthur L. Levy, MD
Associate Professor of Medicine
Yale Cancer Center
Yale University School of Medicine
New Haven, CT

Dawn E. Tiedemann, AOCN, APRN
Clinical Nurse Specialist
Hematology-Oncology Associates
Meriden, CT

Preface

The development of effective drugs for the treatment of cancer represents a significant achievement beginning with the discovery of the antimetabolites and alkylating agents in the 1940s and 1950s. The success of that effort can be attributed in large measure to the close collaboration and interaction between basic scientists, synthetic organic chemists, pharmacologists, and clinicians. This tradition continues to flourish, especially as we now enter the world of pharmacogenomics, genomics, and proteomics, and the rapid identification of new molecular targets for drug design and development.

In this, our tenth edition, we have condensed and summarized a wealth of information on chemotherapeutic and biologic agents in current clinical practice into a reference guide that presents essential information in a practical and readable format. The primary indications, drug doses and schedules, toxicities, and special considerations for each agent have been expanded and revised to take into account new information that has been gathered over the past year. We have included three new agents that all have been approved by the FDA.

This drug manual is divided into five chapters. Chapter 1 gives a brief overview of the key principles of cancer chemotherapy and reviews the clinical settings where chemotherapy is used. Chapter 2 reviews individual chemotherapeutic and biologic agents that are in current clinical use; these agents are presented in alphabetical order according to their generic name. In this chapter, specific details are provided regarding drug classification and category, key mechanisms of action and resistance, critical aspects of clinical pharmacology and pharmacokinetics, clinical indications, special precautions and considerations, and toxicity. Chapter 3 includes recommendations for dose modifications that are required in the setting of myelosuppression and/or liver and renal dysfunction. Additionally, relevant information is provided highlighting the teratogenic potential of various agents. Chapter 4 presents a review of the combination drug regimens and selected single-agent regimens for solid tumors and hematologic malignancies that are used commonly in daily clinical practice. This section is organized alphabetically by specific cancer type. Finally, Chapter 5 reviews individual agents used to treat chemotherapy-induced nausea and vomiting, a significant toxicity observed with many of the anticancer agents in current practice, and commonly used antiemetic regimens.

It remains our hope that this book will continue to serve as both an in-depth reference and an immediate source of practical information that can be used by physicians and other healthcare professionals actively involved in the daily care of cancer patients. This drug manual continues to be a work in progress, and our goal is to continue to update it on an annual basis and to incorporate new drugs and treatment strategies that reflect the rapid advances in the field of cancer drug development.

Edward Chu, MD
Vincent T. DeVita, Jr., MD

Acknowledgments

This book represents the efforts of many dedicated people. It reflects my own personal and professional roots in the field of cancer pharmacology and cancer drug development and reaffirms the teaching and support of my colleagues and mentors at Brown University, the National Cancer Institute (NCI), and the Yale Cancer Center. In particular, Bruce Chabner, Paul Calabresi, Robert Parks, Joseph Bertino, and Vince DeVita have had a major influence on my development as a cancer pharmacologist and medical oncologist. While at the NCI, I was fortunate to have been trained under the careful tutelage of Carmen Allegra, Bob Wittes, and Bruce Chabner. Here at Yale, I have been privileged to work with a group of extraordinarily talented individuals including Yung-chi Cheng, William Prusoff, Alan Sartorelli, Richard Edelson, and Vince DeVita, all of whom have graciously shared their scientific insights, wisdom, support, and friendship. I would also like to take this opportunity to thank my co-author, colleague, mentor, and friend Vince DeVita, who recruited me to the Yale Cancer Center and who has been so tremendously supportive of my professional and personal career. I wish to thank my wife, Laurie Harrold, for her love and patience, for her insights as a practicing medical oncologist, and for her help in writing and reviewing various sections of this book. I would also like to thank my parents, Ming and Shih-Hsi Chu for their constant love, support, and encouragement, and for instilling in me the desire, joy, and commitment to become a medical oncologist and cancer pharmacologist. Special thanks go to my colleagues at Jones and Bartlett, particularly Clayton Jones and Chris Davis, for giving me the opportunity to develop this book and for their continued encouragement, support, and patience throughout this entire process. Finally, I wish to dedicate this book to my faithful dogs, Mika and Lexi, and to my two beautiful children, Ashley and Joshua, who have brought me great joy and pride and who have shown me the true meaning of unconditional loyalty and love.

Edward Chu, MD

1

Principles of Cancer Chemotherapy

Vincent T. DeVita, Jr., and Edward Chu

Introduction

The development of chemotherapy in the 1950s and 1960s resulted in curative therapeutic strategies for patients with hematologic malignancies and several types of advanced solid tumors. These advances confirmed the principle that chemotherapy could indeed cure cancer and provided the rationale for integrating chemotherapy into combined modality programs with surgery and radiation therapy in early stages of disease so as to provide clinical benefit. The principal obstacles to the clinical efficacy of chemotherapy have been toxicity to the normal tissues of the body and the development of cellular drug resistance. The development and application of molecular techniques to analyze gene expression of normal and malignant cells at the level of DNA, RNA, and/or protein has helped to identify some of the critical mechanisms through which chemotherapy exerts its antitumor effects and activates the program of cell death. This modern-day technology has also provided insights into the molecular and genetic events within cancer cells that can confer chemosensitivity to drug treatment. This enhanced understanding of the molecular pathways by which chemotherapy exerts its cytotoxic activity and by which genetic change can result in resistance to drug therapy has provided the rationale for developing innovative therapeutic strategies in which molecular, genetic, and biologic therapies can be used in combination to directly attack these novel targets.

The Role of Chemotherapy in the Treatment of Cancer

Chemotherapy is presently used in four main clinical settings: (1) primary induction treatment for advanced disease or for cancers for which there are no other effective treatment approaches, (2) neoadjuvant treatment for patients who present with localized disease, for whom local forms of therapy, such as surgery and/or radiation, are inadequate by themselves, (3) adjuvant treatment to local methods of treatment, including surgery and/or radiation therapy, and (4) direct instillation into sanctuary sites or by site-directed perfusion of specific regions of the body directly affected by the cancer.

Primary induction chemotherapy refers to drug therapy administered as the primary treatment for patients who present with advanced cancer for which no alternative treatment exists. This has been the mainstay approach to treat patients with advanced, metastatic disease, and in most cases, the goals of therapy are to palliate tumor-related symptoms, improve overall quality of life, and prolong time to tumor progression (TTP) and survival. Studies in a wide range of solid tumors have clearly shown that chemotherapy in patients with advanced disease confers survival benefit when compared to supportive care, providing sound rationale for the early initiation of drug treatment. Cancer chemotherapy can be curative in a relatively small subset of patients who present with advanced disease. In adults, these curative cancers include Hodgkin's and non-Hodgkin's lymphoma, germ cell cancer, and choriocarcinoma, while the curative childhood cancers include acute lymphoblastic leukemia, Burkitt's lymphoma, Wilms' tumor, and embryonal rhabdomyosarcoma.

Neoadjuvant chemotherapy refers to the use of chemotherapy for patients who present with localized cancer for which alternative local therapies, such as surgery, exist but are less than completely effective. For chemotherapy to be used as the initial treatment of a cancer, which would be partially curable by either surgery or radiation therapy, there must be documented evidence for its clinical efficacy in the advanced disease setting. At present, neoadjuvant therapy is most often administered in the treatment of anal cancer, bladder cancer, breast cancer, esophageal cancer, laryngeal cancer, locally advanced non–small cell lung cancer (NSCLC), and osteogenic sarcoma. For some of these diseases, such as anal cancer, gastroesophageal cancer, laryngeal cancer, and non–small cell lung cancer, optimal clinical benefit is derived when chemotherapy is administered with radiation therapy either concurrently or sequentially.

One of the most important roles for cancer chemotherapy is as an adjuvant to local treatment modalities such as surgery and/or radiation therapy, and this has been termed adjuvant chemotherapy. The development of disease recurrence, either locally or systemically, following surgery and/or radiation is mainly due to the spread of occult micrometastases. Thus, the goal of adjuvant therapy is to reduce the incidence of both local and systemic recurrence and to improve the overall survival (OS) of patients. In general, chemotherapy regimens with clinical activity against advanced disease may have curative potential following surgical resection of the primary tumor, provided the appropriate dose and schedule are administered. Several well-conducted, randomized phase III clinical studies have documented that adjuvant chemotherapy is effective in prolonging both disease-free survival (DFS) and OS in patients with breast cancer, colon cancer (CRC), gastric cancer, NSCLC, Wilms' tumor, and osteogenic sarcoma. There is also evidence to support the use of adjuvant chemotherapy in patients with anaplastic astrocytomas. Patients with primary malignant melanoma at high risk of metastases derive benefit in terms of improved DFS and OS from adjuvant treatment with the biologic agent α-interferon, although this treatment must be given for one year's duration for maximal clinical efficacy. Finally, the antihormonal agents tamoxifen, anastrozole, and letrozole are effective in the adjuvant therapy of postmenopausal women whose breast tumors express the estrogen receptor. However, because these agents are cytostatic rather than cytocidal, they must be administered on a long-term basis, with the standard recommendation now being 5 years.

Principles of Combination Chemotherapy

With rare exceptions (e.g., choriocarcinoma and Burkitt's lymphoma), single drugs at clinically tolerable doses have been unable to cure cancer. In the 1960s and early 1970s, drug combination regimens were developed based on known biochemical actions of available anticancer drugs rather than on their clinical efficacy. Such regimens were, however, largely ineffective. The era of effective combination chemotherapy began when a number of active drugs from different classes became available for use in combination in the treatment of the acute leukemias and lymphomas. Following this initial success with hematologic malignancies, combination chemotherapy was extended to the treatment of solid tumors.

Combination chemotherapy with conventional cytotoxic agents accomplishes several important objectives not possible with single-agent therapy. First, it provides maximal cell kill within the range of toxicity tolerated by the host for each drug as long as dosing is not compromised. Second, it provides a broader range of interaction between drugs and tumor cells with different genetic abnormalities in a heterogeneous tumor population. Finally, it may prevent and/or slow the subsequent development of cellular drug resistance.

Certain principles have guided the selection of drugs in the most effective drug combinations, and they provide a paradigm for the development of new drug therapeutic programs. First, only drugs known to be partially effective against the same tumor when used alone should be selected for use in combination. If available, drugs that produce some fraction of complete remission are preferred to those that produce only partial responses. Second, when several drugs of a class are available and are equally effective, a drug should be selected on the basis of toxicity that does not overlap with the toxicity of other drugs to be used in the combination. Although such selection leads to a wider range of side effects, it minimizes the risk of a lethal effect caused by multiple insults to the same organ system by different drugs and allows dose intensity to be maximized. In addition, drugs should be used in their optimal dose and schedule, and drug combinations should be given at consistent intervals. Because long intervals between cycles negatively affect dose intensity, the treatment-free interval between cycles should be the shortest possible time necessary for recovery of the most sensitive normal target tissue, which is usually the bone marrow. Finally, there should be a clear understanding of the biochemical, molecular, and pharmacokinetic mechanisms of interaction between the individual drugs in a given combination, to allow for maximal effect. Omission of a drug from a combination may allow overgrowth by a cell line sensitive to that drug alone and resistant to other drugs in the combination. Finally, arbitrary reduction in the dose of an effective drug to add other less effective drugs may dramatically reduce the dose of the most effective agent below the threshold of effectiveness and destroy the capacity of the combination to cure disease in a given patient.

One final issue relates to the optimal duration of chemotherapy drug administration. Several randomized trials in the adjuvant treatment of breast and colorectal cancer have shown that short-course treatment on the order of 6 months is as effective as long-course therapy (12 months). While progressive disease during chemotherapy is a clear indication to stop treatment in the advanced disease setting, the optimal duration of chemotherapy for patients without disease progression has not been well-defined. With the development of novel and more potent drug regimens, the potential risk of cumulative adverse events, such as cardiotoxicity secondary to the anthracyclines and neurotoxicity secondary to the taxanes and the platinum analogs, must also be factored into the decision-making process. There is, however, no evidence of clinical benefit in continuing therapy indefinitely until disease progression. A recent randomized study in advanced CRC comparing continuous and intermittent palliative chemotherapy showed that a policy of stopping and rechallenging with the same chemotherapy provides a reasonable treatment option for patients. Similar observations have been observed in the treatment of advanced, metastatic disease affecting other organ sites, including NSCLC, breast cancer, germ cell cancer, ovarian cancer, and small cell lung cancer. However, for such an intermittent treatment approach to be adopted into clinical practice, several issues need to be addressed. First, the induction chemotherapy regimen must be of sufficient clinical efficacy and duration to ensure that the majority of responses are achieved during the treatment period. Second, there must be a good response to the re-initiation of the same chemotherapy or to the administration of an effective salvage chemotherapy regimen. Third, there should be a sufficient time interval between the termination of primary induction chemotherapy and the onset of progressive disease. Finally, patients who are taken off active chemotherapy must be followed closely to ensure that treatment can be reinstituted at the first sign of disease progression.

The Concept of Dose Intensity

One of the main factors limiting the ability of chemotherapy and/or radiation therapy to achieve cure is effective dosing. The dose-response curve in biologic systems is usually sigmoidal in shape, with a threshold, a lag phase, a linear phase, and a plateau phase. For chemotherapy and radiation therapy, therapeutic selectivity is significantly dependent on the differential between the dose-response curves of normal and tumor tissues. In experimental in vivo models, the dose-response curve is usually steep in the linear phase, and a reduction in dose when the tumor is in the linear phase of the dose-response curve almost always results in a loss in the capacity to cure the tumor effectively before a reduction in the antitumor activity is observed. Thus, although complete remissions continue to be observed with dose reduction as low as 20%, residual tumor cells may not be entirely eliminated, thereby allowing for eventual relapse to occur. Although in vivo systems may not represent the ideal model for human malignancies, the general principles may be applicable to the clinical setting. Because anticancer drugs are associated with toxicity, it is often appealing for clinicians to avoid acute toxicity by simply reducing the dose or by increasing the time interval between each cycle of treatment. Such empiric modifications in dose represent a major reason for treatment failure in patients with drug-sensitive tumors who are receiving chemotherapy in either the adjuvant or advanced disease setting.

A major issue facing clinicians is the ability to deliver effective doses of chemotherapy in a dose-intense manner. Dose intensity was defined as the amount of drug delivered per unit of time and was expressed as milligrams per square meter per week, regardless of the schedule or route of administration. A positive relationship between dose intensity and response rate has been well-documented in several solid tumors, including advanced ovarian, breast, lung, and colon cancers, as well as in hematologic malignancies, including the lymphomas. At present, there are three main approaches to deliver chemotherapy in a dose-intense fashion. The first approach is via dose escalation where the doses of the anticancer agents are increased. Perhaps the best example of this approach is high-dose chemotherapy with stem cell transplantation. The second strategy is to administer anticancer agents in a dose-dense manner by reducing the interval between treatment cycles, and the best example of this approach is the dose-dense adjuvant treatment of early-stage breast cancer. Finally, the third approach is an alternative way to administer dose-dense therapy by sequential scheduling of either single agents, combination regimens, or monotherapy in sequence with combination regimens.

2

Chemotherapeutic and Biologic Drugs

Edward Chu, Laurie J. Harrold, Dawn Tiedemann, and M. Sitki Copur

Albumin-Bound Paclitaxel

Trade Names
Abraxane

Classification
Taxane, anti-microtubule agent

Category
Chemotherapy drug

Drug Manufacturer
Abraxis

Mechanism of Action
- Albumin-bound form of paclitaxel with a mean particle size of about 130 nm. Selective binding of albumin-bound paclitaxel to specific albumin receptors present on tumor cells versus normal cells.
- Active moiety is paclitaxel, which is isolated from the bark of the Pacific yew tree, *Taxus brevifolia*.
- Cell cycle–specific, active in the mitosis (M) phase of the cell cycle.
- High-affinity binding to microtubules enhances tubulin polymerization. Normal dynamic process of microtubule network is inhibited, leading to inhibition of mitosis and cell division.

Mechanism of Resistance
- Alterations in tubulin with decreased binding affinity for drug.

- Multidrug-resistant phenotype with increased expression of P170 glycoprotein. Results in enhanced drug efflux with decreased intracellular accumulation of drug. Cross-resistant to other natural products, including vinca alkaloids, anthracyclines, taxanes, and etoposide.

Absorption

Not orally bioavailable.

Distribution

Distributes widely to all body tissues. Extensive binding (<90%) to plasma and cellular proteins.

Metabolism

Paclitaxel is metabolized extensively by the hepatic P450 microsomal system. About 20% of drug is excreted via fecal elimination. Less than 10% is eliminated as the parent form with the majority being eliminated as metabolites. Renal clearance is relatively minor with less than 1% of drug cleared via the kidneys. The clearance of abraxane is 43% greater than paclitaxel, and the volume of distribution is about 50% higher than paclitaxel. Terminal elimination half-life is on the order of 27 hours.

Indications

FDA-approved for the treatment of breast cancer after failure of combination chemotherapy for metastatic disease or relapse within six months of adjuvant chemotherapy.

Dosage Range

1. Recommended dose is 260 mg/m^2 IV on day 1 every 21 days.

2. An alternative regimen is a weekly schedule of 125 mg/m^2 IV on days 1, 8, and 15 every 28 days.

Drug Interactions

None well characterized to date.

Special Considerations

1. Contraindicated in patients with baseline neutrophil counts of <1,500 cells/mm^3.

2. Closely monitor complete blood count (CBC) with differential on a periodic basis.

3. Abraxane has not been studied in patients with hepatic or renal dysfunction. Use with caution in patients with abnormal liver function, as patients with abnormal liver function may be at higher risk for toxicity.

4. In contrast to paclitaxel, no premedication is required to prevent hypersensitivity reactions prior to administration of abraxane.

5. Abraxane can **NOT** be substituted for or with other paclitaxel formulations as the albumin form of paclitaxel may significantly alter the drug's clinical activity.

6. Closely monitor infusion site for infiltration during drug administration as injection site reactions have been observed.

7. Pregnancy category D. Breast-feeding should be avoided.

Toxicity 1

Myelosuppression with dose-limiting neutropenia and anemia. Thrombocytopenia relatively uncommon.

Toxicity 2

Neurotoxicity mainly in the form of sensory neuropathy with numbness and paresthesias. Dose-dependent effect. In contrast to paclitaxel, abraxane-mediated neuropathy appears to be more readily reversible.

Toxicity 3

Ocular and visual disturbances seen in 13% of patients with severe cases seen in 1%.

Toxicity 4

Asthenia, fatigue, and weakness.

Toxicity 5

Alopecia with loss of total body hair.

Toxicity 6

Nausea/vomiting, diarrhea, and mucositis are the main gastrointestinal (GI) toxicities. Mucositis is generally mild seen in less than 10%. Mild to moderate nausea and vomiting, usually of brief duration.

Toxicity 7

Transient elevations in serum transaminases, bilirubin, and alkaline phosphatase.

Toxicity 8

Injection site reactions.

A

Aldesleukin

Trade Names

Interleukin-2, IL-2, Proleukin

Classification

Immunotherapy, cytokine

Category

Biologic response modifier agent

Drug Manufacturer

Novartis

Mechanism of Action

- Glycoprotein cytokine that functions as a T-cell growth factor.
- Biologic effect of interleukin-2 (IL-2) is mediated by specific binding to the interleukin-2 receptor (IL-2R).
- Precise mechanism by which IL-2 mediates its anticancer activity remains unknown but appears to require an intact immune system.
- Enhances lymphocyte mitogenesis and lymphocyte cytotoxicity.
- Induces lymphokine-activated (LAK) and natural killer (NK) cell activity.
- Induces interferon-γ production.

Mechanism of Resistance

- Up to 75% of patients may develop anti-IL-2 antibodies.
- Increased expression of counter-regulatory factors, such as glucocorticoids, which act to reduce the efficacy of interleukin-2.

Absorption

Not available for oral use and is administered only via the parenteral route. Peak plasma levels are achieved in 5 hours after subcutaneous (SC) administration.

Distribution

After short intravenous (IV) infusion, high plasma concentrations of IL-2 are achieved followed by rapid distribution into the extravascular space.

Metabolism

IL-2 is catabolized by renal tubular cells to amino acids. The major route of elimination is through the kidneys by both glomerular filtration and tubular secretion. The elimination half-life is 85 minutes.

Indications

1. Metastatic renal cell cancer.
2. Metastatic malignant melanoma.

Dosage Range

Renal cell cancer: 600,000 IU/kg IV every 8 hours for a maximum of 14 doses. Following nine days of rest, the schedule is repeated for another 14 doses, for a maximum of 28 doses per course.

Drug Interaction 1

Corticosteroids—May decrease the antitumor efficacy of IL-2 due to its inhibitory effect on the immune system.

Drug Interaction 2

Nonsteroidal anti-inflammatory drugs—May enhance the capillary leak syndrome observed with IL-2.

Drug Interaction 3

Antihypertensives—IL-2 potentiates the effect of antihypertensive medications. For this reason, all antihypertensives should be stopped at least 24 hours before IL-2 treatment.

Special Considerations

1. Use with caution in patients with pre-existing cardiac, pulmonary, central nervous system (CNS), hepatic, and/or renal impairment as there is an increased risk for developing serious and sometimes fatal reactions.

2. Pretreatment evaluation should include CBC; serum chemistries, including liver function tests (LFTs), renal function, and electrolytes; pulmonary function tests (PFTs); and stress thallium.

3. Patients should be monitored closely throughout the entire treatment, including vital signs every 2–4 hours, strict input and output, and daily weights. Continuous cardiopulmonary monitoring is important during therapy.

4. Monitor for capillary leak syndrome (CLS), which begins almost immediately after initiation of therapy. Manifested by hypotension, peripheral edema, ascites, pleural and/or pericardial effusions, weight gain, and altered mental status.

5. Early administration of dopamine (1–5 µg/kg/min) in the setting of CLS may maintain perfusion to the kidneys and preserve renal function.

6. Use with caution in the presence of concurrent medications known to be nephrotoxic and hepatotoxic as IL-2 therapy is associated with both nephrotoxicity and hepatotoxicity.

7. Use with caution in patients with known autoimmune disease as treatment with IL-2 is associated with autoimmune thyroiditis leading to thyroid function impairment.

8. Allergic reactions have been reported in patients receiving iodine contrast media up to 4 months following IL-2 therapy.

9. Pregnancy category C.

Toxicity 1

Flu-like symptoms, including fever, chills, malaise, myalgias, and arthralgias. Observed in all patients.

Toxicity 2

Vascular leak syndrome. Usual dose-limiting toxicity, characterized by weight gain, arrhythmias, and/or tachycardia, hypotension, edema, oliguria and renal insufficiency, pleural effusions, and pulmonary congestion.

Toxicity 3

Myelosuppression with anemia, thrombocytopenia, and neutropenia.

Toxicity 4

Hepatotoxicity presenting as increases in serum bilirubin levels along with changes in serum transaminases. Usually reversible within 4–6 days after discontinuation of IL-2 therapy.

Toxicity 5

Neurologic and neuropsychiatric findings can develop both acutely and chronically during treatment. Somnolence, delirium, and confusion are common but generally resolve after drug termination. Alterations in cognitive function and impaired memory more common with continuous infusion IL-2.

Toxicity 6

Erythema, skin rash, urticaria, and generalized erythroderma may occur within a few days of starting therapy.

Toxicity 7

Alterations in thyroid function, including hyperthyroidism and hypothyroidism.

Alemtuzumab

Trade Names
Campath

Classification
Monoclonal antibody

Category
Biologic response modifier agent

Drug Manufacturer
Genzyme

Mechanism of Action
- Recombinant humanized monoclonal antibody (Campath-1H) directed against the 21–28 kDa cell surface glycoprotein CD52 that is expressed on most normal and malignant B and T lymphocytes, NK cells, monocytes, and macrophages.
- CD52 antigen is not expressed on the surface of hematopoietic stem cells and mature plasma cells.
- Immunologic mechanisms involved in antitumor activity, including antibody-dependent cellular cytotoxicity (ADCC) and/or complement-mediated cell lysis.

Mechanism of Resistance
None yet defined.

Absorption
Alemtuzumab is given only by the IV route.

Distribution
Peak and trough levels rise during the first few weeks of therapy and approach steady-state levels by week 6. However, there is marked variability, and levels correlate roughly with the number of circulating CD52+ B cells.

Metabolism
Metabolism has not been extensively characterized. Half-life is on the order of 12 days with minimal clearance by the liver and kidneys.

Indications
1. Relapsed and/or refractory B-cell chronic lymphocytic leukemia (B-CLL)—Indicated in patients who have been treated with alkylating agents and who have failed fludarabine therapy.
2. T-cell prolymphocytic leukemia—Clinical activity in patients who failed first-line therapy.

Dosage Range

The recommended dose is 30 mg/day IV three times per week for maximum of 12 weeks.

Drug Interactions

None known.

Special Considerations

1. Contraindicated in patients with active systemic infections, underlying immunodeficiency (HIV-positive, AIDS, etc.), or known type I hypersensitivity or anaphylactic reactions to alemtuzumab or any of its components.

2. Patients should be premedicated with acetaminophen, 650 mg PO, and diphenhydramine, 50 mg PO, 30 minutes before drug infusion to reduce the incidence of infusion-related reactions.

3. Alemtuzumab should be initiated at a dose of 3 mg, administered daily as a 2-hour IV infusion. When this daily dose of 3 mg is tolerated, the daily dose can then be increased to 10 mg. Once the 10-mg daily dose is tolerated, the maintenance dose of 30 mg daily can then be initiated. This maintenance dose of 30 mg/day is administered three times each week on alternate days (Monday, Wednesday, and Friday) for a maximum of 12 weeks. Dose escalation to the 30-mg daily dose usually can be accomplished within 7 days. Alemtuzumab should **NOT** be given IV push or bolus.

4. Monitor closely for infusion-related events, which usually occur within the first 30–60 minutes after the start of the infusion and most commonly during the first week of therapy. Pulse, blood pressure, and oral temperature should be measured every 15–30 minutes. Immediate institution of diphenhydramine (50 mg IV), acetaminophen (625 mg PO), hydrocortisone (200 mg IV), and/or vasopressors may be required. Resuscitation equipment should be readily available at bedside.

5. Patients should be placed on anti-infective prophylaxis upon initiation of therapy to reduce the risk of serious opportunistic infections. This should include Bactrim DS, one tablet PO bid three times per week, and famciclovir or equivalent, 250 mg PO bid. Fluconazole may also be included in the regimen to reduce the incidence of fungal infections. If a serious infection occurs while on therapy, alemtuzumab should be stopped immediately and only reinitiated following the complete resolution of the underlying infection.

6. Monitor CBC and platelet counts on a weekly basis during alemtuzumab therapy. Treatment should be stopped for severe hematologic toxicity or in any patient with evidence of autoimmune anemia and/or thrombocytopenia.

7. Most significant antitumor effects of alemtuzumab are observed in peripheral blood, bone marrow, and spleen. Tumor cells usually cleared from blood within 1–2 weeks of initiation of therapy, while normalization in bone marrow may take up to 6–12 weeks. Lymph nodes, especially those that are large and bulky, seem to be less responsive to therapy.

8. Pregnancy category C. Should be given to a pregnant woman only if clearly indicated. Breast-feeding should be avoided during treatment and for at least 3 months following the last dose of drug.

Toxicity 1

Infusion-related symptoms, including fever, chills, nausea and vomiting, urticaria, skin rash, fatigue, headache, diarrhea, dyspnea, and/or hypotension. Usually occur within the first week of initiation of therapy.

Toxicity 2

Significant immunosuppressive agent with an increased incidence of opportunistic infections, including *Pneumocystis carinii*, cytomegalovirus (CMV), herpes zoster, *Candida*, *Cryptococcus*, and *Listeria* meningitis. Prophylaxis with anti-infective agents is indicated as outlined above. Recovery of CD4 and CD8 counts is slow and may take over 1 year to return to normal.

Toxicity 3

Myelosuppression with neutropenia most common, but anemia and thrombocytopenia also observed. In rare instances, pancytopenia with marrow hypoplasia occurs, which can be fatal.

Altretamine

Trade Names

Hexalen, Hexamethylmelamine, HMM

Classification

Nonclassic alkylating agent

Category

Chemotherapy drug

Drug Manufacturer

MGI Pharma

Mechanism of Action

- Triazine derivative that requires biochemical activation in the liver for its antitumor activity.
- Exact mechanism(s) of action unclear but appears to act like an alkylating agent. Forms cross-links with DNA resulting in inhibition of DNA synthesis and function.
- May also inhibit RNA synthesis.

Mechanism of Resistance

- Mechanisms of resistance have not been well characterized.
- Does not exhibit cross-resistance to other classic alkylating agents and does not exhibit multidrug-resistant phenotype.

Absorption

Oral absorption is extremely variable secondary to extensive first-pass metabolism in the liver. Peak plasma levels are achieved 0.5–3 hours after an oral dose.

Distribution

Widely distributed throughout the body, with highest concentrations found in tissues with high fat content. About 90% of drug is bound to plasma proteins.

Metabolism

Extensively metabolized in the liver by the microsomal P450 system. Less than 1% of parent compound is excreted in urine. About 60% of drug is eliminated in urine as demethylated metabolites (pentamethylmelamine and tetramethylmelamine) within the first 24 hours. The terminal elimination half-life is on the order of 4–10 hours.

Indications

Ovarian cancer—Active in advanced disease and in persistent and/or recurrent tumors following first-line therapy with a cisplatin- and/or alkylating agent-based regimen.

Dosage Range

Usual dose is 260 mg/m²/day PO for either 14 or 21 days on a 28-day schedule. Total daily dose is given in four divided doses after meals and bedtime.

Drug Interaction 1

Cimetidine—Cimetidine increases the half-life and subsequent toxicity of altretamine. In contrast, ranitidine does not affect drug metabolism.

Drug Interaction 2

Phenobarbital—Phenobarbital may decrease the half-life and toxicity of altretamine.

Drug Interaction 3

Monamine oxidase (MAO) inhibitors—Concurrent use of MAO inhibitors with altretamine may result in significant orthostatic hypotension.

Special Considerations

1. Closely monitor patient for signs of neurologic toxicity.
2. Vitamin B6 (pyridoxine) may be used to decrease the incidence and severity of neurologic toxicity. However, antitumor activity may be compromised with vitamin B6 treatment.
3. Pregnancy category D.

Toxicity 1

Nausea and vomiting. Mild to moderate, observed in 30% of patients. Worsens with increasing cumulative doses of drug.

Toxicity 2

Myelosuppression. Dose-limiting toxicity. Leukocyte and platelet nadirs occur at 3–4 weeks with recovery by day 28. Anemia occurs in 20% of patients.

Toxicity 3

Neurotoxicity in the form of somnolence, mood changes, lethargy, depression, agitation, hallucinations, and peripheral neuropathy. Observed in about 25% of patients.

Toxicity 4

Hypersensitivity, skin rash.

Toxicity 5

Elevations in LFTs, mainly alkaline phosphatase.

Toxicity 6

Flu-like syndrome in the form of fever, malaise, arthralgias, and myalgias.

Toxicity 7

Abdominal cramps and diarrhea are occasionally observed.

Amifostine

Amifostine
(prodrug)

$NH_2-(CH_2)_3-NH-(CH_2)_2-S-PO_3H_2$

membrane-bound
alkaline phosphatase

$NH_2-(CH_2)_3-NH-(CH_2)_2-SH$

WR-1065
(active form)

Trade Names
Ethyol, WR2721

Classification
Organic thiophosphate analog

Category
Chemoprotective drug

Drug Manufacturer
MedImmune

Mechanism of Action

- Organic thiophosphate analog originally developed by Walter Reed Army Institute.
- Inactive in its parent form and serves as a prodrug.
- Requires activation by the enzyme alkaline phosphatase to the active, free thiol metabolite WR1065. This enzyme is expressed on the plasma membrane surface of endothelial cells lining blood vessels and on the surface of proximal renal tubular cells.
- Activation occurs to a greater extent in normal cells when compared to tumor cells because of a higher level of expression of alkaline phosphatase.
- Free thiol acts as a potent scavenger of oxygen free radicals and superoxide anions to inactivate the reactive species of cisplatin and radiation.
- Does not adversely affect the antitumor activity of cisplatin and/or radiation.

Absorption
Amifostine is not orally bioavailable. Approximately 50% of drug bioavailable after SC injection.

Distribution

Amifostine is confined primarily to the intravascular compartment. Rapidly cleared from plasma with a distribution half-life of <1 minute and <10% of drug remains in plasma 6 minutes after drug administration. The active metabolite of the drug is widely distributed in body tissues, but it does not cross the blood-brain barrier or distribute into skeletal muscle.

Metabolism

Rapidly metabolized by the enzyme alkaline phosphatase to the active, free thiol metabolite WR1065. Activation occurs to a much greater extent in normal cells versus tumor cells given the higher levels of alkaline phosphatase, higher pH, and increased vascularity in normal cells. The elimination half-life is 8 minutes, and <5% of drug is excreted in urine either as the parent form or as amifostine metabolites.

Indications

1. Reduce the incidence of nephrotoxicity in patients with ovarian cancer receiving cisplatin-based chemotherapy.

2. Reduce the incidence of moderate to severe xerostomia in patients undergoing postoperative radiation treatment for head and neck cancer, where the radiation port includes a significant portion of the parotid glands.

Dosage Range

1. Recommended dose for reduction of cumulative renal toxicity is 910 mg/m^2 IV, administered once daily 30 minutes before cisplatin chemotherapy.

2. Recommended dose for reduction of xerostomia is 200 mg/m^2 administered once daily 15–30 minutes before radiation therapy.

3. Alternative regimen for head and neck cancer patients is 500 mg SC administered once daily 20 minutes before radiation therapy.

Drug Interactions

None well characterized to date.

Special Considerations

1. Patients should be given antiemetics before drug treatment, because amifostine is a moderate to severe emetogenic agent. Antiemetic cocktail should include a 5-HT3 inhibitor (granisetron or ondansetron), benadryl, and decadron.

2. Patients should be well hydrated before drug treatment and be kept in a supine position during the infusion.

3. Antihypertensive medications should be stopped at least 24 hours before starting therapy, because amifostine induces hypotension.

4. Blood pressure and vital signs of patients must be monitored every 5 minutes during the infusion and 10 minutes after the infusion. In the event of hypotension, the infusion should be stopped immediately, and the patient treated with IV fluids and/or pressors. Treatment can resume if the blood pressure has returned to normal within 5 minutes and the patient remains asymptomatic.

5. Infuse amifostine over a period of 15 minutes when used before chemotherapy and over 3 minutes when used before radiation, as longer infusion times are associated with an increased risk of side effects.

6. SC administration is associated with a lower incidence of nausea/vomiting and hypotension and is a more convenient treatment option.

7. Pregnancy category C. Breast-feeding should be avoided.

Toxicity 1

Nausea and vomiting are common and may be severe.

Toxicity 2

Hypotension occurs in up to 60% of patients. Usually asymptomatic. Mean time of onset is 14 minutes into the infusion. Blood pressure usually returns to normal within 5–15 minutes.

Toxicity 3

Infusion-related reaction in the form of flushing, chills, dizziness, somnolence, and sneezing.

Toxicity 4

Hypocalcemia develops in <1% of patients and usually is clinically asymptomatic. Amifostine affects the release of parathyroid hormone.

Aminoglutethimide

Trade Names

Cytadren

Classification

Adrenal steroid inhibitor

Category

Hormonal agent

Drug Manufacturer

Novartis

Mechanism of Action

- Nonsteroidal inhibitor of corticosteroid biosynthesis.
- Produces a chemical adrenalectomy with a decreased synthesis of estrogens, androgens, glucocorticoids, and mineralocorticoids.

Absorption

Excellent bioavailability via the oral route. Peak plasma concentrations occur within 1–1.5 hours after ingestion.

Distribution

Approximately 25% of the drug is bound to plasma proteins. Significant reduction in distribution with prolonged treatment.

Metabolism

Metabolized in the liver by the cytochrome P450 system with N-acetylaminoglutethimide being the major metabolite. Metabolism is under genetic control, and acetylator status of patients is important. About 40%–50% of the drug is excreted unchanged in the urine. Initial half-life of drug is about 13 hours but decreases to 7 hours with chronic treatment, suggesting that the drug may accelerate its own rate of degradation.

Indications

1. Breast cancer—Hormone-responsive, advanced disease.
2. Prostate cancer—Hormone-responsive, advanced disease.

Dosage Range

Usual dose is 250 mg PO qid (1,000 mg total).

Drug Interaction 1

Warfarin, phenytoin, phenobarbital, theophylline, medroxyprogesterone, and digoxin—Aminoglutethimide enhances the metabolism of warfarin, phenytoin, phenobarbital, theophylline, medroxyprogesterone, and digoxin, thereby decreasing their clinical activity.

Drug Interaction 2

Dexamethasone—Aminoglutethimide enhances the metabolism of dexamethasone but not hydrocortisone.

Special Considerations

1. Administer hydrocortisone along with aminoglutethimide to prevent adrenal insufficiency. The use of higher doses during the initial 2 weeks of therapy reduces the frequency of adverse events. For example, start at 100 mg PO daily for the first 2 weeks, then 40 mg PO daily in divided doses. Higher doses of steroid replacement may be required under conditions of stress such as surgery, trauma, or acute infection.

2. Closely monitor patient for signs and symptoms of hypothyroidism. Monitor thyroid function tests on a regular basis.

3. Monitor for signs and symptoms of orthostatic hypotension. May need to add fludrocortisone (Florinef) 0.1–0.2 mg PO qd.

4. Monitor patient for signs of somnolence and lethargy. Severe cases may warrant immediate discontinuation of drug.

5. Discontinue drug if skin rash persists for more than 1 week.

6. Pregnancy category D.

Toxicity 1

Maculopapular skin rash. Usually seen in the first week of therapy. Self-limited with resolution in 5–7 days, and discontinuation of therapy not necessary.

Toxicity 2

Fatigue, lethargy, and somnolence. Occur in 40% of patients, and onset is within the first week of therapy. Dizziness, nystagmus, and ataxia are less common (10% of patients).

Toxicity 3

Mild nausea and vomiting.

Toxicity 4

Hypothyroidism.

Toxicity 5

Adrenal insufficiency. Occurs in the absence of hydrocortisone replacement. Presents as postural hypotension, hyponatremia, and hyperkalemia.

Toxicity 6

Myelosuppression. Leukopenia and thrombocytopenia rarely occur.

Anastrozole

Trade Names
Arimidex

Classification
Nonsteroidal aromatase inhibitor

Category
Hormonal agent

Drug Manufacturer
AstraZeneca

Mechanism of Action
- Potent and selective nonsteroidal inhibitor of aromatase.
- Inhibits the synthesis of estrogens by inhibiting the conversion of adrenal androgens (androstenedione and testosterone) to estrogens (estrone, estrone sulfate, and estradiol). Serum estradiol levels are suppressed by 90% within 14 days, and nearly completely suppressed after 6 weeks of therapy.
- No inhibitory effect on adrenal corticosteroid or aldosterone biosynthesis.

Mechanism of Resistance
None characterized.

Absorption
Excellent bioavailability via the oral route, with 85% of a dose absorbed within 2 hours of ingestion. Absorption is not affected by food.

Distribution
Widely distributed throughout the body. About 40% of drug is bound to plasma proteins.

Metabolism
Extensively metabolized in the liver (up to 85%) by N-dealkylation, hydroxylation, and glucuronidation, to inactive forms. Half-life of drug is

about 50 hours. Steady-state levels of drug are achieved after 7 days of a once-daily administration. The major route of elimination is fecal, with renal excretion accounting for only 10% of drug clearance.

Indications

1. Metastatic breast cancer—First-line treatment of postmenopausal women with hormone-receptor positive or hormone-receptor unknown disease. FDA-approved.

2. Metastatic breast cancer—Postmenopausal women with hormone-receptor positive, advanced disease, and progression while on tamoxifen therapy.

3. Adjuvant treatment of postmenopausal women with hormone-receptor positive, early-stage breast cancer. FDA-approved.

Dosage Range

1. Metastatic breast cancer: Recommended dose is 1 mg PO qd for both first- and second-line therapy.

2. Early-stage breast cancer: Recommended dose is 1 mg PO qd for adjuvant therapy. The optimal duration of therapy is unknown. In the ATAC trial, anastrozole was given for 5 years.

Drug Interactions

None known.

Special Considerations

1. No dose adjustments are required for patients with either hepatic or renal dysfunction.

2. Caution patients about the risk of hot flashes.

3. No need for glucocorticoid and/or mineralocorticoid replacement.

4. Closely monitor women with osteoporosis or at risk of osteoporosis by performing bone densitometry at the start of therapy and at regular intervals. Treatment or prophylaxis for osteoporosis should be initiated when appropriate.

5. Pregnancy category D.

Toxicity 1

Asthenia is most common toxicity and occurs in up to 20% of patients.

Toxicity 2

Mild nausea and vomiting. Constipation or diarrhea can also occur.

Toxicity 3

Hot flashes. Occurs in 10% of patients.

Toxicity 4

Dry, scaling skin rash.

Toxicity 5

Arthralgias occur in 10% to 15% of patients involving hands, knees, hips, lower back, and shoulders. Early morning stiffness is usual presentation.

Toxicity 6

Headache.

Toxicity 7

Peripheral edema in 7% of patients.

Toxicity 8

Flu-like syndrome in the form of fever, malaise, and myalgias.

Arsenic trioxide (As$_2$O$_3$)

Trade Names

Trisenox

Classification

Natural product

Category

Chemotherapy and differentiating agent

Drug Manufacturer

Cephalon

Mechanism of Action

- Precise mechanism of action has not been fully elucidated.

- Induces differentiation of acute promyelocytic leukemic cells by degrading the chimeric PML/RAR-α protein, resulting in release of the maturation block at the promyelocyte stage of myelocyte differentiation.

- Induces apoptosis through a mitochondrial-dependent pathway, resulting in release of cytochrome C and subsequent caspase activation.

- Direct antiproliferative activity by arresting cells at either the G1-S or G2-M checkpoints.

- Inhibits the process of angiogenesis through apoptosis of endothelial cells and/or inhibition of production of critical angiogenic factors, including vascular endothelial growth factor.

Mechanism of Resistance

None well characterized to date.

Absorption

Arsenic trioxide is given only by the IV route.

Distribution

Widely distributes in liver, kidneys, heart, lung, hair, nails, and skin.

Metabolism

The clinical pharmacology of arsenic trioxide has not been well characterized. Metabolism occurs via reduction of pentavalent arsenic to trivalent arsenic and methylation reactions mediated by methyltransferase enzymes that occur primarily in the liver. However, the methyltransferases appear to be distinct from the liver microsomal P450 system. The methylated trivalent arsenic metabolite is excreted mainly in the urine.

Indications

Acute promyelocytic leukemia (APL)—FDA-approved for induction of remission and consolidation in patients with APL who are refractory to or have relapsed following first-line therapy with all-trans retinoic acid (ATRA) and anthracycline-based chemotherapy and whose APL is characterized by the presence of the t(15;17) translocation or PML/RAR-α gene expression.

Dosage Range

1. Induction therapy—0.15 mg/kg/day IV for a maximum of 60 days.
2. Consolidation therapy—Should be initiated 3 weeks after completion of induction treatment and only in those patients who achieve a complete bone marrow remission. The recommended dosage is 0.15 mg/kg/day IV for 5 days/week for a total of 5 weeks.

Drug Interaction 1

Medications that can prolong the QT interval such as antiarrhythmics—Increased risk of prolongation of the QT interval and subsequent arrhythmias when arsenic trioxide is administered concomitantly.

Drug Interaction 2

Amphotericin B—Increased risk of prolonged QT interval and Torsade de Pointes ventricular arrhythmia in patients receiving amphotericin and induction therapy with arsenic trioxide.

Special Considerations

1. Contraindicated in patients who are hypersensitive to arsenic.
2. Use with caution in patients who are on agents that prolong the QT interval, in those who have a history of Torsade de Pointes, pre-existing QT interval prolongation, untreated sinus node dysfunction, high-degree atrioventricular block, or in those who may be severely dehydrated or malnourished at baseline.
3. Use with caution in patients with renal impairment as renal excretion is the main route of elimination of arsenic.
4. Before initiation of therapy, all patients should have a baseline electrocardiogram (EKG) performed and serum electrolytes, including potassium, calcium, magnesium, blood urea nitrogen (BUN), and creatinine, should be evaluated. Any pre-existing electrolyte abnormalities should be corrected before starting therapy.
5. Serum electrolytes should be closely monitored during therapy. Serum potassium concentrations should be maintained above 4 mEq/L and magnesium concentrations above 1.8 mg/dL.
6. Therapy should be stopped when the QT interval >500 millisecond and only resumed when the QT interval drops to below 460 millisecond, all electrolyte abnormalities are corrected, and cardiac monitoring shows no evidence of arrhythmias.

7. Monitor closely for new-onset fever, dyspnea, weight gain, abnormal respiratory symptoms, and/or physical findings, or chest x-ray abnormalities, because 30% of patients will develop the APL differentiation syndrome. This syndrome can be fatal, and high-dose steroids with dexamethasone 10 mg IV bid should be started immediately and continued for 3–5 days. While this syndrome more commonly occurs with median baseline white blood cells of 5,000 mm^3, it can occur in the absence of leukocytosis. In most cases, therapy can be resumed once the syndrome has completely resolved.

8. Monitor CBC every other day and bone marrow cytology every 10 days during induction therapy.

9. Pregnancy category D. Breast-feeding should be avoided as arsenic is excreted in breast milk.

Toxicity 1

Fatigue.

Toxicity 2

Prolonged QT interval (>500 msec) on EKG seen in 40%–50% of patients. Does not usually increase upon repeat exposure to arsenic trioxide, and QT interval returns to baseline following termination of therapy. Torsade de Pointes ventricular arrhythmia and/or complete AV block can be observed in this setting.

Toxicity 3

APL differentiation syndrome. Occurs in about 30% of patients and is characterized by fever, dyspnea, skin rash, fluid retention and weight gain, pleural and/or pericardial effusions. This syndrome is identical to the retinoic acid syndrome observed with retinoid therapy.

Toxicity 4

Leukocytosis is observed in 50%–60% of patients with a gradual increase in WBC that peaks between 2 and 3 weeks after starting therapy. Usually resolves spontaneously without treatment and/or complications.

Toxicity 5

Light-headedness most commonly observed during drug infusion. Headache and insomnia.

Toxicity 6

Mild nausea and vomiting, abdominal pain, and diarrhea.

Toxicity 7

Musculoskeletal pain.

Toxicity 8

Mild hyperglycemia.

Toxicity 9

Peripheral neuropathy.

Toxicity 10

Carcinogen and teratogen.

A

Asparaginase

Trade Names

Elspar, L-Asparaginase

Classification

Enzyme

Category

Chemotherapy drug

Drug Manufacturer

Merck

Mechanism of Action

- Purified from *Escherichia coli* and/or *Erwinia chrysanthemi*.
- Tumor cells lack asparagine synthetase and thus require exogenous sources of L-Asparagine.
- L-Asparaginase hydrolyzes circulating L-Asparagine to aspartic acid and ammonia.
- Depletion of the essential amino acid L-Asparagine results in rapid inhibition of protein synthesis. Cytotoxicity of drug correlates well with inhibition of protein synthesis.

Mechanism of Resistance

- Increased expression of the L-Asparagine synthetase gene. This facilitates the cellular production of L-Asparagine from endogenous sources.
- Formation of antibodies against L-Asparaginase, resulting in inhibition of function.

Absorption

L-Asparaginase is not orally bioavailable.

Distribution

Remains in the vascular compartment after IV administration. After intramuscular (IM) injection, peak plasma levels are reached within 14–24 hours. Peak plasma levels after IM injection are 50% lower than those achieved with IV injection. Plasma protein binding is on the order of 30%. The apparent volume of distribution is about 70%–80% of the plasma volume. Cerebrospinal fluid (CSF) penetration is negligible (<1% of plasma level).

Metabolism

Metabolism is not well characterized. Minimal urinary and/or biliary excretion occurs. Plasma half-life depends on formulation of drug: 40–50 hours for *E. coli*–derived L-Asparaginase and 3–5 days for polyethylene glycol (PEG)-Asparaginase.

Indications

Acute lymphocytic leukemia.

Dosage Range

1. Dose varies depending on specific regimens. L-Asparaginase is given at a dose of 6,000–10,000 IU/m^2 IM every 3 days for a total of nine doses. Treatment with L-Asparaginase is started after completion of other chemotherapy drugs used in the induction therapy of acute lymphoblastic leukemia (vincristine, prednisone, and doxorubicin).

2. L-Asparaginase is given less commonly as a single agent at a dose of 200 IU/kg IV for 28 consecutive days.

Drug Interaction 1

Methotrexate—L-Asparaginase can inhibit the cytotoxic effects of methotrexate and thus rescue from methotrexate antitumor activity and host toxicity. It is recommended that these drugs be administered 24 hours apart.

Drug Interaction 2

Vincristine—L-Asparaginase inhibits the clearance of vincristine resulting in increased host toxicity, especially neurotoxicity. Vincristine should be administered 12–24 hours before L-Asparaginase.

Special Considerations

1. An intradermal skin test dose of 2 IU should be performed before the initial administration of L-Asparaginase or whenever the dose is being repeated more than 1 week from the immediately previous one. The patient should be observed for at least 1 hour before the full dose is given. A negative dermal test does not completely rule out the possibility of an allergic reaction.

2. Monitor patient for allergic reactions and/or anaphylaxis. Contraindicated in patients with a prior history of anaphylactic reaction. L-Asparaginase isolated from the *Erwinia* species may be tried in patients previously treated with *E. coli* asparaginase, but allergic reactions may still occur.

3. L-Asparaginase is a contact irritant in both powder and solution forms. The drug must be handled and administered with caution.

4. Induction treatment of acute lymphoblastic leukemia with L-Asparaginase may induce rapid lysis of blast cells. Prophylaxis against tumor lysis syndrome with vigorous IV hydration, urinary alkalinization, and allopurinol is recommended for all patients.

5. Contraindicated in patients with either active pancreatitis or a history of pancreatitis. If pancreatitis develops while on therapy, L-Asparaginase should be stopped immediately.

6. Close monitoring of LFTs, amylase, coagulation tests, and fibrinogen levels.

7. L-Asparaginase can interfere with thyroid function tests. This effect is probably due to a marked reduction in serum concentration of thyroxine-binding globulin, which is observed within 2 days after the first dose. Levels of thyroxine-binding globulin return to normal within 4 weeks of the last dose.

8. Pregnancy category C.

Toxicity 1

Hypersensitivity reaction. Occurs in up to 25% of patients. Mild form manifested by skin rash and urticaria. Anaphylactic reaction may be life-threatening and presents as bronchospasm, respiratory distress, and hypotension. Resuscitation drugs and equipment should be readily available at bedside before drug treatment.

Toxicity 2

Fever, chills, nausea, and vomiting. Acute reaction observed in about two-thirds of patients.

Toxicity 3

Mild elevation in LFTs, including serum bilirubin, alkaline phosphatase, and SGOT. Common and usually transient. Liver biopsy reveals fatty changes.

Toxicity 4

Increased risk of both bleeding and clotting. Alterations in clotting with decreased levels of clotting factors, including fibrinogen, factors IX and XI, antithrombin III, proteins C and S, plasminogen, and α-2-antiplasmin. Observed in over 50% of patients.

Toxicity 5

Pancreatitis develops in up to 10% of patients. Usually manifested as transient increase in serum amylase levels with quick resolution upon cessation of therapy.

Toxicity 6

Neurologic toxicity, including lethargy, confusion, agitation, hallucinations, and/or coma. These side effects may require treatment discontinuation. Severe neurotoxicity resembles ammonia toxicity.

Toxicity 7

Myelosuppression is mild and rarely observed.

Toxicity 8

Decreased serum levels of insulin, lipoproteins, and albumin.

Toxicity 9

Renal toxicity. Usually mild and manifested by mild elevations in BUN and creatinine, proteinuria, and elevated serum acid levels.

A

Azacitidine

NH_2

HO

OH OH

Trade Name

Vidaza

Classification

Antimetabolite, hypomethylating agent

Category

Chemotherapy drug

Drug Manufacturer

Celgene

Mechanism of Action

- Cytidine analog.
- Cell cycle–specific with activity in the S-phase.
- Requires activation to the nucleotide metabolite azacitidine triphosphate.
- Incorporation of azacitidine triphosphate into RNA, resulting in inhibition of RNA processing and function.
- Incorporation of azacitidine triphosphate into DNA, resulting in inhibition of DNA methyltransferases, which then leads to a loss of DNA methylation and gene reactivation. Aberrantly silenced genes, such as tumor suppressor genes, are reactivated and expressed.

Mechanism of Resistance

None well characterized to date.

Absorption

Not available for oral use and is administered via the SC and IV route. The bioavailability of SC azacitidine is 89% relative to IV azacitidine.

Distribution

The distribution in humans has not been fully characterized. Does cross blood-brain barrier.

Metabolism

The precise route of elimination and metabolic fate of azacitidine is not well characterized in humans. In vitro studies suggest that azacitidine may be metabolized by the liver. One of the elimination pathways is via deamination by cytidine deaminase, found principally in the liver but also in plasma, granulocytes, intestinal epithelium, and peripheral tissues. Urinary excretion is the main route of elimination of the parent drug and its metabolites. The half-lives of azacitidine and its metabolites are approximately 4 hours.

Indications

FDA-approved for treatment of patients with myelodysplastic syndromes (MDS), including refractory anemia, refractory anemia with ringed sideroblasts, refractory anemia with excess blasts, refractory anemia with excess blasts in transformation, and chronic myelomonocytic leukemia.

Dosage Range

Recommended dose is 75 mg/m^2 SC/IV daily for 7 days. Cycles should be repeated every 4 weeks.

Drug Interactions

None characterized to date.

Special Considerations

1. Patients should be treated for a minimum of four cycles, as it may take longer than four cycles for clinical benefit.

2. Patients should be pretreated with effective antiemetics to prevent nausea/vomiting.

3. Monitor complete blood counts on a regular basis during therapy.

4. Use with caution in patients with underlying kidney dysfunction. If unexplained elevations in BUN or serum creatinine occur, the next cycle should be delayed, and the subsequent dose should be reduced by 50%. If unexplained reductions in serum bicarbonate levels to <20 mEq/L occur, the subsequent dose should be reduced by 50%.

5. Pregnancy category D. Breast-feeding should be avoided.

Toxicity 1

Myelosuppression with neutropenia and thrombocytopenia.

Toxicity 2

Fatigue and anorexia.

Toxicity 3

GI toxicity in the form of nausea/vomiting, constipation, and abdominal pain.

A

Toxicity 4

Renal toxicity with elevations in serum creatinine, renal tubular acidosis, and hypokalemia.

Toxicity 5

Peripheral edema.

Bendamustine

Cl-CH$_2$-CH$_2$ \
Cl-CH$_2$-CH$_2$ —N [benzimidazole ring structure] N=CH—N \
CH$_3$

Trade Names
Treanda

Classification
Alkylating agent

Category
Chemotherapy drug

Drug Manufacturer
Cephalon

Mechanism of Action
- Bifunctional alkylating agent consisting of a purine benzimidazole ring and a nitrogen mustard moiety.
- Forms cross-links with DNA resulting in single- and double-strand breaks and inhibition of DNA synthesis and function.
- Inhibits mitotic checkpoints and induces mitotic catastrophe, leading to cell death.
- Cell cycle–nonspecific. Active in all phases of the cell cycle.

Mechanism of Resistance
- Increased activity of DNA repair enzymes.
- Increased expression of sulfhydryl proteins, including glutathione and glutathione-related enzymes.
- Cross-resistance between bendamustine and other alkylating agents is only partial.

Absorption
High oral bioavailability on the order of 90%. No oral formulation is currently available, and as such, it is administered only by the IV route.

Distribution
Bendamustine is highly protein bound (>95%), mainly to albumin. Protein binding is not affected by elderly age or low serum albumin levels.

Metabolism

Metabolized in the liver via hydrolysis to both active and inactive forms. Two active minor metabolites, M3 and M4, are mainly formed by CYP1A2 enzymes. Parent drug and its metabolites are eliminated to a large extent by the kidneys, and 45% of parent drug is excreted in urine. The elimination half-life of the parent compound is approximately 40 minutes.

Indications

1. FDA-approved for the treatment of chronic lymphocytic leukemia (CLL).

2. FDA-approved for the treatment of indolent B-cell non-Hodgkin's lymphoma that has progressed during or within 6 months of treatment with rituximab or a rituximab containing regimen.

Dosage Range

1. CLL treatment-naïve—100 mg/m^2 IV on days 1 and 2 every 28 days. May give up to a total of six cycles.

2. Non-Hodgkin's lymphoma—120 mg/m^2 IV on days 1 and 2 every 21 days. May give up to a total of eight cycles.

Drug Interactions

Inhibitors or inducers of CYP1A2—Concurrent use of bendamustine with CYP1A2 inhibitors (ciprofloxacin, fluvoxamine) or CYP1A2 inducers (omeprazole, smoking) may alter bendamustine metabolism and subsequent drug levels.

Special Considerations

1. Use with caution in patients with mild or moderate renal impairment. Bendamustine should not be used in patients with CrCl <40 mL/min.

2. Use with caution in patients with mild hepatic impairment. Should not be used in setting of moderate (SGOT or SGPT 2.5–10 × ULN and total bilirubin 1.5–3 × ULN) or severe (total bilirubin >3 × ULN) hepatic impairment.

3. Monitor for tumor lysis syndrome, especially within the first treatment cycle. Consider using allopurinol during the first 1 to 2 weeks of bendamustine therapy in patients at high risk.

4. Closely monitor CBCs on a periodic basis. Treatment delays and/ or dose reduction may be warranted. Prior to starting the next cycle of therapy, the ANC should be ≥1,000/mm^3 and the platelet count ≥75,000/mm^3.

5. Closely monitor for hypersensitivity infusion reactions, and discontinuation of therapy should be considered in patients who experience grade 3 or 4 infusion reactions.

6. Bendamustine therapy should be held or discontinued in the setting of severe or progressive skin reactions.

7. Pregnancy category D.

Toxicity 1

Myelosuppression: May warrant treatment delay or dose reduction. Monitor closely and restart treatment based on ANC and platelet count recovery.

Toxicity 2

Mild nausea and vomiting.

Toxicity 3

Hypersensitivity reactions presenting with fever, chills, pruritus, and rash. Anaphylactoid and severe anaphylactic reactions have occurred rarely.

Toxicity 4

Pyrexia, fatigue, and asthenia.

Toxicity 5

Tumor lysis syndrome typically occurs within the first treatment cycle and in high-risk patients.

Toxicity 6

Skin rash, toxic skin reactions, and bullous exanthema occur in <10% of patients.

Bevacizumab

B

Avastin

Classification
Monoclonal antibody, anti-VEGF-antibody

Category
Biologic response modifier agent

Drug Manufacturer
Genentech

Mechanism of Action

- Recombinant humanized monoclonal antibody directed against the vascular endothelial growth factor (VEGF). Binds to all isoforms of VEGF-A. VEGF is a pro-angiogenic growth factor that is overexpressed in a wide range of solid human cancers, including colorectal cancer.

- Precise mechanism(s) of action remains unknown.

- Binding of VEGF prevents its subsequent interaction with VEGFR-receptors on the surface of endothelial cells and tumors, and in so doing, results in inhibition of VEGFR-signaling.

- Inhibits formation of new blood vessels in primary tumor and metastatic tumors.

- Inhibits tumor blood vessel permeability and reduces interstitial tumoral pressures, and in so doing, may enhance blood flow delivery within tumor.

- Restores antitumor response by enhancing dendritic cell function.

- Immunologic mechanisms may also be involved in antitumor activity, and they include recruitment of ADCC and/or complement-mediated cell lysis.

Mechanism of Resistance
- None have been characterized to date.

Distribution
Distribution in body is not well characterized. The predicted time to reach steady-state levels is on the order of 100 days.

Metabolism

Metabolism of bevacizumab has not been extensively characterized. Half-life is on the order of 17–21 days with minimal clearance by the liver or kidneys.

Indications

1. Metastatic colorectal cancer—FDA-approved for use in combination with any intravenous 5-fluorouracil-based chemotherapy in first-line therapy.

2. Metastatic colorectal cancer—FDA-approved for use in combination with FOLFOX-4 in second-line therapy.

3. Non–small cell lung cancer—FDA-approved for non-squamous, non–small cell lung cancer in combination with carboplatin/paclitaxel.

4. Breast cancer—FDA-approved for metastatic HER2-negative breast cancer in combination with paclitaxel for patients who have not received chemotherapy.

5. Glioblastoma—FDA-approved as a single agent for glioblastoma with progressive disease following prior therapy.

6. Renal cell cancer—FDA-approved in combination with interferon-α for metastatic renal cell cancer.

Dosage Range

1. Recommended dose for the first-line treatment of advanced colorectal cancer is 5 mg/kg IV in combination with intravenous 5-FU–based chemotherapy on an every 2-week schedule.

2. Recommended dose for the second-line treatment of advanced colorectal cancer in combination with FOLFOX-4 is 10 mg/kg IV on an every 2-week schedule.

3. Can also be administered at 7.5 mg/kg IV every 3 weeks when used in combination with capecitabine-based regimens for advanced colorectal cancer.

4. Recommended dose for advanced non–small cell lung cancer is 15 mg/kg IV every 3 weeks.

5. Recommended dose for metastatic breast cancer is 10 mg/kg IV every 2 weeks.

6. Recommended dose for glioblastoma is 10 mg/kg IV every 2 weeks.

7. Recommended dose for renal cell cancer is 10 mg/kg IV every 2 weeks.

Drug Interactions

No formal drug interactions have been well characterized to date.

Special Considerations

1. Patients should be warned of the increased risk of arterial thromboembolic events, including myocardial infarction and stroke. Risk factors are age >65 years and history of angina, stroke, and prior arterial thromboembolic events. This represents a black-box warning.

2. Patients should be warned of the potential for serious and, in some cases, fatal hemorrhage resulting from hemoptysis in patients with non–small cell lung cancer. These events have been mainly observed in patients with a central, cavitary, and/or necrotic lesion involving the pulmonary vasculature and have occurred suddenly. Patients with recent hemoptysis (>1/2 tsp of red blood) should not receive bevacizumab. This represents a black-box warning.

3. Bevacizumab treatment can result in the development of GI perforations and wound dehiscence, which in some cases has resulted in death. These events represent a black-box warning for the drug. Caution should be exercised in treating patients who have undergone recent surgical and/or invasive procedures, and bevacizumab should be given at least 28 days after any surgical and/or invasive intervention. In patients who have undergone surgical resection of the liver, bevacizumab should not be given for at least 6 to 8 weeks after the surgical procedure.

4. Bevacizumab treatment can result in the development of wound dehiscence, which in some cases can be fatal. This represents a black-box warning.

5. Carefully monitor for infusion-related symptoms. May need to treat with benadryl and acetaminophen.

6. Use with caution in patients with uncontrolled hypertension as bevacizumab can result in grade 3 hypertension in about 10% of patients. Should be permanently discontinued in patients who develop hypertensive crisis. In most cases, however, hypertension is well-managed with increasing the dose of the anti-hypertensive medication and/or with the addition of another anti-hypertensive medication.

7. Bevacizumab should be terminated in patients who develop the nephrotic syndrome. Therapy should be interrupted for proteinuria >2 grams/24 hours and resumed when <2 grams/24 hours.

8. Bevacizumab treatment can result in reversible posterior leukoencephalopathy syndrome (RPLS), as manifested by headache, seizure, lethargy, confusion, blindness and other visual side effects, as well as other neurologic disturbances. This syndrome can occur from 16 hours to 1 year after initiation of therapy, usually resolves or improves within days, and magnetic resonance imaging is necessary to confirm the diagnosis.

9. There are no recommended dose reductions for bevacizumab. In the setting of adverse events, bevacizumab should be discontinued or temporarily interrupted.

10. Pregnancy category B.

Toxicity 1

Gastrointestinal perforations and wound healing complications.

Toxicity 2

Bleeding complications with epistaxis being most commonly observed. Serious life-threatening pulmonary hemorrhage occur in rare cases in patients with non–small cell lung cancer as outlined above in Special Considerations.

Toxicity 3

Increased risk of arterial thromboembolic events, including myocardial infarction, angina, and stroke. There is also an increased incidence of venous thromboembolic events.

Toxicity 4

Hypertension occurs in up to 20%–30% of patients with grade 3 hypertension observed in 10%–15% of patients. Usually well controlled with oral anti-hypertensive medication.

Toxicity 5

Proteinuria with nephrotic syndrome developing in up to 5% of patients.

Toxicity 6

Infusion-related symptoms with fever, chills, urticaria, flushing, fatigue, headache, bronchospasm, dyspnea, angioedema, and hypotension. Relatively uncommon (<5%).

Toxicity 7

CNS events with dizziness and depression. Posterior leukoencephalopathy syndrome occurs rarely (<0.1%), presenting with headache, seizure, lethargy, confusion, blindness, and other visual disturbances.

Bexarotene

$$H_3C \quad CH_3 \quad CH_2$$

Trade Names
Targretin

Classification
Retinoid

Category
Differentiating agent

Drug Manufacturer
Ligand

Mechanism of Action
- Selectively binds and activates retinoid X receptors (RXRs).
- RXRs form heterodimers with various other receptors, including retinoic acid receptors (RARs), vitamin D receptors, and thyroid receptors. Once activated, these receptors function as transcription factors, which then regulate the expression of various genes involved in controlling cell differentiation, growth, and proliferation.
- Precise mechanism by which bexarotene exerts its antitumor activity in cutaneous T-cell lymphoma (CTCL) remains unknown.

Absorption
Well absorbed by the GI tract. Peak plasma levels observed 2 hours after oral administration.

Distribution
Distribution is not well characterized. Highly bound to plasma proteins (>99%).

Metabolism
Extensive metabolism occurs in the liver via the cytochrome P450 system to both active and inactive metabolites. Both parent drug and its metabolites are eliminated primarily through the hepatobiliary system and in feces. Renal clearance is minimal accounting for <1%. The elimination half-life is about 7 hours.

Indications

Treatment of cutaneous manifestations of CTCL in patients who are refractory to at least one prior systemic therapy.

Dosage Range

Recommended initial dose is 300 mg/m^2/day PO. Should be taken as a single dose with food.

Drug Interaction 1

Gemfibrozil—Gemfibrozil inhibits metabolism of bexarotene by the liver P450 system resulting in increased plasma concentrations. Concurrent administration of gemfibrozil with bexarotene is not recommended.

Drug Interaction 2

Inhibitors of cytochrome P450 system—Drugs that inhibit the liver P450 system, such as ketoconazole, itraconazole, and erythromycin, may cause an increase in plasma concentrations of bexarotene.

Drug Interaction 3

Inducers of cytochrome P450 system—Drugs that induce the liver P450 system, such as rifampin, phenytoin, and phenobarbital, may cause a reduction in plasma bexarotene concentrations.

Special Considerations

1. Use with caution in patients with abnormal liver function. Monitor liver function tests at baseline and during therapy. Treatment should be discontinued when LFTs are 3-fold higher than the upper limit of normal.

2. Use with caution in diabetic patients who are on insulin, agents enhancing insulin secretion, or insulin sensitizers as bexarotene therapy can enhance their effects resulting in hypoglycemia.

3. Use with caution in patients with history of lipid disorders as significant alterations in lipid profile are observed with bexarotene therapy. Lipid profile should be obtained at baseline, weekly until the lipid response is established, and at 8-week intervals.

4. Thyroid function tests should be obtained at baseline and during therapy as bexarotene is associated with hypothyroidism.

5. Use with caution in patients with known hypersensitivity to retinoids.

6. Patients should be advised to limit vitamin A supplementation to <1,500 IU/day to avoid potential additive toxic effects with bexarotene.

7. Patients should be advised to avoid exposure to sunlight as bexarotene is associated with photosensitivity.

8. Patients who experience new-onset visual difficulties should have an ophthalmologic evaluation as bexarotene is associated with retinal

complications, development of new cataracts, and/or worsening of pre-existing cataracts.

9. Pregnancy category X. Must not be given to a pregnant woman or to a woman who intends to become pregnant. If a woman becomes pregnant while on therapy, bexarotene must be stopped immediately.

Toxicity 1

Hypertriglyceridemia and hypercholesterolemia are common. Reversible upon dose reduction, cessation of therapy, or when anti-lipemic therapy is begun (gemfibrozil is not recommended, see Drug Interaction 1).

Toxicity 2

Hypothyroidism develops in 50% of patients.

Toxicity 3

Headache and asthenia.

Toxicity 4

Myelosuppression with leukopenia more common than anemia.

Toxicity 5

Nausea, abdominal pain, and diarrhea.

Toxicity 6

Skin rash, dry skin, and rarely alopecia.

Toxicity 7

Dry eyes, conjunctivitis, blepharitis, cataracts, corneal lesions, and visual field defects.

Bicalutamide

$$NH-\overset{O}{\underset{}{C}}-\overset{OH}{\underset{CH_3}{C}}-CH_2-SO_2-\langle\ \rangle-F$$

$C_{18}H_{14}N_2O_4F_4S$

CF$_3$

CN

Trade Names

Casodex

Classification

Antiandrogen

Category

Hormonal drug

Drug Manufacturer

AstraZeneca

Mechanism of Action

- Nonsteroidal, antiandrogen agent that binds to androgen receptor and inhibits androgen uptake as well as inhibits androgen binding in nucleus in androgen-sensitive prostate cancer cells.
- Affinity to androgen receptor is 4-fold greater than flutamide.

Mechanism of Resistance

- Decreased expression of androgen receptor.
- Mutation in androgen receptor leading to decreased binding affinity to bicalutamide.

Absorption

Well absorbed by the GI tract. Peak plasma levels observed 1–2 hours after oral administration. Absorption is not affected by food.

Distribution

Distribution is not well characterized. Extensively bound to plasma proteins (96%).

Metabolism

Extensive metabolism occurs in the liver via oxidation and glucuronidation by cytochrome P450 enzymes to inactive metabolites. Both parent drug and its metabolites are cleared in urine and feces. The elimination half-life is long, on the order of several days.

Indications

Stage D2 metastatic prostate cancer.

Dosage Range

Recommended dose is 50 mg PO once daily either alone or in combination with a luteinizing hormone–releasing hormone (LHRH) analog.

Drug Interactions

Warfarin—Bicalutamide can displace warfarin from their protein-binding sites leading to increased anticoagulant effect. Coagulation parameters (PT and INR) must be followed closely, and dose adjustments may be needed.

Special Considerations

1. Use with caution in patients with abnormal liver function. Monitor LFTs at baseline and during therapy.

2. Caution patients about the potential for hot flashes. Consider the use of clonidine 0.1–0.2 mg PO daily, Megace 20 mg PO bid, or soy tablets one tablet PO tid for prevention and/or treatment.

3. Instruct patients on the potential risk of altered sexual function and impotence.

4. Pregnancy category D.

Toxicity 1

Hot flashes, decreased libido, impotence, gynecomastia, nipple pain, and galactorrhea. Occur in 50% of patients.

Toxicity 2

Constipation observed in 10% of patients. Nausea, vomiting, and diarrhea occur rarely.

Toxicity 3

Transient elevations in serum transaminases are rare.

Bleomycin

Trade Names

Blenoxane

Classification

Antitumor antibiotic

Category

Chemotherapy drug

Drug Manufacturer

Bristol-Myers Squibb

Mechanism of Action

- Small peptide with a molecular weight of 1,500.
- Contains a DNA-binding region and an iron-binding region at opposite ends of the molecule.
- Iron is absolutely necessary as a cofactor for free radical generation and bleomycin's cytotoxic activity.
- Cytotoxic effects result from the generation of activated oxygen free radical species, which causes single- and double-strand DNA breaks and eventual cell death.

Mechanism of Resistance

- Increased expression of DNA repair enzymes resulting in enhanced repair of DNA damage.
- Decreased drug accumulation through altered uptake of drug.

Absorption

Oral bioavailability of bleomycin is poor. After IM administration, peak levels are obtained in about 60 minutes but reach only one-third the levels achieved after an IV dose. When administered in the intrapleural space for the treatment of malignant pleural effusion (pleurodesis), approximately 45%–50% of the drug is absorbed into the systemic circulation.

Distribution

Distributes into intra- and extra-cellular fluid. Less than 10% of drug bound to plasma proteins.

Metabolism

After IV administration, there is a rapid biphasic disappearance from the circulation. The terminal half-life is approximately 3 hours in patients with normal renal function. Bleomycin is rapidly inactivated in tissues, especially the liver and kidney, by the enzyme bleomycin hydrolase. Elimination of bleomycin is primarily via the kidneys, with 50%–70% of a given dose being excreted unchanged in urine. Patients with impaired renal function may experience increased drug accumulation and are at risk for increased toxicity. Dose reductions are required in the presence of renal dysfunction.

Indications

1. Hodgkin's and non-Hodgkin's lymphoma.

2. Germ cell tumors.

3. Head and neck cancer.

4. Squamous cell carcinomas of the skin, cervix, and vulva.

5. Sclerosing agent for malignant pleural effusion and ascites.

Dosage Range

1. Hodgkin's lymphoma: 10 units/m^2 IV on days 1 and 15 every 28 days, as part of the ABVD regimen.

2. Testicular cancer: 30 units IV on days 2, 9, and 16 every 21 days, as part of the PEB regimen.

3. Intracavitary instillation into pleural space: 60 units/m^2.

Drug Interaction 1

Oxygen—High concentrations of oxygen may enhance the pulmonary toxicity of bleomycin. FIO_2 should be maintained at no higher than 25% when possible.

Drug Interaction 2

Phenothiazines—Phenothiazines enhance the activity of bleomycin by competing with liver P450 enzymes.

Drug Interaction 3

Cisplatin—Cisplatin decreases renal clearance of bleomycin and, in so doing, may enhance toxicity.

Drug Interaction 4

Radiation therapy—Radiation therapy enhances the pulmonary toxicity of bleomycin.

Special Considerations

1. PFTs with special focus on DLCO and vital capacity should be obtained at baseline and before each cycle of therapy. A decrease of >15% in PFTs should mandate the immediate discontinuation of bleomycin, even in the absence of clinical symptoms. Increased risk of pulmonary toxicity when cumulative dose >400 units.

2. Chest x-ray should be obtained at baseline and before each cycle of therapy to monitor for evidence of infiltrates and/or interstitial lung findings.

3. Monitor for clinical signs of pulmonary dysfunction, including shortness of breath, dyspnea, decreased O_2 saturation, and decreased lung expansion.

4. Use with caution in patients with impaired renal function because drug clearance may be reduced. Doses should be reduced in the presence of renal dysfunction. Baseline creatinine clearance should be obtained, and renal status should be monitored before each cycle.

5. Patients with lymphoma may be at increased risk for developing an anaphylactic reaction. This complication can be immediate or delayed. An anaphylaxis kit that includes epinephrine, antihistamines, and corticosteroids should be readily available at bedside during bleomycin administration.

6. Premedicate patients with acetaminophen 30 minutes before administration of drug and every 6 hours for 24 hours if fever and chills are noted.

7. Patients undergoing surgery must inform the surgeon and anesthesiologist of prior treatment with bleomycin. High concentrations of forced inspiratory oxygen (FIO2) at the time of surgery may enhance the pulmonary toxicity of bleomycin.

Toxicity 1

Skin reactions are the most common side effects and include erythema, hyperpigmentation of the skin, striae, and vesiculation. Skin peeling, thickening of the skin and nail beds, hyperkeratosis, and ulceration can also occur. These manifestations usually occur in the second and third week after treatment, when the cumulative dose has reached 150–200 units. Alopecia is common.

Toxicity 2

Pulmonary toxicity is dose-limiting. Occurs in 10% of patients. Usually presents as pneumonitis with cough, dyspnea, dry inspiratory crackles, and infiltrates on chest x-ray. This complication is both dose- and age-related.

Increased incidence in patients >70 years of age and with cumulative doses >400 units. Rarely progresses to pulmonary fibrosis but can be fatal in about 1% of patients. PFTs are the most sensitive approach to follow, with specific focus on DLCO and vital capacity. A decrease of 15% or more in the PFTs should mandate immediate stoppage of the drug.

Toxicity 3

Hypersensitivity reaction in the form of fever and chills observed in up to 25% of patients. True anaphylactoid reactions are rare but more common in patients with lymphoma.

Toxicity 4

Vascular events, including myocardial infarction, stroke, and Raynaud's phenomenon, are rarely reported.

Toxicity 5

Myelosuppression is relatively mild.

Bortezomib

Trade Names

VELCADE®

Classification

Proteosome inhibitor

Category

Chemotherapy drug

Drug Manufacturer

Millennium: The Takeda Oncology Company

Mechanism of Action

- Reversible inhibitor of the 26S proteosome.

- The 26S proteosome is a large protein complex that degrades ubiquinated proteins. This pathway plays an essential role in regulating the intracellular concentrations of various cellular proteins.

- Inhibition of the 26S proteosome prevents the targeted proteolysis of ubiquinated proteins, and disruption of this normal pathway can affect multiple signaling pathways within the cell, leading to cell death.

- Results in down-regulation of the NF-κB pathway. NF-κB is a transcription factor that stimulates the production of various growth factors, including IL-6, cell adhesion molecules, and anti-apoptotic proteins, all of which contribute to cell growth and chemoresistance. Inhibition of the NF-κB pathway by bortezomib leads to inhibition of cell growth and restores chemosensitivity.

Mechanism of Resistance

None well characterized to date.

B

Absorption

Bortezomib is given only by the intravenous route.

Distribution

Volume of distribution not well characterized. About 80% of drug bound to plasma proteins.

Metabolism

Bortezomib has a mean elimination half-life of 76 to 108 hours upon multiple dosing with the 1.3 mg/m$_2$ dose. It is metabolized by the liver cytochrome P450 system. The major metabolic pathway is deboronation, forming two deboronated metabolites. The deboronated metabolites are inactive as 26S proteosome inhibitors. Elimination pathways for bortezomib have not been well characterized.

Indications

VELCADE® (bortezomib) for Injection is indicated for the treatment of patients with multiple

myeloma.

Dosage Range

Recommended dose for relapsed multiple myeloma and mantle cell lymphoma is 1.3 mg/m^2 administered by IV twice weekly for 2 weeks (on days 1, 4, 8, and 11) followed by a 10-day rest period (days 12–21).

Drug Interactions

Ketoconazole: Co-administration of ketoconazole, a potent CYP3A inhibitor, increased the exposure of bortezomib. Therefore, patients should be closely monitored when given bortezomib in combination with potent CYP3A4 inhibitors (e.g. 556 ketoconazole, ritonavir). Patients who are concomitantly receiving VELCADE and drugs that are inhibitors or inducers of cytochrome P450 3A4 should be closely monitored for either toxicities or reduced efficacy.

Special Considerations

1. Contraindicated in patients with hypersensitivity to boron, bortezomib, and/or mannitol.

2. Use with caution in patients with impaired liver function, because drug metabolism and/or clearance may be reduced. No formal dose recommendations in this setting, although patients should be closely monitored for toxicities.

3. The pharmacokinetics of VELCADE are not influenced by the degree of renal impairment. Therefore, dosing adjustments of VELCADE are not necessary for patients with renal insufficiency. Since dialysis may reduce VELCADE concentrations, the drug should be administered after the dialysis procedure.

4. Use with caution in patients with a history of syncope, patients who are on anti-hypertensive medications, and patients who are dehydrated, because bortezomib can cause orthostatic hypotension.

5. Bortezomib should be withheld at the onset of any grade 3 non-hematologic toxicity, excluding neuropathy, or any grade 4 hematologic toxicities. After symptoms have resolved, therapy can be restarted with a 25% dose reduction. With respect to neuropathy, the dose of bortezomib should be reduced to 1.0 mg/m^2 with grade 1 peripheral neuropathy with pain or grade 2 peripheral neuropathy. In the presence of grade 2 neurotoxicity, therapy should be withheld until symptoms have resolved and restarted at a dose of 0.7 mg/m^2 along with changing the treatment schedule to once per week. In the presence of grade 4 neurotoxicity, therapy should be discontinued.

6. Pregnancy category D.

Toxicity 1

Fatigue, malaise, and generalized weakness. Usually observed during the first and second cycles of therapy.

Toxicity 2

GI toxicity in the form of nausea/vomiting and diarrhea.

Toxicity 3

Myelosuppression with thrombocytopenia and neutropenia.

Toxicity 4

Peripheral sensory neuropathy, although a mixed sensorimotor neuropathy has also been observed. Symptoms may improve and/or return to baseline upon discontinuation of bortezomib.

Toxicity 5

Fever (>38°C) in up to 40% of patients.

Toxicity 6

Orthostatic hypotension in up to 12% of patients.

Busulfan

$$CH_3 - \overset{\overset{O}{\|}}{\underset{\underset{O}{\|}}{S}} - O - CH_2CH_2CH_2CH_2O - \overset{\overset{O}{\|}}{\underset{\underset{O}{\|}}{S}} - CH_3$$

Trade Names
Myleran, Busulfex

Classification
Alkylating agent

Category
Chemotherapy drug

Drug Manufacturer
GlaxoSmithKline

Mechanism of Action
- Methanesulfonate-type bifunctional alkylating agent.
- Interacts with cellular thiol groups and nucleic acids to form DNA-DNA and DNA-protein cross-links. Cross-linking of DNA results in inhibition of DNA synthesis and function.
- Cell cycle–nonspecific, active in all phases of the cell cycle.

Mechanism of Resistance
- Decreased cellular uptake of drug.
- Increased intracellular thiol content due to glutathione or glutathione-related enzymes.
- Enhanced activity of DNA repair enzymes.

Absorption
Excellent oral bioavailability with peak levels in serum occurring within 2–4 hours after administration. About 30% of drug is bound to plasma proteins.

Distribution
Distributes rapidly in plasma with broad tissue distribution. Crosses the blood-brain barrier and also crosses the placental barrier.

Metabolism
Metabolized primarily in the liver by the cytochrome P450 system. Metabolites, including sulfoxane, 3-hydroxysulfoxane, and methanesulfonic acid, are excreted in urine, with 50%–60% excreted within 48 hours. Metabolism may be influenced by circadian rhythm with higher clearance

rates observed in the evening, especially in younger patients. The terminal half-life is 2.5 hours.

Indications

1. Chronic myelogenous leukemia (CML) (standard dose).
2. Bone marrow/stem cell transplantation for refractory leukemia, lymphoma (high dose). Use in combination with cyclophosphamide as conditioning regimen prior to allogeneic stem cell transplantation for CML.

Dosage Range

1. CML: Usual dose for remission induction is 4–8 mg/day PO. Dosing on a weight basis is 1.8 mg/m^2/day. Maintenance dose is usually 1–3 mg/day PO.
2. Transplant setting: 4 mg/kg/day IV for four days to a total dose of 16 mg/kg.

Drug Interaction 1

Acetaminophen—Acetaminophen may decrease busulfan metabolism in the liver when given 72 hours before busulfan, resulting in enhanced toxicity.

Drug Interaction 2

Itraconazole—Itraconazole reduces busulfan metabolism by up to 20%.

Drug Interaction 3

Phenobarbital and phenytoin—Phenobarbital and phenytoin increase busulfan metabolism in the liver by inducing the activity of the liver microsomal system.

Special Considerations

1. Monitor CBC while on therapy. When the total WBC count has declined to approximately 15,000/mm^3, busulfan should be withheld until the nadir is reached and the counts begin to rise above this level. A decrease in the WBC count may not be seen during the first 10–15 days of therapy, and it may continue to fall for more than one month even after the drug has been stopped.
2. Monitor patients for pulmonary symptoms as busulfan can cause interstitial pneumonitis.
3. Ingestion of busulfan on an empty stomach may decrease the risk of nausea and vomiting.
4. Pregnancy category D. Breast-feeding should be avoided.

Toxicity 1

Myelosuppression with pancytopenia is dose-limiting toxicity.

Toxicity 2

Nausea/vomiting and diarrhea are common (>80% of patients) but generally mild with standard doses. Anorexia is also frequently observed.

Toxicity 3

Mucositis is dose-related and may require interruption of therapy in some instances.

Toxicity 4

Hyperpigmentation of skin, especially in hand creases and nail beds. Skin rash and pruritus also observed.

Toxicity 5

Impotence, male sterility, amenorrhea, ovarian suppression, menopause, and infertility.

Toxicity 6

Pulmonary symptoms, including cough, dyspnea, and fever, can be seen after long-term therapy. Interstitial pulmonary fibrosis, referred to as "busulfan lung", is a rare but severe side effect of therapy. May occur 1–10 years after discontinuation of therapy.

Toxicity 7

Adrenal insufficiency occurs rarely.

Toxicity 8

Hepatotoxicity with elevations in LFTs. Hepato-veno-occlusive disease is observed with high doses of busulfan (>16 mg/day) used in transplant setting.

Toxicity 9

Insomnia, anxiety, dizziness, and depression are the most common neurologic side effects. Seizures can occur, usually with high-dose therapy.

Toxicity 10

Increased risk of secondary malignancies, especially acute myelogenous leukemia, with long-term chronic use.

Capecitabine

$$HN-C(=O)-O-(CH_2)_4-CH_3$$

carboxylesterase
(liver)

capecitabine

5-fluoro-5′-deoxycytidine
(5′-DFCR)

cytidine
deaminase
(liver, tumors)

dThdPase
(tumors)

5-fluoro-5′-deoxyuridine
(5′-DFUR)

5-fluorouracil
(5-FU)

Trade Names

Xeloda

Classification

Antimetabolite

Category

Chemotherapy drug

Drug Manufacturer

Roche

Mechanism of Action

- Fluoropyrimidine carbamate prodrug form of 5-fluorouracil (5-FU).
  Capecitabine itself is inactive.

- Activation to cytotoxic forms is a complex process that involves 3 successive enzymatic steps. Metabolized in liver to 5'-deoxy-5-fluorocytidine (5'-DFCR) by the carboxylesterase enzyme and then to 5'-deoxy-5-fluorouridine (5'-DFUR) by cytidine deaminase (found in liver and in tumor tissues). Subsequently converted to 5-FU by the enzyme thymidine phosphorylase, which is expressed in higher levels in tumor versus normal tissue.
- Inhibition of the target enzyme thymidylate synthase by the 5-FU metabolite FdUMP.
- Incorporation of 5-FU metabolite FUTP into RNA resulting in alterations in RNA processing and/or translation.
- Incorporation of 5-FU metabolite FdUTP into DNA resulting in inhibition of DNA synthesis and function.
- Inhibition of TS leads to accumulation of dUMP and subsequent misincorporation of dUTP into DNA, resulting in inhibition of DNA synthesis and function.

Mechanism of Resistance

- Increased expression of thymidylate synthase.
- Decreased levels of reduced folate substrate 5,10-methylenetetrahdrofolate for thymidylate synthase reaction.
- Decreased incorporation of 5-FU into RNA.
- Decreased incorporation of 5-FU into DNA.
- Increased activity of DNA repair enzymes, uracil glycosylase, and dUTPase.
- Decreased expression of mismatch repair enzymes (hMLH1, hMSH2).
- Increased salvage of physiologic nucleosides including thymidine.
- Increased expression of dihydropyrimidine dehydrogenase.
- Alterations in thymidylate synthase with decreased binding affinity of enzyme for FdUMP.

Absorption

Capecitabine is readily absorbed by the GI tract. Peak plasma levels are reached in 1.5 hours, while peak 5-FU levels are achieved at 2 hours after oral administration. The rate and extent of absorption are reduced by food.

Distribution

Plasma protein binding of capecitabine and its metabolites is less than 60%. Primarily bound to albumin (35%).

Metabolism

Capecitabine undergoes extensive enzymatic metabolism to 5-FU. After being absorbed as an intact molecule from the GI tract, it undergoes an initial hydrolysis reaction in the liver catalyzed by carboxylesterase to 5'-DFCR. In the next step, 5'-DFCR is converted in the liver and other tissues to 5'-DFUR by the enzyme cytidine deaminase. Finally, 5'-DFUR is converted to 5-FU by the enzyme thymidine phosphorylase in tumor tissue as well as in normal tissues expressing this enzyme. Selective accumulation of 5-FU within tumor tissue (colorectal) vs. normal tissue (colon) (3.2 x) and plasma (21.4 x) has been demonstrated in a population of colorectal cancer patients requiring definitive surgical resection who received capecitabine preoperatively.

Catabolism accounts for >85% of drug metabolism. Dihydropyrimidine dehydrogenase is the main enzyme responsible for the catabolism of 5-FU, and it is present in liver and extrahepatic tissues such as GI mucosa, WBCs, and the kidneys. Greater than 90% of an administered dose of drug and its metabolites is cleared in the urine. The major metabolite excreted in urine is α-fluoro-β-alanine (FBAL). Only 3% of the drug is cleared by fecal elimination. The elimination half-life of both capecitabine and 5-FU is 45 minutes.

Indications

1. Metastatic breast cancer—FDA-approved when used in combination with docetaxel for the treatment of patients with metastatic breast cancer after failure of prior anthracycline-containing chemotherapy.

2. Metastatic breast cancer—FDA-approved as monotherapy in patients refractory to both paclitaxel- and anthracycline-based chemotherapy or when anthracycline therapy is contraindicated.

3. Metastatic colorectal cancer—FDA-approved as first-line therapy when fluoropyrimidine therapy alone is preferred.

4. Stage III colon cancer—FDA-approved as adjuvant therapy when fluoropyrimidine therapy alone is preferred. Approved in Europe in combination with oxaliplatin as part of the XELOX regimen.

Dosage Range

1. Recommended dose is 1,250 mg/m² PO bid (morning and evening) for 2 weeks with 1 week rest. For combination therapy (capecitabine in combination with docetaxel) with docetaxel being dosed at 75 mg/m² day 1 of a 21-day cycle.

2. May decrease dose of capecitabine to 850–1000 mg/m² bid on days 1–14 to reduce risk of toxicity without compromising efficacy. [See section Special Considerations (8).]

3. An alternative dosing schedule for capecitabine monotherapy is 1,250–1,500 mg/m² PO bid for 1 week on and 1 week off. This schedule appears to be well tolerated, with no compromise in clinical efficacy.

4. Capecitabine should be used at lower doses (850–1000 mg/m² bid on days 1–14) when used in combination with other cytotoxic agents, such as oxaliplatin.

Drug Interaction 1

Capecitabine-warfarin interaction: Patients receiving concomitant capecitabine and oral coumarin-derivative anticoagulant therapy should have their coagulation parameters (PT and INR) monitored frequently in order to adjust the anticoagulant dose accordingly. A clinically important capecitabine-warfarin drug interaction has been documented. Altered coagulation parameters and/or bleeding, including death, have been reported in patients taking capecitabine concomitantly with coumarin-derivative anticoagulants such as warfarin and phenprocoumon. Post-marketing reports have shown clinically significant increases in PT and INR in patients who were stabilized on anticoagulants at the time capecitabine was introduced. These events occurred within several days and up to several months after initiating capecitabine therapy and, in a few cases, within 1 month after stopping capecitabine. These events occurred in patients with and without liver metastases. Age greater than 60 and a diagnosis of cancer independently predispose patients to an increased risk of coagulopathy.

Drug Interaction 2

Aluminum hydroxide, magnesium hydroxide—Concomitant use of aluminum hydroxide– or magnesium hydroxide–containing antacids may increase the bioavailability of capecitabine by 16%–35%.

Drug Interaction 3

Phenytoin—Capecitabine may increase phenytoin blood levels and subsequent phenytoin toxicity. Dose adjustment of phenytoin may be necessary.

Drug Interaction 4

Leucovorin—Leucovorin enhances the toxicity of capecitabine.

Special Considerations

1. Capecitabine should be taken with a glass of water within 30 minutes after a meal.

2. Contraindicated in patients with known hypersensitivity to 5-FU.

3. Contraindicated in patients with known dihydropyrimidine dehydrogenase (DPD) deficiency.

4. No dose adjustments are necessary in patients with mild to moderate liver dysfunction. However, patients should be closely monitored.

5. In the setting of moderate renal dysfunction (baseline creatinine clearance, 30–50 mL/min), a 25% dose reduction is recommended. Patients should be closely monitored as they may be at greater risk for increased toxicity. Contraindicated in patients with severe renal impairment (creatinine clearance <30 mL/min).

6. Patients should be monitored for diarrhea and its associated sequelae, including dehydration, fluid imbalance, and infection. Elderly

patients (>80 years of age) are especially vulnerable to the GI toxicity of capecitabine. Moderate to severe diarrhea (>grade 2) is an indication to interrupt therapy immediately. Subsequent doses should be reduced accordingly.

7. Drug therapy should be stopped immediately in the presence of grades 2 to 4 hyperbilirubinemia until complete resolution or a decrease in intensity to grade 1.

8. Drug therapy should be stopped immediately in the presence of grades 2 or higher adverse event until complete resolution or a decrease in intensity to grade 1. Treatment should continue at 75% of the initial starting dose for grade 2 or 3 toxicity. For grade 4 toxicities, if the physician chooses to continue treatment, treatment should continue at 50% of the initial starting dose.

9. Patients who experience unexpected, severe grade 3 or 4 myelosuppression, GI toxicity, and/or neurologic toxicity upon initiation of therapy may have an underlying deficiency in dihydropyrimidine dehydrogenase. Therapy must be discontinued immediately, and further testing to identify the presence of this pharmacogenetic syndrome should be considered.

10. Vitamin B6 (pyridoxine, 50 mg PO bid) may be used to prevent and/or reduce the incidence and severity of hand-foot syndrome. Dose may be increased to 100 mg PO bid if symptoms do not resolve within 3–4 days.

11. Celecoxib at a dose of 200 mg PO bid may be effective in preventing and/or reducing the incidence and severity of hand-foot syndrome. A low-dose nicotine patch has also been found to be effective in this setting.

12. In patients with the hand-foot syndrome, the affected skin should be well hydrated using a bland and mild moisturizer. Instruct patients to soak affected hands and feet in cool to tepid water for 10 minutes, then apply petroleum jelly onto the wet skin. The use of lanolin-containing salves or ointments such as Bag-Balm emollient may help.

13. Pregnancy category D. Breast-feeding should be avoided.

Toxicity 1

Diarrhea. Dose-limiting, observed in up to 55% of patients. Similar to GI toxicity observed with continuous infusion 5-FU. Mucositis, loss of appetite, dehydration also noted.

Toxicity 2

Hand-foot syndrome (palmar-plantar erythrodysesthesia). Severe hand-foot syndrome is seen in 15–20% of patients. Characterized by tingling, numbness, pain, erythema, dryness, rash, swelling, increased pigmentation, and/or pruritus of the hands and feet. Similar to dermatologic toxicity observed with continuous infusion 5-FU.

Toxicity 3

Nausea and vomiting. Occur in 15%–53% of patients.

Toxicity 4

Elevations in serum bilirubin (20%–40%), alkaline phosphatase, and hepatic transaminases (SGOT, SGPT). Usually transient and clinically asymptomatic.

Toxicity 5

Myelosuppression is observed less frequently than with IV 5-FU. Leukopenia more common than thrombocytopenia.

Toxicity 6

Neurologic toxicity manifested by confusion, cerebellar ataxia, and rarely encephalopathy.

Toxicity 7

Cardiac symptoms of chest pain, EKG changes, and serum enzyme elevation. Rare event but increased risk in patients with prior history of ischemic heart disease.

Toxicity 8

Tear-duct stenosis, acute and chronic conjunctivitis.

Carboplatin

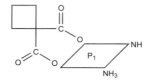

Trade Names
Paraplatin, CBDCA

Classification
Platinum analog

Category
Chemotherapy drug

Drug Manufacturer
Bristol-Myers Squibb

Mechanism of Action
- Covalently binds to DNA with preferential binding to the N-7 position of guanine and adenine.
- Reacts with two different sites on DNA to produce cross-links, either intrastrand (<90%) or interstrand (<5%). Formation of DNA adducts results in inhibition of DNA synthesis and function as well as inhibition of transcription.
- Binding to nuclear and cytoplasmic proteins may result in cytotoxic effects.
- Cell cycle–nonspecific agent.

Mechanism of Resistance
- Reduced accumulation of carboplatin due to alterations in cellular transport.
- Increased inactivation by thiol-containing proteins such as glutathione and glutathione-related enzymes.
- Enhanced DNA repair enzyme activity (e.g., ERCC-1).
- Deficiency in mismatch repair (MMR) enzymes (e.g., hMLH1, hMSH2).

Absorption
Not absorbed by the oral route.

Distribution

Widely distributed in body tissues. Crosses the blood-brain barrier and enters the CSF. Does not bind to plasma proteins and has an apparent volume of distribution of 16 L.

Metabolism

Carboplatin does not undergo significant metabolism. As observed with cisplatin, carboplatin undergoes aquation reaction in the presence of low concentrations of chloride. This reaction is 100-fold slower with carboplatin when compared to cisplatin. Carboplatin is extensively cleared by the kidneys, with about 60%–70% of drug excreted in urine within 24 hours. The elimination of carboplatin is slower than that of cisplatin, with a terminal half-life of 2–6 hours.

Indications

1. Ovarian cancer.
2. Germ cell tumors.
3. Head and neck cancer.
4. Small cell and non–small cell lung cancer.
5. Bladder cancer.
6. Relapsed and refractory acute leukemia.
7. Endometrial cancer.

Dosage Range

1. Dose of carboplatin is usually calculated to a target area under the curve (AUC) based on the glomerular filtration rate (GFR).
2. Calvert formula is used to calculate dose: Total dose (mg) = (target AUC) × (GFR + 25). *Note: Dose is in mg **NOT** mg/m^2.
3. Target AUC is usually between 5 and 7 mg/mL/min for previously untreated patients. In previously treated patients, lower AUCs (between 4 and 6 mg/mL/min) are recommended. AUCs >7 are not associated with improved response rates.
4. Bone marrow/stem cell transplant setting: Doses up to 1,600 mg/m^2 divided over several days.

Drug Interaction 1

Myelosuppressive agents—Increased risk of myelosuppression when carboplatin is combined with other myelosuppressive drugs.

Drug Interaction 2

Paclitaxel—Carboplatin should be administered after paclitaxel when carboplatin and paclitaxel are used in combination. This sequence prevents delayed paclitaxel excretion and increased host toxicity.

Special Considerations

1. Use with caution in patients with abnormal renal function. Dose reduction is required in the setting of renal dysfunction. Baseline creatinine clearance must be obtained. Renal status must be closely monitored during therapy.

2. Although carboplatin is not as emetogenic as cisplatin, pretreatment with antiemetic agents is strongly recommended.

3. Avoid needles or IV administration sets containing aluminum because precipitation of drug may occur.

4. Contraindicated in patients with a history of severe allergic reactions to cisplatin, other platinum compounds, or mannitol.

5. In contrast to cisplatin, IV hydration pretreatment and post-treatment are not necessary. However, patients should still be instructed to maintain adequate oral hydration.

6. Hemodialysis clears carboplatin at 25% of the rate of renal clearance. Peritoneal dialysis is unable to remove carboplatin.

7. Risk of hypersensitivity reactions increases from 1% to 27% in patients receiving more than seven courses of carboplatin-based therapy. For such patients, a 0.02-mL intradermal injection of an undiluted aliquot of their planned carboplatin dose should be administered 1 hour before each cycle of carboplation. This skin test identifies patients in whom carboplatin may be safely administered.

8. Pregnancy category D.

Toxicity 1

Myelosuppression is significant and dose-limiting. Dose-dependent, cumulative toxicity is more severe in elderly patients. Thrombocytopenia is most commonly observed, with nadir by day 21.

Toxicity 2

Nausea and vomiting. Delayed nausea and vomiting can also occur, albeit rarely. Significantly less emetogenic than cisplatin.

Toxicity 3

Renal toxicity. Significantly less common than with cisplatin and rarely symptomatic.

Toxicity 4

Peripheral neuropathy is observed in less than 10% of patients. Patients older than 65 years and/or previously treated with cisplatin may be at higher risk for developing neurologic toxicity.

Toxicity 5

Mild and reversible elevation of liver enzymes, particularly alkaline phosphatase and SGOT.

Toxicity 6

Allergic reaction. Can occur within a few minutes of starting therapy. Presents mainly as skin rash, urticaria, and pruritus. Bronchospasm and hypotension are uncommon.

Toxicity 7

Amenorrhea, azoospermia, impotence, and sterility.

Toxicity 8

Alopecia is uncommon.

Carmustine

$$CI - CH_2 - CH_2 - N - \overset{\overset{\displaystyle O}{\displaystyle \|}}{C} - NH - CH_2 - CH_2 - CI$$
$$\underset{NO}{|}$$

Trade Names

BCNU, Bischloroethylnitrosourea

Classification

Alkylating agent

Category

Chemotherapy drug

Drug Manufacturer

Bristol-Myers Squibb

Mechanism of Action

- Nitrosourea analog.
- Cell cycle–nonspecific.
- Chloroethyl metabolites interfere with the synthesis of DNA, RNA, and protein.

Mechanism of Resistance

- Decreased cellular uptake of drug.
- Increased intracellular thiol content due to glutathione or glutathione-related enzymes.
- Enhanced activity of DNA repair enzymes.

Absorption

Not absorbed via the oral route.

Distribution

Lipid-soluble drug with broad tissue distribution. Crosses the blood-brain barrier, reaching concentrations >50% of those in plasma.

Metabolism

After IV infusion, carmustine is rapidly taken up into tissues and degraded. Extensively metabolized in the liver. Approximately 60%–70% of drug is excreted in urine in its metabolite form, while 10% is excreted as respiratory CO_2. Short serum half-life of only 15–20 minutes.

Indications

1. Brain tumors—Glioblastoma multiforme, brain stem glioma, medulloblastoma, astrocytoma, and ependymoma.
2. Hodgkin's lymphoma.
3. Non-Hodgkin's lymphoma.
4. Multiple myeloma.
5. Glioblastoma multiforme—implantable BCNU-impregnated wafer (Gliadel).

Dosage Range

1. Usual dose is 200 mg/m² IV every 6 weeks. Dose can sometimes be divided over 2 days.
2. Higher doses (450–600 mg/m²) are used with stem cell rescue.
3. Implantable BCNU-impregnated wafers: Up to eight wafers are placed into the surgical resection site after excision of the primary brain tumor.

Drug Interaction 1

Cimetidine—Cimetidine enhances the toxicity of carmustine.

Drug Interaction 2

Amphotericin B—Amphotericin B enhances the cellular uptake of carmustine, thus resulting in increased host toxicity, including renal toxicity.

Drug Interaction 3

Digoxin—Carmustine may decrease the plasma levels of digoxin.

Drug Interaction 4

Phenytoin—Carmustine may decrease the plasma levels of phenytoin.

Special Considerations

1. Administer carmustine slowly over a period of 1–2 hours to avoid intense pain and/or burning at the site of injection. Strategies to decrease pain and/or burning include diluting the drug, slowing the rate of administration, or placing ice above the IV injection site.
2. Monitor CBC while on therapy. Repeated cycles should not be given before 6 weeks, given the delayed and potentially cumulative myelosuppressive effects of carmustine.
3. PFTs should be obtained at baseline and monitored periodically during therapy. There is an increased risk of pulmonary toxicity in patients with a baseline forced vital capacity (FVC) or DLCO below 70% of predicted.
4. Pregnancy category D.

Toxicity 1

Myelosuppression is dose-limiting. Nadir typically occurs at 4–6 weeks after therapy and may persist for 1–3 weeks.

Toxicity 2

Nausea and vomiting may occur within 2 hours after a dose of drug and can last for up to 4–6 hours.

Toxicity 3

Facial flushing and a burning sensation at the IV injection site. Skin contact with drug may cause brownish discoloration and pain.

Toxicity 4

Hepatotoxicity with transient elevations in serum transaminases develops in up to 90% of patients within 1 week of therapy. With high-dose therapy, hepato-veno-occlusive disease may be observed in 5%–20% of patients.

Toxicity 5

Impotence, male sterility, amenorrhea, ovarian suppression, menopause, and infertility. Gynecomastia is occasionally observed.

Toxicity 6

Pulmonary toxicity is uncommon at low doses. At cumulative doses greater than 1,400 mg/m^2, interstitial lung disease and pulmonary fibrosis in the form of an insidious cough, dyspnea, pulmonary infiltrates, and/or respiratory failure may develop.

Toxicity 7

Renal toxicity is uncommon at total cumulative doses of less than 1,000 mg/m^2.

Toxicity 8

Increased risk of secondary malignancies, especially acute myelogenous leukemia and myelodysplasia.

Cetuximab

Trade Names

Erbitux

Classification

Monoclonal antibody, anti-EGFR-antibody

Category

Biologic response modifier agent

Drug Manufacturer

Bristol-Myers Squibb and ImClone/Eli Lilly

Mechanism of Action

- Recombinant chimeric IgG1 monoclonal antibody directed against the epidermal growth factor receptor (EGFR). EGFR is overexpressed in a broad range of human solid tumors, including colorectal cancer, head and neck cancer, non–small cell lung cancer, pancreatic cancer, and breast cancer.
- Precise mechanism(s) of action remains unknown.
- Binds with nearly 10-fold higher affinity to EGFR than normal ligands EGF and TGF-α, which then results in inhibition of EGFR. Prevents both homodimerization and heterodimerization of the EGFR, which leads to inhibition of autophosphorylation and inhibition of EGFR signaling.
- Inhibition of the EGFR signaling pathway results in inhibition of critical mitogenic and anti-apoptotic signals involved in proliferation, growth, invasion/metastasis, angiogenesis.
- Inhibition of the EGFR pathway enhances the response to chemotherapy and/or radiation therapy.
- Immunologic mechanisms may also be involved in antitumor activity, and they include recruitment of ADCC and/or complement-mediated cell lysis.

Mechanism of Resistance

- Mutations in EGFR leading to decreased binding affinity to cetuximab.
- Decreased expression of EGFR.
- Presence of KRAS mutations, which mainly occur in codons 12 and 13.
- Presence of BRAF mutations.
- Activation/induction of alternative cellular signaling pathways, such as PI3K/Akt and IGF-1R.

Distribution

Distribution in the body is not well characterized.

Metabolism

Metabolism of cetuximab has not been extensively characterized. Half-life is on the order of 5–7 days with minimal clearance by the liver or kidneys, as has been observed for other monoclonal antibodies and peptides used in the clinic.

Indications

1. FDA-approved for the treatment of EGFR-expressing colorectal cancer in combination with irinotecan in irinotecan-refractory disease or as monotherapy in patients who are deemed to be irinotecan-intolerant. The use of cetuximab is not recommended for the treatment of mCRC with KRAS mutations.

2. Approved in Europe in combination with cytotoxic chemotherapy in the front-line treatment of wild-type KRAS mCRC.

3. Head and neck cancer—used in combination with radiation therapy for the treatment of locally or regionally advanced squamous cell cancer of the head and neck. FDA-approved.

4. Pancreatic cancer—remains investigational.

5. Non–small cell lung cancer—remains investigational. Awaiting FDA approval.

6. Breast cancer—remains investigational.

Dosage Range

Loading dose of 400 mg/m² IV administered over 120 minutes, followed by maintenance dose of 250 mg/m² IV given on a weekly basis.

An alternative dosing schedule is 500 mg/m² IV every 2 weeks with no need for a loading dose.

Drug Interactions

None well characterized to date.

Special Considerations

1. Cetuximab should be used with caution in patients with known hypersensitivity to murine proteins and/or any individual components.

2. The level of EGFR expression does not accurately predict for cetuximab clinical activity. As such, EGFR testing should not be required for the clinical use of cetuximab.

3. KRAS testing should be performed in all patients being considered for cetuximab therapy. Only patients with wild-type KRAS should be

treated with cetuximab either as monotherapy or in combination with cytotoxic chemotherapy.

4. Development of skin toxicity appears to be a surrogate marker for cetuximab clinical activity.

5. Use with caution in patients with underlying interstitial lung disease as these patients are at increased risk for developing worsening of their interstitial lung disease.

6. In patients who develop a skin rash, topical antibiotics such as Cleocin gel or either oral Cleocin and/or oral minocycline may help. Patients should be warned to avoid sunlight exposure.

7. About 90% of patients experience severe infusion reactions with the first infusion despite the use of prophylactic antihistamine therapy. However, some patients may experience infusion reactions with later infusions.

8. Electrolyte status should be closely monitored, especially serum magnesium and calcium levels, as hypomagnesemia and hypocalcemia have been observed with cetuximab treatment.

9. Pregnancy category C. Breast-feeding should be avoided.

Toxicity 1

Infusion-related symptoms with fever, chills, urticaria, flushing, fatigue, headache, bronchospasm, dyspnea, angioedema, and hypotension. Occurs in 40%–50% of patients, although severe reactions occur in less than 1%. Usually mild to moderate in severity and observed most commonly with administration of the first infusion.

Toxicity 2

Pruritus, dry skin with mainly a pustular, acneiform skin rash. Presents mainly on the face and upper trunk. Improves with continued treatment and resolves upon cessation of therapy.

Toxicity 3

Pulmonary toxicity in the form of interstitial lung disease (ILD) manifested by increased cough, dyspnea, and pulmonary infiltrates. Observed in less than 1% of patients and more frequent in patients with underlying pulmonary disease.

Toxicity 4

Hypomagnesemia.

Toxicity 5

Asthenia and generalized malaise observed in nearly 50% of patients.

Toxicity 6

Paronychial inflammation with swelling of the lateral nail folds of the toes and fingers. Occurs with prolonged use.

Chlorambucil

$$Cl\diagdown N \diagup \bigcirc \diagup CH_2CH_2CH_2CO_2H$$
$$Cl\diagup$$

Trade Names
Leukeran

Classification
Alkylating agent

Category
Chemotherapy drug

Drug Manufacturer
GlaxoSmithKline

Mechanism of Action
- Aromatic analog of nitrogen mustard.
- Functions as a bifunctional alkylating agent.
- Forms cross-links with DNA resulting in inhibition of DNA synthesis and function.
- Cell cycle–nonspecific. Active in all phases of the cell cycle.

Mechanism of Resistance
- Decreased cellular uptake of drug.
- Increased activity of DNA repair enzymes.
- Increased expression of sulfhydryl proteins, including glutathione and glutathione-related enzymes.

Absorption
Oral bioavailability is approximately 75% when taken with food. Maximum plasma levels are achieved within 1–2 hours after oral administration. Extensively bound to plasma proteins.

Distribution
Distribution of chlorambucil has not been well studied.

Metabolism
Metabolized extensively by the liver cytochrome P450 system to both active and inactive forms. Parent drug and its metabolites are eliminated by the kidneys, and 60% of drug metabolites are excreted in urine within 24 hours. The terminal elimination half-life is 1.5–2.5 hours for the parent drug and about 2.5–4 hours for drug metabolites.

Indications

1. Chronic lymphocytic leukemia (CLL).
2. Non-Hodgkin's lymphoma.
3. Hodgkin's lymphoma.
4. Waldenstrom's macroglobulinemia.

Dosage Range

CLL: 0.1–0.2 mg/kg PO daily for 3–6 weeks as required. This dose is for initiation of therapy. For maintenance therapy, a dose of 2–4 mg PO daily is recommended.

Drug Interactions

Phenobarbital, phenytoin, and other drugs that stimulate the liver P450 system—Concurrent use of chlorambucil with these drugs may increase its metabolic activation, leading to increased formation of toxic metabolites.

Special Considerations

1. Careful review of patient's medication list is required.
2. Contraindicated within 1 month of radiation and/or cytotoxic therapy, recent smallpox vaccine, and seizure history.
3. Use with caution when combined with allopurinol or colchicine as drug-induced hyperuricemia may be exacerbated.
4. Closely monitor CBCs. Discontinuation of chlorambucil is not necessary at the first sign of a reduction in the WBC. However, fall may continue for 10 days or more after the last dose.
5. Therapy should be discontinued promptly if generalized skin rash develops as this side effect may rapidly progress to erythema multiforme, toxic epidermal necrolysis, or Stevens-Johnson syndrome.
6. Pregnancy category D.

Toxicity 1

Myelosuppression is dose-limiting. Leukopenia and thrombocytopenia observed equally, with delayed and prolonged nadir occurring 25–30 days and recovery by 40–45 days. Usually reversible, but irreversible bone marrow failure can occur.

Toxicity 2

Mild nausea and vomiting are common.

Toxicity 3

Hyperuricemia.

Toxicity 4

Pulmonary fibrosis and pneumonitis are dose-related and potentially life-threatening. Relatively rare event.

Toxicity 5

Seizures. Children with nephrotic syndrome and patients receiving large cumulative doses are at increased risk. Patients with a history of seizure disorder may be especially prone to seizures.

Toxicity 6

Skin rash, urticaria on face, scalp, and trunk with spread to legs seen in the early stages of therapy. Stevens-Johnson syndrome and toxic epidermal neurolysis are rare events.

Toxicity 7

Amenorrhea, oligospermia/azoospermia, and sterility.

Toxicity 8

Increased risk of secondary malignancies, including acute myelogenous leukemia.

C Cisplatin

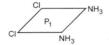

Trade Names

Cis-diamminedichloroplatinum, CDDP, Platinol

Classification

Platinum analog

Category

Chemotherapy drug

Drug Manufacturer

Bristol-Myers Squibb

Mechanism of Action

- Covalently binds to DNA with preferential binding to the N-7 position of guanine and adenine.
- Reacts with two different sites on DNA to produce cross-links, either intrastrand (>90%) or interstrand (<5%). Formation of DNA adducts results in inhibition of DNA synthesis and function as well as inhibition of transcription.
- Binding to nuclear and cytoplasmic proteins may result in cytotoxic effects.

d(GpG) adduct

$$H_3N \diagdown \diagup NH_3$$
$$Pt$$
$$5' - G - G - 3'$$
$$3' - C - C - 5'$$

d(ApG) adduct

$$H_3N \diagdown \diagup NH_3$$
$$Pt$$
$$5' - A - G - 3'$$
$$3' - T - C - 5'$$

d(GpXpG) adduct

$$H_3N \diagdown \diagup NH_3$$
$$Pt$$
$$5' - G - X - G - 3'$$
$$3' - C - X - C - 5'$$

Interstrand cross-link

$$H_3N \diagdown \diagup NH_3$$
$$Pt$$
$$- G - \diagup C -$$
$$- C - G -$$

Mechanism of Resistance

- Increased inactivation by thiol-containing proteins such as glutathione and glutathione-related enzymes.

- Increased DNA repair enzyme activity (e.g., ERCC-1).
- Deficiency in mismatch repair enzymes (e.g., hMHL1, hMSH2).
- Decreased drug accumulation due to alterations in cellular transport.

Absorption

Not absorbed orally. Systemic absorption is rapid and complete after intraperitoneal (IP) administration.

Distribution

Widely distributed to all tissues with highest concentrations in the liver and kidneys. Less than 10% remaining in the plasma 1 hour after infusion.

Metabolism

Plasma concentrations of cisplatin decay rapidly, with a half-life of approximately 20–30 minutes following bolus administration. Within the cytoplasm of the cell, low concentrations of chloride (4 mM) favor the aquation reaction whereby the chloride atom is replaced by a water molecule, resulting in a highly reactive species. Platinum clearance from plasma proceeds slowly after the first 2 hours due to covalent binding with serum proteins, such as albumin, transferrin, and γ-globulin. Approximately 10%–40% of a given dose of cisplatin is excreted in the urine in 24 hours, with 35%–50% being excreted in the urine after 5 days of administration. Approximately 15% of the drug is excreted unchanged.

Indications

1. Testicular cancer.
2. Ovarian cancer.
3. Bladder cancer.
4. Head and neck cancer.
5. Esophageal cancer.
6. Small cell and non–small cell lung cancer.
7. Non-Hodgkin's lymphoma.
8. Trophoblastic neoplasms.

Dosage Range

1. Ovarian cancer: 75 mg/m^2 IV on day 1 every 21 days as part of the cisplatin/paclitaxel regimen, and 100 mg/m^2 on day 1 every 21 days as part of the cisplatin/cyclophosphamide regimen.
2. Testicular cancer: 20 mg/m^2 IV on days 1–5 every 21 days as part of the PEB regimen.
3. Non–small cell lung cancer: 60–100 mg/m^2 IV on day 1 every 21 days as part of the cisplatin/etoposide or cisplatin/gemcitabine regimens.
4. Head and neck cancer: 20 mg/m^2/day IV continuous infusion for 4 days.

Drug Interaction 1

Phenytoin—Cisplatin decreases pharmacologic effect of phenytoin. For this reason, phenytoin dose may need to be increased with concurrent use with cisplatin.

Drug Interaction 2

Amifostine, mesna—The nephrotoxic effect of cisplatin is inactivated by amifostine and mesna.

Drug Interaction 3

Aminoglycosides, amphotericin B, other nephrotoxic agents—Increased renal toxicity with concurrent use of cisplatin and aminoglycosides, amphotericin B, and/or other nephrotoxic agents.

Drug Interaction 4

Etoposide, methotrexate, ifosfamide, bleomycin—Cisplatin reduces the renal clearance of etoposide, methotrexate, ifosfamide, and bleomycin, resulting in the increased accumulation of each of these drugs.

Drug Interaction 5

Etoposide—Cisplatin may enhance the antitumor activity of etoposide.

Drug Interaction 6

Radiation therapy—Cisplatin acts as a radiosensitizing agent.

Drug Interaction 7

Paclitaxel—Cisplatin should be administered after paclitaxel when cisplatin and paclitaxel are used in combination. This sequence prevents delayed paclitaxel excretion and increased host toxicity.

Drug Interaction 8

Aminoglycosides, furosemide—Risk of ototoxicity is increased when cisplatin is combined with aminoglycosides and loop diuretics such as furosemide.

Special Considerations

1. Contraindicated in patients with known hypersensitivity to cisplatin or other platinum analogs.

2. Use with caution in patients with abnormal renal function. Dose of drug must be reduced in the setting of renal dysfunction. Creatinine clearance should be obtained at baseline and before each cycle of therapy. Carefully monitor renal function (BUN and creatinine) as well as serum electrolytes (Na, Mg, Ca, K) during treatment.

3. Fluid status of patient is critical. Patients must be hydrated before, during, and post drug administration. Usual approach is to give at least one liter before and one liter post drug treatment of 0.9% sodium chloride with 20 mEq of KCl. With higher doses of drug,

more aggressive hydration should be considered with at least two liters of fluid administered before drug. In this setting, urine output should be greater than 100 cc/hr. Furosemide diuresis may be used after every two liters of fluid.

4. Use with caution in patients with hearing impairment or pre-existing peripheral neuropathy. Baseline audiology exam and periodic evaluation during therapy are recommended to monitor the effects of drug on hearing. Contraindicated in patients with pre-existing hearing deficit.

5. Cisplatin is a potent emetogenic agent. Give antiemetic premedication to prevent cisplatin-induced nausea and vomiting. Prophylaxis against delayed emesis (>24 hours after the drug administration) is also recommended. A combination of a 5-HT3 antagonist (e.g., ondansetron or granisetron) and dexamethasone is standard therapy for prevention of nausea and vomiting.

6. Avoid aluminum needles when administering the drug because precipitate may form, resulting in decreased potency.

7. Cisplatin is inactivated in the presence of alkaline solutions containing sodium bicarbonate.

Toxicity 1

Nephrotoxicity. Dose-limiting toxicity in up to 35%–40% of patients. Effects on renal function are dose-related and usually observed at 10–20 days after therapy. Generally reversible. Electrolyte abnormalities, mainly hypomagnesemia, hypocalcemia, and hypokalemia, are common. Hyperuricemia rarely occurs.

Toxicity 2

Nausea and vomiting. Two forms are observed: acute (within the first 24 hours) and delayed (>24 hours). Early form begins within 1 hour of starting cisplatin therapy and may last for 8–12 hours. The delayed form can last for 3–5 days.

Toxicity 3

Myelosuppression. Occurs in 25%–30% of patients, with WBCs, platelets, and RBCs equally affected. Leukopenia and thrombocytopenia are more pronounced at higher doses. Coombs-positive hemolytic anemia rarely observed.

Toxicity 4

Neurotoxicity usually in the form of peripheral sensory neuropathy. Paresthesias and numbness in a classic stocking-glove pattern. Tends to occur after several cycles of therapy and risk increases with cumulative doses. Loss of motor function, focal encephalopathy, and seizures also observed. Neurologic effects may be irreversible.

Toxicity 5

Ototoxicity with high-frequency hearing loss and tinnitus.

Toxicity 6

Hypersensitivity reactions consisting of facial edema, wheezing, bronchospasm, and hypotension. Occur within a few minutes of drug administration.

Toxicity 7

Ocular toxicity manifested as optic neuritis, papilledema, and cerebral blindness. Altered color perception may be observed in rare cases.

Toxicity 8

Transient elevation in LFTs, mainly SGOT and serum bilirubin.

Toxicity 9

Metallic taste of foods and loss of appetite.

Toxicity 10

Vascular events, including myocardial infarction, arteritis, cerebrovascular accidents, and thrombotic microangiopathy. Raynaud's phenomenon has been reported.

Toxicity 11

Azoospermia, impotence, and sterility.

Toxicity 12

Alopecia.

Toxicity 13

Inappropriate secretion of antidiuretic hormone (SIADH).

Cladribine

Trade Names

2-Chlorodeoxyadenosine, 2-CdA, Leustatin

Classification

Antimetabolite

Category

Chemotherapy drug

Drug Manufacturer

Ortho Biotech

Mechanism of Action

- Purine deoxyadenosine analog with high specificity for lymphoid cells.
- Presence of the 2-chloro group on adenine ring renders cladribine resistant to breakdown by adenosine deaminase.
- Antitumor activity against both dividing and resting cells.
- Metabolized intracellularly to 5'-triphosphate form (Cld-ATP), which is the presumed active species.
- Triphosphate metabolite incorporates into DNA resulting in inhibition of DNA chain extension and inhibition of DNA synthesis and function.
- Inhibition of ribonucleotide reductase.
- Depletes nicotine adenine dinucleotide (NAD) concentration, resulting in depletion of ATP.
- Induction of apoptosis (programmed cell death).

Mechanism of Resistance

- Decreased expression of the activating enzyme deoxycytidine kinase resulting in decreased formation of cytotoxic cladribine metabolites.

- Increased expression of 5'-nucleotidase, which dephosphorylates cladribine nucleotide metabolites Cld-AMP and Cld-ATP.

Absorption

Oral absorption is variable with about 50% of drug orally bioavailable. About 97% of drug is bioavailable after SC injection.

Distribution

Widely distributed throughout the body. About 20% of drug is bound to plasma proteins. Crosses the blood-brain barrier, but CSF concentrations reach only 25% of those in plasma.

Metabolism

Extensively metabolized intracellularly to nucleotide metabolite forms. Intracellular concentrations of phosphorylated metabolites exceed those in plasma by several hundred-fold. Terminal half-life is on the order of 5–7 hours. Cleared by the kidneys via a cation organic carrier system. Renal clearance is approximately 50%, with 20%–35% of drug eliminated unchanged.

Indications

1. Hairy cell leukemia.

2. Chronic lymphocytic leukemia.

3. Non-Hodgkin's lymphoma (low-grade).

Dosage Range

Usual dose is 0.09 mg/kg/day IV via continuous infusion for 7 days. One course is usually administered. If patient does not respond to one course, it is unlikely that a response will be seen with a second course of therapy.

Drug Interactions

None known.

Special Considerations

1. Use with caution in patients with abnormal renal function.

2. Closely monitor for signs of infection. Patients are at increased risk for opportunistic infections, including herpes, fungus, and *Pneumocystis carinii*.

3. Closely monitor for signs of tumor lysis syndrome. Increased risk in patients with a high tumor cell burden.

4. Allopurinol should be given before initiation of therapy to prevent hyperuricemia.

5. Pregnancy category D.

Toxicity 1

Myelosuppression. Dose-limiting toxicity. Neutropenia more commonly observed than anemia or thrombocytopenia. Leukocyte nadir occurs at 7–14 days, with recovery in 3–4 weeks.

Toxicity 2

Immunosuppression. Decrease in CD4+ and CD8+ cells occurs in most patients. Increased risk of opportunistic infections, including fungus, herpes, and *Pneumocystis carinii*. Complete recovery of CD4+ counts to normal may take up to 40 months.

Toxicity 3

Fever occurs in 40%–50% of patients. Most likely due to release of pyrogens and/or cytokines from tumor cells. Associated with fatigue, malaise, myalgias, arthralgias, and chills. Incidence decreases with continued therapy.

Toxicity 4

Mild nausea and vomiting observed in less than 30% of patients.

Toxicity 5

Tumor lysis syndrome. Rare event, most often in the setting of high tumor cell burden.

Toxicity 6

Skin reaction at the site of injection.

C

Clofarabine

$$\text{(chemical structure of clofarabine)}$$

Trade Names

Clolar

Classification

Antimetabolite

Category

Chemotherapy drug

Drug Manufacturer

Genzyme

Mechanism of Action

- Purine deoxyadenosine nucleoside analog.

- Presence of the 2-fluoro group on the sugar ring renders clofarabine resistant to breakdown by adenosine deaminase.

- Cell cycle–specific with activity in the S-phase.

- Requires intracellular activation to the cytotoxic triphosphate nucleotide metabolite.

- Incorporation of clofarabine triphosphate into DNA resulting in chain termination and inhibition of DNA synthesis and function.

- Clofarabine triphosphate inhibits DNA polymerases α, ß, and γ, which, in turn, interferes with DNA chain elongation, DNA synthesis, and DNA repair.

- Clofarabine triphosphate disrupts the mitochondrial membrane, leading to release of cytochrome C and the induction of apoptosis.

- Inhibits the enzyme ribonucleotide reductase, resulting in decreased levels of essential deoxyribonucleotides for DNA synthesis and function.

Mechanism of Resistance

- Decreased activation of drug through decreased expression of the anabolic enzyme deoxycytidine kinase.
- Decreased transport of drug into cells.
- Increased expression of CTP synthetase activity resulting in increased concentrations of competing physiologic nucleotide substrate dCTP.

Absorption

Not absorbed via the oral route.

Distribution

Approximately 50% bound to plasma proteins, primarily to albumin.

Metabolism

Extensively metabolized intracellularly to nucleotide metabolite forms. Clofarabine has high affinity for the activating enzyme deoxycytidine kinase and is a more efficient substrate for this enzyme than the normal substrate deoxycytidine. Renal clearance is approximately 50%–60%. The pathways of non-renal elimination remain unknown. The terminal elimination half-life is on the order of 5 hours.

Indications

FDA-approved for the treatment of pediatric patients 1–21 years of age with relapsed or refractory acute lymphoblastic leukemia after at least two prior regimens.

Dosage Range

Recommended dose is 52 mg/m^2 IV over 2 hours daily for 5 days every 2–6 weeks.

Drug Interactions

None well characterized to date.

Special Considerations

1. Use with caution in patients with abnormal liver and/or renal function. Closely monitor liver and renal function during therapy.

2. As clofarabine is excreted mainly by the kidneys, drugs with known renal toxicity should be avoided during the five days of drug treatment.

3. Concomitant use of medications known to cause liver toxicity should be avoided.

4. Patients should be closely monitored for evidence of tumor lysis syndrome and systemic inflammatory response syndrome (SIRS)/ capillary leak syndrome, which result from rapid reduction in peripheral leukemic cells following drug treatment. The use

of hydrocortisone 100 mg/m^2 IV on days 1–3 may prevent the development of SIRS or capillary leak.

5. Pregnancy category D.

Toxicity 1

Myelosuppression is dose-limiting with neutropenia, anemia, and thrombocytopenia.

Toxicity 2

Capillary leak syndrome/SIRS with tachypnea, tachycardia, pulmonary edema, and hypotension. Pericardial effusion observed in up to 35% of patients, but usually minimal to small and not hemodynamically significant.

Toxicity 3

Nausea/vomiting and diarrhea are most common GI side effects.

Toxicity 4

Hepatic dysfunction with elevation of serum transaminases and bilirubin. Usually occur within 1 week and reversible with resolution in 14 days.

Toxicity 5

Increased risk of opportunistic infections, including fungal, viral, and bacterial infections.

Toxicity 6

Renal toxicity with elevation in serum creatinine observed in up to 10% of patients.

Toxicity 7

Cardiac toxicity as manifested by left ventricular dysfunction and tachycardia.

Cyclophosphamide

Trade Names
Cytoxan, CTX

Classification
Alkylating agent

Category
Chemotherapy drug

Drug Manufacturer
Bristol-Myers Squibb

Mechanism of Action
- Inactive in its parent form.
- Activated by the liver cytochrome P450 microsomal system to the cytotoxic metabolites phosphoramide mustard and acrolein.
- Cyclophosphamide metabolites form cross-links with DNA resulting in inhibition of DNA synthesis and function.
- Cell cycle–nonspecific agent, active in all phases of the cell cycle.

Mechanism of Resistance
- Decreased cellular uptake of drug.
- Decreased expression of drug-activating enzymes of the liver P450 system.
- Increased expression of sulfhydryl proteins including glutathione and glutathione-associated enzymes.
- Increased expression of aldehyde dehydrogenase resulting in enhanced enzymatic detoxification of drug.
- Enhanced activity of DNA repair enzymes.

Absorption
Well-absorbed by the GI tract with a bioavailability of nearly 90%.

Distribution
Distributed throughout the body, including brain and CSF. Also distributed in milk and saliva. Minimal binding of parent drug to plasma

proteins; however, about 60% of the phosphoramide mustard metabolite is bound to plasma proteins.

Metabolism

Extensively metabolized in the liver by the cytochrome P450 system to both active and inactive forms. The active forms are 4-hydroxycyclophosphamide, phosphoramide mustard, and acrolein. Parent drug and its metabolites are eliminated exclusively in urine. The elimination half-life ranges from 4 to 6 hours.

Indications

1. Breast cancer.
2. Non-Hodgkin's lymphoma.
3. Chronic lymphocytic leukemia.
4. Ovarian cancer.
5. Bone and soft tissue sarcoma.
6. Rhabdomyosarcoma.
7. Neuroblastoma and Wilms' tumor.

Dosage Range

1. Breast cancer: When given orally, the usual dose is 100 mg/m^2 PO on days 1–14 given every 28 days. When administered IV, the usual dose is 600 mg/m^2 given every 21 days as part of the AC or CMF regimens.

2. Non-Hodgkin's lymphoma: Usual dose is 400–600 mg/m^2 IV on day 1 every 21 days, as part of the CVP regimen, and 750 mg/m^2 on day 1 every 21 days, as part of the CHOP regimen.

3. High-dose bone marrow transplantation: Usual dose in the setting of bone marrow transplantation is 60 mg/kg IV for 2 days.

Drug Interaction 1

Phenobarbital, phenytoin, and other drugs that stimulate the liver P450 system—Increase the rate of metabolic activation of cyclophosphamide to its cytotoxic metabolites.

Drug Interaction 2

Anticoagulants—Cyclophosphamide increases the effect of anticoagulants, and thus the dose of anticoagulants may need to be decreased depending on the coagulation parameters, PT/INR.

cyclophosphamide

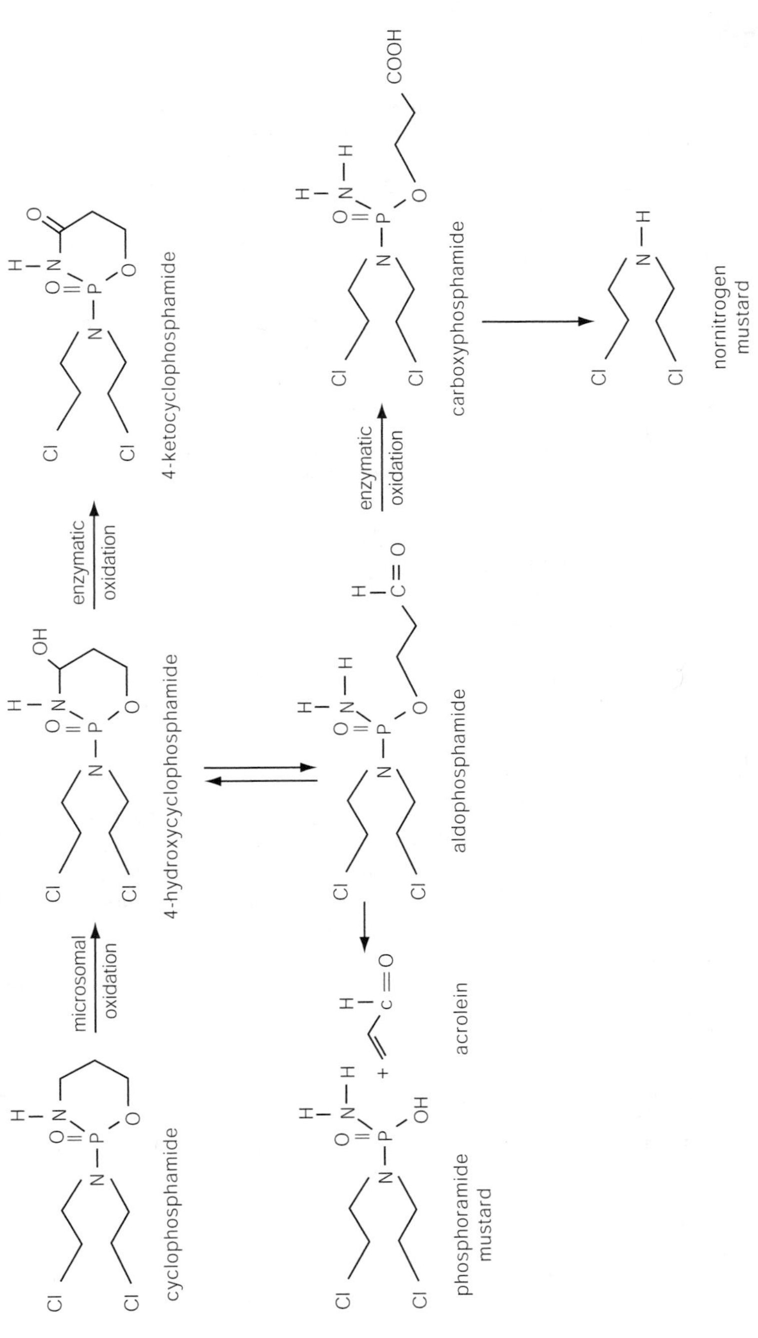

4-hydroxycyclophosphamide

4-ketocyclophosphamide

aldophosphamide

carboxyphosphamide

nornitrogen mustard

phosphoramide mustard

acrolein

microsomal oxidation

enzymatic oxidation

enzymatic oxidation

Drug Interaction 3

Digoxin—Cyclophosphamide decreases the plasma levels of digoxin by activating its metabolism in the liver.

Drug Interaction 4

Doxorubicin—Cyclophosphamide may increase the risk of doxorubicin-induced cardiotoxicity.

Special Considerations

1. Use with caution in patients with abnormal renal function. Dose should be reduced in the setting of renal dysfunction. Creatinine clearance should be obtained at baseline and before each cycle of therapy.

2. Administer oral form of drug during the daytime.

3. Encourage fluid intake of at least 2–3 L/day to reduce the risk of hemorrhagic cystitis. High-dose therapy requires administration of IV fluids for hydration.

4. Encourage patients to empty bladder several times daily (on average, every 2 hours) to reduce the risk of bladder toxicity.

5. Pregnancy category D.

Toxicity 1

Myelosuppression is dose-limiting. Mainly leukopenia with nadir occurring at 7–14 days with recovery by day 21. Thrombocytopenia may occur, usually with high-dose therapy.

Toxicity 2

Bladder toxicity in the form of hemorrhagic cystitis, dysuria, and increased urinary frequency occurs in 5%–10% of patients. Time of onset is variable and may begin within 24 hours of therapy or may be delayed for up to several weeks. Usually reversible upon discontinuation of drug. Uroprotection with mesna and hydration must be used with high-dose therapy to prevent bladder toxicity.

Toxicity 3

Nausea and vomiting. Usually dose-related, occurs within 2–4 hours of therapy, and may last up to 24 hours. Anorexia is fairly common.

Toxicity 4

Alopecia generally starting 2–3 weeks after starting therapy. Skin and nails may become hyperpigmented.

Toxicity 5

Amenorrhea with ovarian failure. Sterility may be permanent.

Toxicity 6

Cardiotoxicity is observed with high-dose therapy.

Toxicity 7

Increased risk of secondary malignancies, including acute myelogenous leukemia and bladder cancer, especially in patients with chronic hemorrhagic cystitis.

Toxicity 8

Immunosuppression with an increased risk of infections.

Toxicity 9

SIADH.

Toxicity 10

Hypersensitivity reaction with rhinitis and irritation of the nose and throat. Usually self-resolving in 1–3 days, but steroids and/or diphenhydramine may be required.

Cytarabine

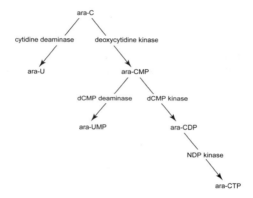

Trade Names

Cytosine arabinoside, Ara-C

Classification

Antimetabolite

Category

Chemotherapy drug

Drug Manufacturer

Bedford Laboratories

Mechanism of Action

- Deoxycytidine analog originally isolated from the sponge *Cryptothethya crypta*.
- Cell cycle–specific with activity in the S-phase.
- Requires intracellular activation to the nucleotide metabolite ara-CTP. Antitumor activity of cytarabine is determined by a balance between intracellular activation and degradation and the subsequent formation of cytotoxic ara-CTP metabolites.

- Incorporation of ara-CTP into DNA resulting in chain termination and inhibition of DNA synthesis and function.
- Ara-CTP inhibits several DNA polymerases α, β, and γ, which then interferes with DNA synthesis, DNA repair, and DNA chain elongation.
- Ara-CTP inhibits the enzyme ribonucleotide reductase, resulting in decreased levels of essential deoxyribonucleotides required for DNA synthesis and function.

Mechanism of Resistance

- Decreased activation of drug through decreased expression of the anabolic enzyme deoxycytidine kinase.
- Increased breakdown of drug by the catabolic enzymes, cytidine deaminase and deoxycytidylate (dCMP) deaminase.
- Decreased transport of drug into cells.
- Increased expression of CTP synthetase activity resulting in increased concentrations of competing physiologic nucleotide substrate dCTP.

Absorption

Poor oral bioavailability (~20%) as a result of extensive deamination within the GI tract.

Distribution

Rapidly cleared from the bloodstream after IV administration. Distributes rapidly into tissues and total body water. Crosses the blood-brain barrier with CSF levels reaching 20%–40% of those in plasma. Binding to plasma proteins has not been well characterized.

Metabolism

Undergoes extensive metabolism, with approximately 70%–80% of drug being recovered in the urine as the ara-U metabolite within 24 hours. Deamination occurs in liver, plasma, and peripheral tissues. The principal enzyme involved in drug catabolism is cytidine deaminase, which converts ara-C into the inactive metabolite ara-U. dCMP-deaminase converts ara-CMP into ara-UMP, and this represents an additional catabolic pathway of the drug. The terminal elimination half-life is 2–6 hours. The half-life of ara-C in CSF is somewhat longer, ranging from 2 to 11 hours, due to the relatively low activity of cytidine deaminase present in CSF.

Indications

1. Acute myelogenous leukemia.
2. Acute lymphocytic leukemia.
3. Chronic myelogenous leukemia.
4. Leptomeningeal carcinomatosis.
5. Non-Hodgkin's lymphoma.

Dosage Range

Several different doses and schedules have been used:

1. Standard dose: 100 mg/m²/day IV on days 1–7 as a continuous IV infusion, in combination with an anthracycline as induction chemotherapy for AML.

2. High-dose: 1.5–3.0 g/m² IV q 12 hours for 3 days as a high-dose, intensification regimen for AML.

3. SC: 20 mg/m² SC for 10 days per month for 6 months, associated with IFN-α for treatment of CML.

4. Intrathecal: 10–30 mg intrathecal (IT) up to three times weekly in the treatment of leptomeningeal carcinomatosis secondary to leukemia or lymphoma.

Drug Interaction 1

Gentamicin—Cytarabine antagonizes the efficacy of gentamicin.

Drug Interaction 2

5-Fluorocytosine—Cytarabine inhibits the efficacy of 5-fluorocytosine by preventing its cellular uptake.

Drug Interaction 3

Digoxin—Cytarabine decreases the oral bioavailability of digoxin, thereby decreasing its efficacy. Digoxin levels should be monitored closely while on therapy.

Drug Interaction 4

Alkylating agents, cisplatin, and ionizing radiation—Cytarabine enhances the cytotoxicity of various alkylating agents (cyclophosphamide, carmustine), cisplatin, and ionizing radiation by inhibiting DNA repair mechanisms. Concurrent use of high-dose cytarabine and cisplatin may increase risk of ototoxicity.

Drug Interaction 5

Methotrexate—Pretreatment with methotrexate enhances the formation of ara-CTP metabolites resulting in enhanced cytotoxicity.

Drug Interaction 6

Fludarabine, hydroxyurea—Pretreatment with fludarabine and/or hydroxyurea potentiates the cytotoxicity of cytarabine by enhancing the formation of cytotoxic ara-CTP metabolites.

Drug Interaction 7

GM-CSF, interleukin-3—Cytokines including GM-CSF and interleukin-3 enhance cytarabine-mediated apoptosis mechanisms.

Drug Interaction 8

L-Asparaginase—Increased risk of pancreatitis when L-asparaginase is given before cytarabine.

Special Considerations

1. Monitor CBCs on a regular basis during therapy.

2. Use with caution in patients with abnormal liver and/or renal function. Dose modification should be considered in this setting as patients are at increased risk for toxicity. Monitor hepatic and renal function during therapy.

3. Alkalinization of the urine (pH >7.0), allopurinol, and vigorous IV hydration are recommended to prevent tumor lysis syndrome in patients with acute myelogenous leukemia.

4. High-dose therapy should be administered over a 1- to 2-hour period.

5. Conjunctivitis is observed with high-dose therapy as the drug is excreted in tears. Patients should be treated with hydrocortisone eye drops (2 drops OU qid for 10 days) on the night before the start of therapy.

6. Pregnancy category D.

Toxicity 1

Myelosuppression is dose-limiting. Leukopenia and thrombocytopenia are common. Nadir usually occurs by days 7–10, with recovery by days 14–21. Megaloblastic anemia has also been observed.

Toxicity 2

Nausea and vomiting. Mild to moderate emetogenic agent with increased severity observed with high-dose therapy. Anorexia, diarrhea, and mucositis usually occur 7–10 days after therapy.

Toxicity 3

Cerebellar ataxia, lethargy, and confusion. Neurotoxicity develops in up to 10% of patients. Onset usually 5 days after drug treatment and lasts up to 1 week. In most cases, CNS toxicities are mild and reversible. Risk factors for neurotoxicity include high-dose therapy, age older than 40, abnormal renal function with serum creatinine 1.2 mg/dL, and abnormal liver function.

Toxicity 4

Transient hepatic dysfunction with elevation of serum transaminases and bilirubin. Most often associated with high-dose therapy.

Toxicity 5

Acute pancreatitis.

Toxicity 6

Ara-C syndrome. Described in pediatric patients and represents an allergic reaction to cytarabine. Characterized by fever, myalgia, malaise, bone pain, maculopapular skin rash, conjunctivitis, and occasional chest pain. Usually occurs within 12 hours of drug infusion. Steroids appear to be effective in treating and/or preventing the onset of this syndrome.

Toxicity 7

Pulmonary complications include non-cardiogenic pulmonary edema, acute respiratory distress, and *Streptococcus viridans* pneumonia. Observed with high-dose therapy.

Toxicity 8

Erythema of skin, alopecia, and hidradenitis are usually mild and self-limited. Hand-foot syndrome observed rarely with high-dose therapy.

Toxicity 9

Conjunctivitis and keratitis. Associated with high-dose regimens.

Toxicity 10

Seizures, alterations in mental status, and fever may be observed within the first 24 hours after IT administration.

Dacarbazine

Trade Names
DIC, DTIC-Dome, Imidazole Carboxamide

Classification
Nonclassic alkylating agent

Category
Chemotherapy drug

Drug Manufacturer
Ben Venue Laboratories, Bayer

Mechanism of Action
- Cell cycle–nonspecific drug.
- Initially developed as a purine antimetabolite, but its antitumor activity is not mediated via inhibition of purine biosynthesis.
- Metabolic activation is required for antitumor activity.
- While the precise mechanism of cytotoxicity is unclear, this drug methylates nucleic acids and inhibits DNA, RNA, and protein synthesis.

Mechanism of Resistance
- Increased activity of DNA repair enzymes such as O6-alkylguanine-DNA alkyltransferase (AGAT).

Absorption
Slow and variable oral absorption. For this reason, IV administration preferred.

Distribution
Volume of distribution exceeds total body water content, and drug is widely distributed in body tissues. About 20% of drug is loosely bound to plasma proteins.

Metabolism
Metabolized in the liver by the microsomal P450 system to active metabolites (MTIC, AIC). The elimination half-life of the drug is 5 hours.

D

About 40%–50% of the parent drug is excreted unchanged in urine within 6 hours, and tubular secretion appears to predominate. No specific guidelines for dacarbazine dosing in the setting of hepatic and/or renal dysfunction. However, dose modification should be considered in patients with moderately severe hepatic and/or renal dysfunction.

Indications

1. Metastatic malignant melanoma.
2. Hodgkin's lymphoma.
3. Soft tissue sarcomas.
4. Neuroblastoma.

Dosage Range

1. Hodgkin's lymphoma: 375 mg/m^2 IV on days 1 and 15 every 28 days, as part of the ABVD regimen.
2. Melanoma: 220 mg/m^2 IV on days 1–3 and days 22–24 every 6 weeks, as part of the Dartmouth regimen. As a single agent, 250 mg/ m^2 IV for 5 days or 800–1,000 mg/m^2 IV every 3 weeks.

Drug Interaction 1

Heparin, lidocaine, and hydrocortisone—Incompatible with dacarbazine.

Drug Interaction 2

Phenytoin, phenobarbital—Decreased efficacy of dacarbazine when administered with phenytoin and phenobarbital as these drugs induce dacarbazine metabolism by the liver P450 system.

Special Considerations

1. Dacarbazine is a potent vesicant, and it should be carefully administered to avoid the risk of extravasation.
2. Dacarbazine is a highly emetogenic agent. Use of aggressive antiemetics before drug administration to decrease risk of nausea and vomiting.
3. Patients should avoid sun exposure for several days after dacarbazine therapy.
4. Pregnancy category C.

Toxicity 1

Myelosuppression. Dose-limiting toxicity. Leukopenia and thrombocytopenia are equally affected with nadir occurring at 21–25 days.

Toxicity 2

Nausea and vomiting can be severe, usually occurring within 1–3 hours and lasting for up to 12 hours. Aggressive antiemetic therapy strongly recommended. Anorexia is common, but diarrhea occurs rarely.

Toxicity 3

Flu-like syndrome in the form of fever, chills, malaise, myalgias, and arthralgias. May last for several days after therapy.

Toxicity 4

Pain and/or burning at the site of injection.

Toxicity 5

CNS toxicity in the form of paresthesias, neuropathies, ataxia, lethargy, headache, confusion, and seizures has all been observed.

Toxicity 6

Increased risk of photosensitivity.

Toxicity 7

Teratogenic, mutagenic, and carcinogenic.

D

Dactinomycin-D

Trade Names

Actinomycin-D, Cosmegen

Classification

Antitumor antibiotic

Category

Chemotherapy drug

Drug Manufacturer

Merck

Mechanism of Action

- Product of the *Streptomyces* species.

- Consists of a tricyclic phenoxazone chromophore, which is linked to two short, identical cyclic polypeptides.

- Chromophore moiety preferentially binds to guanine-cytidine base pairs. Binding to single- and double-stranded DNA results in inhibition of DNA synthesis and function.

- Formation of oxygen free radicals results in single- and double-stranded DNA breaks and subsequent inhibition of DNA synthesis and function.

- Inhibition of RNA and protein synthesis may also contribute to the cytotoxic effects.

Mechanism of Resistance

- Reduced cellular uptake of drug, resulting in decreased intracellular drug accumulation.

- Increased expression of the multidrug-resistant gene with elevated P170 protein levels leads to increased drug efflux and decreased intracellular drug accumulation.

Absorption

Poor oral bioavailability and is administered only via the IV route.

Distribution

After an IV bolus injection, dactinomycin rapidly disappears from the circulation in about 2 minutes. Concentrates in nucleated blood cells. Does not cross the blood-brain barrier. Appears to be highly bound to plasma proteins.

Metabolism

Clinical pharmacology is not well characterized. Metabolized only to small extent. Most of drug is eliminated in unchanged form by biliary (50%) and renal (20%) excretion. Terminal elimination half-life ranges from 30 to 40 hours.

Indications

1. Wilms' tumor.
2. Rhabdomyosarcoma.
3. Germ cell tumors.
4. Gestational trophoblastic disease.
5. Ewing's sarcoma.

Dosage Range

1. Adults: 0.4–0.45 mg/m^2 IV on days 1–5 every 2–3 weeks.
2. Children: 0.015 mg/kg/day (up to a maximum dose of 0.5 mg/day) IV on days 1–5 over a period of 16–45 weeks depending on the specific regimen.

Drug Interactions

None known.

Special Considerations

1. Administer drug slowly by IV push to avoid extravasation.
2. Contraindicated in patients actively infected with chickenpox or herpes zoster as generalized infection may result in death.
3. Use with caution in patients either previously treated with radiation therapy or currently receiving radiation therapy. Increased risk of radiation recall skin reaction.
4. Patients should be cautioned against sun exposure while on therapy.
5. Pregnancy category C. May be excreted in breast milk.

Toxicity 1

Myelosuppression. Dose-limiting and severe. Leukopenia and thrombocytopenia equally observed. Nadir occurs at days 8–14 after administration.

Toxicity 2

Nausea and vomiting. Onset within the first 2 hours of therapy, lasts for up to 24 hours, and may be severe.

Toxicity 3

Mucositis and/or diarrhea. Usually occurs within 5–7 days and can be severe.

Toxicity 4

Alopecia is common.

Toxicity 5

Hyperpigmentation of skin, erythema, and increased sensitivity to sunlight. Radiation recall reaction with erythema and desquamation of skin observed with prior or concurrent radiation therapy.

Toxicity 6

Potent vesicant. Tissue damage occurs with extravasation of drug.

Toxicity 7

Elevation of serum transaminases in less than 15% of patients. Dose- and schedule-dependent. Hepato-veno-occlusive disease observed rarely with higher doses and daily schedule.

Darbepoetin alfa

D

Trade Names
Aranesp

Classification
Colony-stimulating growth factor, cytokine

Category
Biologic response modifier agent

Drug Manufacturer
Amgen

Mechanism of Action
- Glycoprotein produced by recombinant DNA techniques. Has the same biologic effects as endogenous erythropoietin.
- It is a 165-amino acid protein that differs from recombinant human erythropoietin in containing five N-linked oligosaccharide chains, while recombinant human erythropoietin contains three chains. The additional carbohydrate chains increase the approximate molecular weight from 30,000 to 37,000 daltons.
- Stimulates division and differentiation of red blood cells in the bone marrow.
- Does not possess antitumor activity.

Absorption
Administered either by the IV or SC route. Following SC injection, absorption is slow and rate-limiting. Peak concentrations are observed about 34 hours post SC administration, while peak concentrations are 90 hours post SC administration in cancer patients. The bioavailability of darbepoetin in chronic renal failure patients after SC injection is 37%.

Distribution
Distributes into total plasma volume. Binding to plasma proteins is not known. Steady-state serum levels are achieved within 4 weeks.

Metabolism
Metabolism is not entirely clear, although catabolism in liver and bone marrow appears to play a role. About 10% of the drug is cleared in urine in unchanged form. The terminal half-life in patients with chronic renal failure is 49 hours, which is about 3-fold longer than erythropoietin when administered by either the IV or SC route and is about 40 hours in cancer patients receiving chemotherapy.

D

Indications

1. Chemotherapy-induced anemia in patients with non-myeloid malignancies.

2. Anemia associated with chronic renal failure, including patients on dialysis and those not on dialysis.

Dosage Range

1. Chemotherapy-induced anemia: Recommended starting dose is 2.25 mg/kg administered as a weekly SC injection. The dose should be adjusted for each patient to achieve and maintain a target hemoglobin level of 12 g/dL. If there is less than a 1 g/dL increase in hemoglobin after 6 weeks of therapy, the dose of darbepoetin should be increased to 4.5 mg/kg. If the hemoglobin increases by more than 1 g/dL in a 2-week period or if the hemoglobin exceeds 12 g/dL, the dose should be reduced by 25%. If the hemoglobin level exceeds 13 g/dL, doses should be held until the hemoglobin falls to 11 g/dL. At that point, therapy should be restarted at a dose that is 40% lower than the previous dose.

2. Alternative treatment schedules include 100 mg/week, 200 mg every 2 weeks, or 300 mg every 3 weeks.

3. Chronic renal failure: recommended starting dose is 0.45 mg/kg body weight administered as a single IV or SC injection once weekly.

Drug Interactions

None characterized.

Special Considerations

1. Contraindicated in patients with uncontrolled hypertension.

2. Use with caution in patients with a history of hypertension and/or cardiovascular disease. Patients should be advised of the importance of close compliance with anti-hypertensive therapy and dietary restriction. The dose of darbepoetin should be reduced or withheld if the blood pressure cannot be effectively controlled by pharmacologic and/or dietary measures.

3. Contraindicated in patients with known hypersensitivity to mammalian-derived products.

4. Contraindicated in patients with known hypersensitivity to the active substance and/or any of the excipients.

5. Use with caution in patients with known porphyria as exacerbation has been observed in patients treated with erythropoietin.

6. Obtain baseline erythropoietin levels before start of therapy. The optimal response is observed in cancer patients with endogenous levels ≤200 U/mL. A baseline serum ferritin level and transferrin saturation should also be obtained. Transferrin saturation should

be at least 20%, and ferritin should be at least 100 mg/mL. Patients may benefit from concomitant treatment with iron supplementation, ferrous sulfate one tablet PO bid or tid or with IV iron.

7. Contraindicated in patients receiving myelosuppressive chemotherapy if the intent of treatment is cure. Remains indicated when myelosuppressive chemotherapy is intended for palliation.

8. The lowest dose of darbepoetin should be used to increase gradually the need for hemoglobin concentrations to the lowest level sufficient to avoid the need for red blood cell transfusions. Increases in dose should not be made more frequently than once a month. The dose of darbepoetin should be adjusted for each patient to achieve and maintain a target hemoglobin level not to exceed 12 g/dL. If the hemoglobin level is increasing and approaching 12 g/dL, the dose should be reduced by 25%.

9. Patients should be closely monitored to ensure that the hemoglobin levels are not greater than 12 g/dL. An increased risk of death and serious cardiovascular events, including myocardial infarction, heart failure, stroke, and thrombosis, has been observed in this setting (this represents a black-box warning).

10. Blood counts should be monitored on a weekly basis during darbepoetin therapy. If the increase in hemoglobin is less than 1 g/dL after 4 weeks of therapy, the dose of darbepoetin can be increased by 25% of the previous dose. Further increases may be made at 4-week intervals until the specified hemoglobin level is achieved.

11. The starting weekly dose of darbepoetin should be estimated on the basis of the weekly erythropoietin dose at the time of substitution. Due to the longer half-life, darbepoetin should be administered once a week if a patient was receiving erythropoietin 2–3 times weekly and should be administered once every 2 weeks if a patient was receiving erythropoietin once per week.

12. Patients should be warned that there is a rare risk of transmission of viral diseases with a remote risk of transmission of Creutzfeldt-Jakob disease (CJD).

13. Pregnancy category C. Breast-feeding should be avoided as it is not known whether darbepoetin is excreted in human milk.

Toxicity 1

Hypertension is common but usually mild.

Toxicity 2

Diarrhea and occasional nausea and vomiting.

Toxicity 3

Local pain at injection site.

Toxicity 4

Headache, fever, fatigue, asthenia, arthralgias, and myalgias.

Toxicity 5

Rare cases of allergic reactions, including skin rash and urticaria.

Dasatinib

Trade Name

Sprycel, BMS-354825

Classification

Signal transduction inhibitor

Category

Chemotherapy drug

Drug Manufacturer

Bristol-Meyers Squibb

Mechanism of Action

- Potent inhibitor of the BCR-ABL kinase and SRC family of kinases (SRC, LCK, YES, FYN), c-KIT, and PDGFR-β.
- Differs from imatinib in that it binds to the active and inactive conformations of the ABL kinase domain and overcomes imatinib resistance resulting from BCR-ABL mutations.

Mechanism of Resistance

- Single point mutation within the ATP-binding pocket of the ABL tyrosine kinase (T315I).

Absorption

Dasatinib has good oral bioavailability. Rapidly absorbed following oral administration. Peak plasma concentrations are observed between 30 minutes and 6 hours of oral ingestion.

Distribution

Extensive distribution in the extravascular space. Binding of parent drug and its active metabolite to plasma proteins in the range of 90%–95%.

Metabolism

Metabolized in the liver primarily by CYP3A4 liver microsomal enzymes. Other liver P450 enzymes, such as UGT, play a relatively minor role in metabolism. Approximately 85% of an administered dose is eliminated in feces within 10 days. The terminal half-life of the parent drug is in the order of 4 to 6 hours.

Indications

1. FDA-approved for the treatment of adults with chronic phase (CP), accelerated phase (AP), or myeloid or lymphoid (MB or LB) phase CML with resistance or intolerance to imatinib.

2. FDA-approved for the treatment of adults with Ph+ ALL with resistance or intolerance to prior therapy.

Dosage Range

Recommended dose is 70 mg PO bid.

An alternative starting dose is 100 mg PO once daily in patients with chronic-phase CML resistant or intolerant to prior therapy including imatinib.

Drug Interaction 1

Dasatinib is an inhibitor of CYP3A4 and may decrease the metabolic clearance of drugs that are metabolized by CYP3A4.

Drug Interaction 2

Drugs such as ketoconazole, itraconazole, erythromycin, and clarithromycin decrease the rate of metabolism of dasatinib, resulting in increased drug levels and potentially increased toxicity.

Drug Interaction 3

Drugs such as rifampin, Dilantin, phenobarbital, carbamazepine, and St. John's wort increase the rate of metabolism of dasatinib, resulting in its inactivation.

Drug Interaction 4

Solubility of dasatinib is pH-dependent. In the presence of famotidine, proton-pump inhibitors, and/or antacids, dasatinib concentrations are reduced.

Special Considerations

1. Oral dasatinib tablets can be taken with or without food, but must not be crushed or cut.

2. Important to review patient's list of medications as dasatinib has several potential drug–drug interactions.

3. Patients should be warned about not taking the herbal medicine St. John's wort while on dasatinib therapy.

4. Monitor CBC on a weekly basis for the first 2 months and periodically thereafter.

5. Use with caution when patients are on aspirin, NSAIDs, or anti-coagulation as there is an increased risk of bleeding.

6. Closely monitor electrolyte status, especially calcium and phosphate levels, as oral calcium supplementation may be required.

7. Sexually active patients on dasatinib therapy should use adequate contraception.

8. Avoid grapefruit and grapefruit juice while on dasatinib therapy.

9. Pregnancy category D.

Toxicity 1

Myelosuppression with thrombocytopenia, neutropenia, and anemia.

Toxicity 2

Bleeding complications in up to 40% of patients resulting from platelet dysfunction.

Toxicity 3

Fluid retention occurs in 50% of patients, with peripheral edema and pleural effusions. Usually mild to moderate in severity.

Toxicity 4

GI toxicity in the form of diarrhea, nausea/vomiting, and abdominal pain.

Toxicity 5

Fatigue, asthenia, and anorexia.

Toxicity 6

Elevations in serum transaminases and/or bilirubin.

Toxicity 7

Hypocalcemia and hypophosphatemia.

Toxicity 8

Cardiac toxicity in the form of heart failure and QTc prolongation. Occurs rarely (3% to 4%).

Daunorubicin

Trade Names

Daunomycin, Cerubidine, Rubidomycin

Classification

Antitumor antibiotic

Category

Chemotherapy drug

Drug Manufacturer

Ben Venue and Bedford Laboratories

Mechanism of Action

- Cell cycle–nonspecific agent.
- Intercalates into DNA resulting in inhibition of DNA synthesis and function.
- Inhibits transcription through inhibition of DNA-dependent RNA polymerase.
- Inhibits topoisomerase II by forming a cleavable complex with DNA and topoisomerase II to create uncompensated DNA helix torsional tension, leading to eventual DNA breaks.
- Formation of cytotoxic oxygen free radicals results in single- and double-stranded DNA breaks with inhibition of DNA synthesis and function.

Mechanism of Resistance

- Increased expression of the multidrug-resistant gene with elevated P170 levels, which leads to increased drug efflux and decreased intracellular drug accumulation.
- Decreased expression of topoisomerase II.
- Mutation in topoisomerase II with decreased binding affinity to drug.
- Increased expression of sulfhydryl proteins, including glutathione and glutathione-dependent enzymes.

Absorption

Daunorubicin is not absorbed orally.

Distribution

Significantly more lipid-soluble than doxorubicin. Widely distributed to tissues with high concentrations in heart, liver, lungs, kidneys, and spleen. Does not cross the blood-brain barrier. Extensively binds to plasma proteins (60%–70%).

Metabolism

Metabolism in the liver with formation of one of its primary metabolites, daunorubicinol, which has antitumor activity. Parent compound and its metabolites are excreted mainly through the hepatobiliary system into feces. Renal clearance accounts for only 10%–20% of drug elimination. The half-life of the parent drug is 20 hours, while the half-life of the daunorubicinol metabolite is 30–40 hours.

Indications

1. Acute myelogenous leukemia—Remission induction and relapse.
2. Acute lymphoblastic leukemia—Remission induction and relapse.

Dosage Range

1. AML: 45 mg/m^2 IV on days 1–3 of the first course of induction therapy and on days 1 and 2 on subsequent courses. Used in combination with continuous infusion ara-C.
2. ALL: 45 mg/m^2 IV on days 1–3 in combination with vincristine, prednisone, and L-asparaginase.
3. Single agent: 40 mg/m^2 IV every 2 weeks.

Drug Interaction 1

Dexamethasone, heparin—Daunorubicin is incompatible with dexamethasone and heparin as a precipitate will form.

Drug Interaction 2

Dexrazoxane—Cardiotoxic effects of daunorubicin are inhibited by the iron-chelating agent dexrazoxane (ICRF-187, Zinecard).

Special Considerations

1. Use with caution in patients with abnormal liver function. Dose reduction is required in the setting of liver dysfunction.
2. Because daunorubicin is a vesicant, administer slowly over 60 minutes with a rapidly flowing IV. Careful administration of the drug, usually through a central venous catheter, is necessary as the drug is a strong vesicant. Close monitoring is necessary to avoid extravasation. If extravasation is suspected, immediately stop infusion, withdraw

fluid, elevate extremity, and apply ice to involved site. May administer local steroids. In severe cases, consult a plastic surgeon.

3. Monitor cardiac function before (baseline) and periodically during therapy with either MUGA radionuclide scan or echocardiogram to assess left ventricular ejection fraction. Risk of cardiotoxicity is higher in patients >70 years of age, in patients with prior history of hypertension or pre-existing heart disease, and in patients previously treated with anthracyclines or prior radiation therapy to the chest. Cumulative doses of >550 mg/m^2 are associated with increased risk for cardiotoxicity.

4. Use with caution in patients previously treated with radiation therapy as daunorubicin can cause a radiation recall skin reaction.

5. Patients should be cautioned to avoid sun exposure and to wear sun protection when outside.

6. Patients should be warned about the potential for red-orange discoloration of urine that may occur for 1–2 days after drug administration.

7. Pregnancy category D. Breast-feeding should be avoided.

Toxicity 1

Myelosuppression. Dose-limiting toxicity with leukopenia being more common than thrombocytopenia. Nadir occurs at 10–14 days with recovery by day 21.

Toxicity 2

Nausea and vomiting. Usually mild, occurring in 50% of patients within 1–2 hours of treatment.

Toxicity 3

Mucositis and diarrhea are common within the first week of treatment but not dose-limiting.

Toxicity 4

Cardiotoxicity. Acute form presents within the first 2–3 days as arrhythmias and/or conduction abnormalities, EKG changes, pericarditis, and/or myocarditis. Usually transient and mostly asymptomatic.

Chronic form associated with a dose-dependent, dilated cardiomyopathy and congestive heart failure. Incidence increases with cumulative doses greater than 550 mg/m^2.

Toxicity 5

Strong vesicant. Extravasation can lead to tissue necrosis and chemical thrombophlebitis at the injection site.

Toxicity 6

Hyperpigmentation of nails, rarely skin rash, and urticaria. Radiation recall skin reaction can occur at prior sites of irradiation. Increased hypersensitivity to sunlight.

Toxicity 7

Alopecia is universal. Usually reversible within 5–7 weeks after termination of treatment.

Toxicity 8

Red-orange discoloration of urine. Lasts 1–2 days after drug administration.

Daunorubicin liposome

Trade Names

DaunoXome

Classification

Antitumor antibiotic

Category

Chemotherapy drug

Drug Manufacturer

Diatos

Mechanism of Action

- Liposomal encapsulation of daunorubicin.
- Protected from chemical and enzymatic degradation, displays reduced plasma protein binding, and shows decreased uptake in normal tissues when compared to parent compound, daunorubicin.
- Penetrates tumor tissue into which daunorubicin is released, possibly through increased permeability of tumor neovasculature to liposome particles.
- Cell cycle–nonspecific agent.
- Intercalates into DNA resulting in inhibition of DNA synthesis and function.
- Inhibits transcription through inhibition of DNA-dependent RNA polymerase.
- Inhibits topoisomerase II by forming a cleavable complex with DNA and topoisomerase II to create uncompensated DNA helix torsional tension, leading to eventual DNA breaks.
- Formation of oxygen free radicals results in single- and double-stranded DNA breaks with subsequent inhibition of DNA synthesis and function.

Mechanism of Resistance

- Increased expression of the multidrug-resistant gene with elevated P170 levels. This leads to increased drug efflux and decreased intracellular drug accumulation.
- Decreased expression of topoisomerase II.
- Mutation in topoisomerase II with decreased binding affinity to drug.
- Increased expression of sulfhydryl proteins, including glutathione and glutathione-dependent enzymes.

Absorption

Daunorubicin liposome is not absorbed orally.

Distribution

Small steady-state volume of distribution (6 L) in contrast to the parent drug, daunorubicin. Distribution is limited mainly to the intravascular compartment. Does not cross the blood-brain barrier. Minimal binding to plasma proteins.

Metabolism

Metabolism in the liver but the primary metabolite, daunorubicinol, is present only in low concentrations. Cleared from plasma at 17 mL/min in contrast to daunorubicin, which is cleared at 240 mL/min. Elimination half-life is about 4–5 hours, far shorter than that of daunorubicin.

Indications

HIV-associated, advanced Kaposi's sarcoma—First-line therapy.

Dosage Range

Usual dose is 40 mg/m^2 IV every 2 weeks.

Drug Interactions

None known.

Special Considerations

1. Use with caution in patients with abnormal liver function. Dose reduction is required in the setting of liver dysfunction.

2. Because the parent drug, daunorubicin, is a vesicant, administer slowly over 60 minutes with a rapidly flowing IV. Careful monitoring is necessary to avoid extravasation. If extravasation is suspected, immediately stop infusion, withdraw fluid, elevate extremity, and apply ice to involved site. May administer local steroids. In severe cases, consult a plastic surgeon.

3. Monitor cardiac function before (baseline) and periodically during therapy with either MUGA radionuclide scan or echocardiogram to assess LVEF. Risk of cardiotoxicity is higher in patients >70 years of age, in patients with prior history of hypertension or pre-existing heart disease, and in patients previously treated with anthracyclines or prior radiation therapy to the chest. Cumulative doses of >320 mg/m^2 are associated with increased risk for cardiotoxicity.

4. Patients may develop back pain, flushing, and chest tightness during the first 5 minutes of infusion. These symptoms are probably related to the lipid component of liposomal daunorubicin. Infusion should be discontinued until symptoms resolve and then resumed at a slower rate.

5. Pregnancy category D.

D

Toxicity 1

Myelosuppression. Dose-limiting toxicity with leukopenia being moderate to severe.

Toxicity 2

Nausea and vomiting. Occur in 50% of patients and are usually mild.

Toxicity 3

Mucositis and diarrhea are common but not dose-limiting.

Toxicity 4

Cardiotoxicity. Acute form presents within the first 2–3 days as arrhythmias and/or conduction abnormalities, EKG changes, pericarditis, and/or myocarditis. Usually transient and mostly asymptomatic.

Chronic form associated with a dose-dependent, dilated cardiomyopathy associated with congestive heart failure. Incidence increases when cumulative doses are greater than 320 mg/m^2.

Toxicity 5

Infusion-related reaction. Occurs within the first 5 minutes of infusion and manifested by back pain, flushing, and tightness in chest and throat. Observed in about 15% of patients and usually with the first infusion. Improves upon termination of infusion and typically does not recur upon reinstitution at a slower infusion rate.

Toxicity 6

Vesicant. Extravasation can lead to tissue necrosis and chemical thrombophlebitis at the site of injection.

Toxicity 7

Hyperpigmentation of nails, rarely skin rash, and urticaria. Radiation recall skin reaction can occur at prior sites of irradiation. Increased hypersensitivity to sunlight.

Toxicity 8

Alopecia. Lower incidence than its parent compound, daunorubicin.

Decitabine

Trade Name

5-Aza-2'-deoxycytidine, Dacogen

Classification

Antimetabolite

Category

Antineoplastic agent, hypomethylating agent

Drug Manufacturer

MGI Pharma

Mechanism of Action

- Deoxycytidine analog.
- Cell cycle–specific with activity in the S-phase.
- Requires activation to the nucleotide metabolite decitabine triphosphate.
- Incorporation of decitabine triphosphate into DNA, results in inhibition of DNA methyltransferases, which then leads to loss of DNA methylation and gene reactivation. Aberrantly silenced genes, such as tumor suppressor genes, are reactivated and expressed.

Mechanism of Resistance

None well characterized to date.

Absorption

Administered only by the IV route.

Distribution

Distribution in humans has not been fully characterized. Does cross blood-brain barrier. Plasma protein binding of decitabine is negligible.

Metabolism

The precise route of elimination and metabolic fate of decitabine is not known in humans. One of the elimination pathways is via deamination by cytidine deaminase, found principally in the liver but also in plasma, granulocytes, intestinal epithelium, and peripheral tissues.

Indications

FDA-approved for treatment of patients with MDS including previously treated and untreated, *de novo* and secondary MDS of all French-American-British subtypes (refractory anemia, refractory anemia with ringed sideroblasts, refractory anemia with excess blasts, refractory anemia with excess blasts in transformation, and chronic myelomonocytic leukemia), and intermediate-1, intermediate-2, and high-risk International Prognostic Scoring System groups.

Dosage Range

1. The recommended dose is 15 mg/m^2 continuous infusion IV over 3 hours repeated every 8 hours for 3 days. Cycles should be repeated every 6 weeks.

2. An alternative schedule is 20 mg/m^2 IV over 1 hour daily for 5 days given every 28 days.

Drug Interactions

None characterized to date.

Special Considerations

1. Patients should be treated for a minimum of 4 cycles. In some cases, a complete or partial response may take longer than 4 cycles.

2. Monitor CBC on a regular basis during therapy. See package insert for recommendations regarding dose adjustments.

3. Decitabine therapy should not be resumed if serum creatinine ≥2 mg/dL, SGPT and/or total bilirubin two times ULN, and ongoing active or uncontrolled infection.

4. Use with caution in patients with underlying liver and/or kidney dysfunction.

5. Pregnancy category D. Breast-feeding should be avoided.

Toxicity 1

Myelosuppression with pancytopenia is dose-limiting.

Toxicity 2

Fatigue and anorexia.

Toxicity 3

GI toxicity in the form of nausea/vomiting, constipation, and abdominal pain.

Toxicity 4

Hyperbilirubinemia.

Toxicity 5

Peripheral edema.

Degarelix

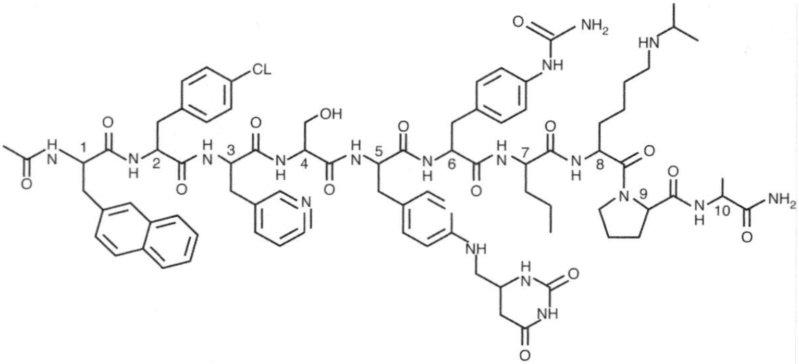

Trade Names

Firmagon

Classification

GnRH antagonist

Category

Hormonal agent

Drug Manufacturer

Ferring

Mechanism of Action

Binds immediately and reversibly to GnRH receptors of the pituitary gland, which leads to inhibition of luteinizing hormone (LH) and follicle stimulating hormone (FSH) production. Causes a rapid and sustained suppression of testosterone without the initial surge that is observed with LHRH agonist therapy.

Absorption

Not orally absorbed because of extensive proteolysis in the hepatobiliary system. Forms a depot upon subcutaneous administration from which degarelix is released into the circulation.

Distribution

Distribution throughout total body water. Approximately 90% of degarelix is bound to plasma proteins.

Metabolism

Metabolism occurs mainly via hydrolysis with excretion of peptide fragments in feces. Approximately 70-80% is eliminated in feces while the remaining 20-30% is eliminated in urine. The elimination half-life is approximately 53 days.

Indications

Advanced prostate cancer.

Dosage Range

Administer 240 mg SC as a starting dose and then 80 mg SC every 28 days.

Drug Interactions

None well-characterized.

Special Considerations

1. Initiation of treatment with degarelix does not induce a transient tumor flare in contrast to LHRH agonists, such as goserelin and leuprolide.

2. Serum testosterone levels decrease to castrate levels within 3 days of initiation of therapy.

3. Use with caution in patients with congenital long QT syndrome, electrolye abnormalities, CHF, and in patients on antiarrhythmic medications, such as quinidine, procainamide, amiodarone, or sotalol, as long-term androgen deprivation therapy prolongs the QT interval.

4. Pregnancy category X.

Toxicity 1

Hot flashes with decreased libido and impotence.

Toxicity 2

Local discomfort at the site of injection with erythema, swelling, and/or induration.

Toxicity 3

Weight gain.

Toxicity 4

Mild elevations in serum transaminases.

Toxicity 5

Fatigue.

D Denileukin diftitox

Trade Names

Ontak, DAB389

Classification

Immunotherapy

Category

Biologic response modifier agent

Drug Manufacturer

Ligand

Mechanism of Action

- Recombinant fusion protein composed of amino acid sequences of human interleukin-2 (IL-2) and the enzymatic and translocation domains of diphtheria toxin.
- Specifically binds to the CD25 component of the IL-2 receptor and then internalized via endocytosis.
- Upon release of diphtheria toxin into cytosol, cellular protein synthesis is inhibited, and cell death via apoptosis occurs.

Absorption

Not available for oral use and is administered only via the IV route.

Distribution

Volume of distribution is similar to that of circulating blood, and the initial distribution half-life is approximately 2–5 minutes.

Metabolism

Metabolized primarily via catabolism by proteolytic degradation pathways. The elimination half-life is 70–80 minutes.

Indications

Persistent or recurrent cutaneous T-cell lymphoma whose malignant cells express the CD25 component of the IL-2 receptor.

Dosage Range

Recommended dose is 9 or 18 µg/kg/day IV on days 1–5 every 21 days.

Drug Interactions

None known.

Special Considerations

1. Expression of CD25 on tumor skin biopsy must be confirmed before administration of denileukin diftitox. A testing service is available and can be reached by calling 1-800-964-5836.

2. Contraindicated in patients with a known hypersensitivity to denileukin diftitox or any of its components including IL-2 and diphtheria toxin.

3. Use with caution in patients with pre-existing cardiac and pulmonary disease as they are at increased risk for developing serious and sometimes fatal reactions.

4. Resuscitative medications, including IV antihistamines, corticosteroids, and epinephrine, and equipment should be readily available at bedside prior to treatment.

5. Monitor serum albumin at baseline and during therapy. Low serum albumin levels place patient at increased risk for vascular leak syndrome. Delay administration of denileukin until the serum albumin is 3 g/dL.

6. Patients should be monitored closely throughout the entire treatment, including vital signs, pre- and post-infusion weights, and evidence of peripheral edema.

7. Premedication with acetaminophen, nonsteroidal anti-inflammatory agents, and antihistamines can help to reduce the incidence and severity of hypersensitivity reactions.

8. Pregnancy category C.

Toxicity 1

Flu-like symptoms with fever, chills, asthenia, myalgias, arthralgias, and headache. Usually mild, transient, and easily manageable.

Toxicity 2

Hypersensitivity reaction manifested by hypotension, back pain, dyspnea, skin rash, chest pain or tightness, tachycardia, dysphagia, and rarely anaphylaxis. Observed in nearly 70% of patients during or within the first 24 hours of drug infusion.

Toxicity 3

Vascular leak syndrome characterized by hypotension, edema, and/or hypoalbuminemia. Usually self-limited process. Pre-existing low serum albumin (<3 g/dL) predisposes patients to this syndrome.

Toxicity 4

Diarrhea may be delayed with prolonged duration. Anorexia along with nausea and vomiting also observed.

Toxicity 5

Myelosuppression is uncommon with anemia occurring more frequently than neutropenia.

Toxicity 6

Hepatotoxicity with elevations in serum transaminases and hypoalbuminemia (albumin <2.3 g/dL) in 15%–20% of patients. Usually occurs during the first course and resolves within 2 weeks of stopping therapy.

Dexrazoxane

Trade Names
Zinecard, ICRF-187

Classification
Iron-chelating agent

Category
Chemoprotective drug

Drug Manufacturer
Pfizer

Mechanism of Action
- Hydrolyzed intracellularly by enzymatic and non-enzymatic mechanisms to yield an EDTA-derived analog.
- Chelator of iron that strips iron from the doxorubicin-iron complex, thereby preventing free radical formation.
- Protects against myocardial toxicity without affecting antitumor activity.
- No pharmacokinetic interaction with anthracycline compounds.

Absorption
Available only for IV use.

Distribution
Rapidly distributed to all body tissues. Not bound to plasma proteins. Peak plasma concentrations are achieved rapidly within 15 minutes of drug infusion.

Metabolism
Metabolism in cells via enzymatic and non-enzymatic mechanisms to yield an EDTA analog. Over 40% of drug is cleared in urine. Plasma elimination half-life is approximately 2–3 hours.

Indications
1. Dexrazoxane is FDA-approved to prevent and/or reduce anthracycline-induced cardiotoxicity in women with metastatic breast

cancer who have received a total cumulative dose of doxorubicin of 300 mg/m² and who would benefit from continued treatment.

2. Dexrazoxane is **NOT** recommended in women who are being started on initial doxorubicin-based therapy.

3. Dexrazoxane is **NOT** recommended in the adjuvant therapy of breast cancer.

Dosage Range

Recommended dose is to give dexrazoxane IV, 30 minutes before doxorubicin, at a ratio of dexrazoxane:doxorubicin of 10:1. For example, with a doxorubicin dose of 50 mg/m², the dose of dexrazoxane should be 500 mg/m².

Drug Interactions

Doxorubicin, epirubicin—Dexrazoxane prevents the cardiotoxicity associated with doxorubicin and epirubicin but may also reduce their respective antitumor activities.

Special Considerations

1. Dexrazoxane should **NOT** be used at the start of doxorubicin therapy as there is evidence to suggest that it may interfere with the antitumor efficacy of doxorubicin leading to decreased response rates observed with the FAC regimen.

2. Monitor cardiac function before (baseline) and periodically during therapy with either MUGA radionuclide scan or echocardiogram to assess LVEF. Treatment with dexrazoxane does not completely eliminate the risk of cardiotoxicity.

3. Sequencing of drugs is important as dexrazoxane should be administered 30 minutes before doxorubicin. Doxorubicin should **NOT** be given before dexrazoxane.

4. Monitor weekly CBC while on therapy. Dexrazoxane may increase the myelosuppressive effects of doxorubicin.

5. Pregnancy category C. Breast-feeding should be avoided.

Toxicity 1

Myelosuppression. Generally mild and reversible.

Toxicity 2

Pain at injection site.

Toxicity 3

Mild nausea and vomiting.

Docetaxel

Trade Names

Taxotere

Classification

Taxane, anti-microtubule agent

Category

Chemotherapy drug

Drug Manufacturer

Sanofi-Aventis

Mechanism of Action

- Semisynthetic taxane. Derived from the needles of the European yew tree.
- High-affinity binding to microtubules enhances tubulin polymerization. Normal dynamic process of microtubule network is inhibited, leading to inhibition of mitosis and cell division.
- Cell cycle–specific agent with activity in the mitotic (M) phase.

Mechanism of Resistance

- Alterations in tubulin with decreased affinity for drug.
- Multidrug-resistant (MDR-1) phenotype with increased expression of P170 glycoprotein. Results in enhanced drug efflux with decreased intracellular accumulation of drug. Cross-resistant to other natural products, including vinca alkaloids, anthracyclines, taxanes, and VP-16.

Absorption

Not administered orally.

Distribution

Distributes widely to all body tissues. Extensive binding (>90%) to plasma and cellular proteins.

Metabolism

Extensively metabolized by the hepatic P450 microsomal system. About 75% of drug is excreted via fecal elimination. Less than 10% is eliminated as the parent compound with the majority being eliminated as metabolites. Renal clearance is relatively minor with less than 10% of drug clearance via the kidneys. Plasma elimination is tri-exponential with a terminal half-life of 11 hours.

Indications

1. Breast cancer—Locally advanced or metastatic breast cancer after failure of prior chemotherapy. FDA-approved.

2. Breast cancer—FDA-approved in combination with doxorubicin and cyclophosphamide for adjuvant treatment of patients with node-positive breast cancer.

3. Non–small cell lung cancer—Locally advanced or metastatic disease after failure of prior platinum-based chemotherapy. FDA-approved.

4. Non–small cell lung cancer—FDA-approved in combination with cisplatin for treatment of patients with locally advanced or metastatic disease who have not previously received chemotherapy.

5. Prostate cancer—FDA-approved in combination with prednisone for androgen-independent (hormone-refractory) metastatic prostate cancer.

6. Gastric cancer—FDA-approved in combination with cisplatin and 5-fluorouracil for advanced gastric cancer, including adenocarcinoma of the gastroesophageal junction, in patients who have not received prior chemotherapy.

7. Head and neck cancer—FDA-approved for use in combination with cisplatin and 5-fluorouracil for induction treatment of patients with inoperable, locally advanced disease.

8. Small cell lung cancer.

9. Refractory ovarian cancer.

10. Bladder cancer.

Dosage Range

1. Metastatic breast cancer: 60, 75, and 100 mg/m^2 IV every 3 weeks or 35–40 mg/m^2 IV weekly for 3 weeks with 1 week of rest.

2. Breast cancer: 75 mg/m^2 IV every 3 weeks in combination with cyclophosphamide and doxorubicin for adjuvant therapy.

3. Non–small cell lung cancer: 75 mg/m² IV every 3 weeks or 35–40 mg/m² IV weekly for 3 weeks with 1 week rest after platinum-based chemotherapy.

4. Non–small cell lung cancer: 75 mg/m² IV every 3 weeks in combination with cisplatin in patients who have not received prior chemotherapy.

5. Metastatic prostate cancer: 75 mg/m² IV every 3 weeks in combination with prednisone.

6. Advanced gastric cancer: 75 mg/m² IV every 3 weeks in combination with cisplatin and 5-FU.

7. Head and neck cancer: 75 mg/m² IV every 3 weeks in combination with cisplatin and 5-FU for induction therapy of locally advanced disease.

Drug Interaction 1

Radiation therapy—Docetaxel acts as a radiosensitizing agent.

Drug Interaction 2

Inhibitors and/or activators of the liver cytochrome P450 CYP3A4 enzyme system—Concurrent use with drugs such as cyclosporine, ketoconazole, and erythromycin may affect docetaxel metabolism and its subsequent antitumor and toxic effects.

Special Considerations

1. Use with caution in patients with abnormal liver function. Patients with abnormal liver function are at significantly higher risk for toxicity, including treatment-related mortality.

2. Closely monitor CBCs, and docetaxel therapy should not be given to patients with neutrophil counts of <1,500 cells/mm³.

3. Patients should receive steroid premedication to reduce the incidence and severity of fluid retention and hypersensitivity reactions. Give dexamethasone 8 mg PO bid for 3 days beginning 1 day before drug administration.

4. Closely monitor patients for allergic and/or hypersensitivity reactions. Usually occur with the first and second treatments. Emergency equipment, including Ambu bag, EKG machine, fluids, pressors, and other drugs for resuscitation, must be at bedside before initiation of treatment.

5. Contraindicated in patients with known hypersensitivity reactions to docetaxel and/or polysorbate 80.

6. Use only glass, polypropylene bottles, or polypropylene or polyolefin plastic bags for drug infusion. Administer only through polyethylene-lined administration sets.

7. Monitor patient's weight, measure daily input and output, and evaluate for peripheral edema.
8. Pregnancy category D. Breast-feeding should be avoided.

Toxicity 1

Myelosuppression. Neutropenia is dose-limiting with nadir at days 7–10 and recovery by day 14. Thrombocytopenia and anemia are also observed.

Toxicity 2

Hypersensitivity reactions with generalized skin rash, erythema, hypotension, dyspnea, and/or bronchospasm. Usually occur within the first 2–3 minutes of an infusion and almost always within the first 10 minutes. Most frequently observed with first or second treatments. Usually prevented by premedication with steroid; overall incidence decreased to less than 3%. When it occurs during drug infusion, treat with hydrocortisone IV, diphenhydramine 50 mg IV, and/or cimetidine 300 mg IV.

Toxicity 3

Fluid retention syndrome. Presents as weight gain, peripheral and/or generalized edema, pleural effusion, and ascites. Incidence increases with total doses >400 mg/m². Occurs in about 50% of patients.

Toxicity 4

Maculopapular skin rash and dry, itchy skin. Most commonly affect forearms and hands. Brown discoloration of fingernails may occur. Observed in up to 50% of patients usually within 1 week after therapy.

Toxicity 5

Alopecia occurs in up to 80% of patients.

Toxicity 6

Mucositis and/or diarrhea seen in 40% of patients. Mild to moderate nausea and vomiting, usually of brief duration.

Toxicity 7

Peripheral neuropathy is less commonly observed with docetaxel than with paclitaxel.

Toxicity 8

Generalized fatigue and asthenia are common, occurring in 60%–70% of patients. Arthralgias and myalgias also observed.

Toxicity 9

Reversible elevations in serum transaminases, alkaline phosphatase, and bilirubin.

Toxicity 10

Vesicant. Phlebitis and/or swelling can be seen at the injection site.

D Doxorubicin

Trade Names

Adriamycin, Hydroxydaunorubicin

Classification

Antitumor antibiotic

Category

Chemotherapy drug

Drug Manufacturer

Bedford Laboratories

Mechanism of Action

- Anthracycline antibiotic isolated from *Streptomyces* species.
- Intercalates into DNA resulting in inhibition of DNA synthesis and function.
- Inhibits transcription through inhibition of DNA-dependent RNA polymerase.
- Inhibits topoisomerase II by forming a cleavable complex with DNA and topoisomerase II to create uncompensated DNA helix torsional tension, leading to eventual DNA breaks.
- Formation of cytotoxic oxygen free radicals results in single- and double-stranded DNA breaks with subsequent inhibition of DNA synthesis and function.

Mechanism of Resistance

- Increased expression of the multidrug-resistant gene with elevated P170 levels, which leads to increased drug efflux and decreased intracellular drug accumulation.
- Decreased expression of topoisomerase II.
- Mutation in topoisomerase II with decreased binding affinity to doxorubicin.

- Increased expression of sulfhydryl proteins, including glutathione and glutathione-dependent proteins.

Absorption

Not absorbed orally.

Distribution

Widely distributed to tissues. Does not cross the blood-brain barrier. About 75% of doxorubicin and its metabolites are bound to plasma proteins.

Metabolism

Metabolized extensively in the liver to the active hydroxylated metabolite, doxorubicinol. About 40%–50% of drug is eliminated via biliary excretion in feces. Less than 10% of drug is cleared by the kidneys. Prolonged terminal half-life of 20–48 hours.

Indications

1. Breast cancer.
2. Hodgkin's and non-Hodgkin's lymphoma.
3. Soft tissue sarcoma.
4. Ovarian cancer.
5. Non–small cell and small cell lung cancer.
6. Bladder cancer.
7. Thyroid cancer.
8. Hepatoma.
9. Gastric cancer.
10. Wilms' tumor.
11. Neuroblastoma.
12. Acute lymphoblastic leukemia.

Dosage Range

1. Single agent: 60–75 mg/m^2 IV every 3 weeks.
2. Single agent: 15–20 mg/m^2 IV weekly.
3. Combination therapy: 45–60 mg/m^2 every 3 weeks.
4. Continuous infusion: 60–90 mg/m^2 IV over 96 hours.

Drug Interaction 1

Dexamethasone, 5-FU, heparin—Doxorubicin is incompatible with dexamethasone, 5-FU, and heparin, as concurrent use will lead to precipitate formation.

Drug Interaction 2

Dexrazoxane—The cardiotoxic effects of doxorubicin are inhibited by the iron-chelating agent dexrazoxane.

Drug Interaction 3

Cyclophosphamide—Increased risk of hemorrhagic cystitis and cardiotoxicity when doxorubicin is given with cyclophosphamide. Important to be able to distinguish between hemorrhagic cystitis and the normal red-orange urine observed with doxorubicin therapy.

Drug Interaction 4

Phenobarbital, phenytoin—Increased plasma clearance of doxorubicin when given concurrently with barbiturates and phenytoin.

Drug Interaction 5

Herceptin, mitomycin-C—Increased risk of cardiotoxicity when doxorubicin is given with Herceptin or mitomycin-C.

Drug Interaction 6

Digoxin—Doxorubicin decreases the oral bioavailability of digoxin.

Drug Interaction 7

6-Mercaptopurine—Increased risk of hepatotoxicity when doxorubicin is given with 6-mercaptopurine.

Special Considerations

1. Use with caution in patients with abnormal liver function. Dose reduction is required in the setting of liver dysfunction.

2. Because doxorubicin is a strong vesicant, administer slowly with a rapidly flowing IV. Avoid using veins over joints or in extremities with compromised venous and/or lymphatic drainage. Use of a central venous catheter is recommended for patients with difficult venous access and mandatory for prolonged infusions. Careful monitoring is necessary to avoid extravasation. If extravasation is suspected, immediately stop infusion, withdraw fluid, elevate extremity, and apply ice to involved site. May administer local steroids. In severe cases, consult a plastic surgeon.

3. Monitor cardiac function before (baseline) and periodically during therapy with either MUGA radionuclide scan or echocardiogram to assess LVEF. Risk of cardiotoxicity is higher in patients >70 years of age, in patients with prior history of hypertension or pre-existing heart disease, in patients previously treated with anthracyclines, or in patients with prior radiation therapy to the chest. Cumulative doses of >450 mg/m² are associated with increased risk for cardiotoxicity.

4. Risk of cardiotoxicity is decreased with weekly or continuous infusion schedules. Use of the iron-chelating agent dexrazoxane (ICRF-187) also is effective at reducing the development of cardiotoxicity.

5. Use with caution in patients previously treated with radiation therapy as doxorubicin can cause radiation recall skin reaction. Increased risk

of skin toxicity when doxorubicin is given concurrently with radiation therapy.

6. Patients should be cautioned to avoid sun exposure and to wear sun protection when outside.
7. Patients should be warned about the potential for red-orange discoloration of urine for 1–2 days after drug administration.
8. Pregnancy category D. Breast-feeding should be avoided.

Toxicity 1

Myelosuppression. Dose-limiting toxicity with leukopenia more common than thrombocytopenia or anemia. Nadir usually occurs at days 10–14 with full recovery by day 21.

Toxicity 2

Nausea and vomiting. Usually mild, occurring in 50% of patients within the first 1–2 hours of treatment.

Toxicity 3

Mucositis and diarrhea. Common but not dose-limiting.

Toxicity 4

Cardiotoxicity. Acute form presents within the first 2–3 days as arrhythmias and/or conduction abnormalities, EKG changes, pericarditis, and/or myocarditis. Usually transient and mostly asymptomatic and not dose-related.

Chronic form results in a dose-dependent, dilated cardiomyopathy associated with congestive heart failure. Risk increases when cumulative doses are greater than 450 mg/m^2.

Toxicity 5

Strong vesicant. Extravasation can lead to tissue necrosis and chemical thrombophlebitis at the site of injection.

Toxicity 6

Hyperpigmentation of nails, rarely skin rash, and urticaria. Radiation recall skin reaction can occur at prior sites of irradiation. Increased hypersensitivity to sunlight.

Toxicity 7

Alopecia. Universal but usually reversible within 3 months after termination of treatment.

Toxicity 8

Red-orange discoloration of urine. Usually occurs within 1–2 days after drug administration.

Toxicity 9

Allergic, hypersensitivity reactions are rare.

Doxorubicin liposome

Trade Names
Doxil

Classification
Antitumor antibiotic

Category
Chemotherapy drug

Drug Manufacturer
Ortho-Biotech

Mechanism of Action

- Liposomal encapsulation of doxorubicin.
- Protected from chemical and enzymatic degradation, reduced plasma protein binding, and decreased uptake in normal tissues.
- Penetrates tumor tissue into which doxorubicin is released.
- Intercalates into DNA resulting in inhibition of DNA synthesis and function.
- Inhibits transcription through inhibition of DNA-dependent RNA polymerase.
- Inhibits topoisomerase II by forming a cleavable complex with DNA and topoisomerase II. This creates uncompensated DNA helix torsional tension, leading to eventual DNA breaks.
- Formation of cytotoxic oxygen free radicals results in single- and double-stranded DNA breaks and subsequent inhibition of DNA synthesis and function.

Mechanism of Resistance

- Increased expression of the multidrug-resistant gene with elevated P170 protein levels, which leads to increased drug efflux and decreased intracellular drug accumulation.
- Decreased expression of topoisomerase II.
- Mutation in topoisomerase II with decreased binding affinity to drug.
- Increased expression of sulfhydryl proteins, including glutathione and glutathione-dependent proteins.

Absorption

Liposomal doxorubicin is not absorbed orally.

Distribution

Mainly confined to the intravascular compartment. In contrast to parent drug, doxorubicin, which has a large V_d (700–1,100 L/m^2), liposomal doxorubicin has a small V_d (2 L/m^2). Does not cross the blood-brain barrier. Binding to plasma proteins has not been well characterized.

Metabolism

Plasma clearance of liposomal doxorubicin is slower than that of doxorubicin, resulting in AUCs that are significantly greater than an equivalent dose of doxorubicin. Prolonged terminal half-life of about 55 hours.

Indications

1. AIDS-related Kaposi's sarcoma—Used in patients with disease that has progressed on prior combination chemotherapy and/or in patients who are intolerant to such therapy.

2. Ovarian cancer—Metastatic disease refractory to both paclitaxel and platinum-based chemotherapy regimens.

3. Multiple myeloma—FDA-approved in combination with bortezomib in patients who have not previously received bortezomib and who have received at least one prior therapy.

Dosage Range

1. Kaposi's sarcoma: 20 mg/m^2 IV every 21 days.

2. Ovarian cancer: 50 mg/m^2 IV every 28 days.

3. Multiple myeloma: 30 mg/m^2 IV on day 4 after bortezomib, which is administered at 1.3 mg/m^2 IV on days 1, 4, 8, and 11, every 21 days.

Drug Interactions

None well characterized to date.

Special Considerations

1. Liposomal doxorubicin should not be substituted for doxorubicin on a mg-per-mg-basis and should be used only where indicated.

2. Use with caution in patients with abnormal liver function. Dose reduction is required in the setting of liver dysfunction.

3. Infusions of liposomal doxorubicin should be given at an initial rate of 1 mg/min over a period of at least 30 minutes to avoid the risk of infusion-associated reactions. This reaction is thought to be related to the lipid component of liposomal doxorubicin. In the event of such a reaction with flushing, dyspnea, or facial swelling, the infusion should be stopped immediately. If symptoms are minor, can restart infusion at 50% the initial rate. Patients should not be rechallenged in the face of a severe hypersensitivity reaction.

4. Careful monitoring is necessary to avoid extravasation. If extravasation is suspected, immediately stop infusion, withdraw fluid,

elevate extremity, and apply ice to involved site. May administer local steroids. In severe cases, consult plastic surgeon.

5. Monitor cardiac function before (baseline) and periodically during therapy with either MUGA radionuclide scan or echocardiogram to assess LVEF. Risk of cardiotoxicity is higher in patients >70 years of age, in patients with prior history of hypertension or pre-existing heart disease, in patients previously treated with anthracyclines, or in patients with prior radiation therapy to the chest.

6. Monitor weekly CBC while on therapy.

7. Patients should be cautioned about the risk of hand-foot syndrome.

8. Patients should be warned about the potential for red-orange discoloration of urine for 1–2 days after drug administration.

9. Pregnancy category D. Breast-feeding should be avoided.

Toxicity 1

Myelosuppression. Dose-limiting toxicity with leukopenia more common than thrombocytopenia or anemia. Nadir usually occurs at days 10–14, with full recovery by day 21.

Toxicity 2

Nausea and vomiting. Usually mild, occurring in 20% of patients.

Toxicity 3

Mucositis and diarrhea. Common but not dose-limiting.

Toxicity 4

Cardiotoxicity. Acute form presents within the first 2–3 days as arrhythmias and/or conduction abnormalities, EKG changes, pericarditis, and/or myocarditis. Usually transient and mostly asymptomatic, and not dose-related.

Chronic form results in a dose-dependent dilated cardiomyopathy associated with congestive heart failure.

Toxicity 5

Skin toxicity manifested as the hand-foot syndrome with skin rash, swelling, erythema, pain, and/or desquamation. Usually mild with onset at 5–6 weeks after the start of treatment. May require subsequent dose reduction. More commonly observed in ovarian cancer patients (37%) than in those with Kaposi's sarcoma (5%).

Toxicity 6

Hyperpigmentation of nails, skin rash, and urticaria. Radiation recall skin reaction can occur at prior sites of irradiation.

Toxicity 7

Alopecia. Common but generally reversible within 3 months after termination of treatment.

Toxicity 8

Infusion reaction with flushing, dyspnea, facial swelling, headache, back pain, tightness in the chest and throat, and/or hypotension. Occurs in about 5%–10% of patients, usually with the first treatment. Upon stopping the infusion, resolves within several hours to a day.

Toxicity 9

Red-orange discoloration of urine. Usually occurs within 1–2 days after drug administration.

Epirubicin

Trade Names

4 Epi-doxorubicin, Ellence

Classification

Antitumor antibiotic

Category

Chemotherapy drug

Drug Manufacturer

Pfizer

Mechanism of Action

- Anthracycline derivative of doxorubicin.
- Intercalates into DNA, which results in inhibition of DNA synthesis and function.
- Inhibits topoisomerase II by forming a cleavable complex with topoisomerase II and DNA.
- Formation of cytotoxic oxygen free radicals, which can cause single- and double-stranded DNA breaks.

Mechanism of Resistance

- Increased expression of the multidrug-resistant gene with enhanced drug efflux. This results in decreased intracellular drug accumulation.
- Decreased expression of topoisomerase II.
- Mutation in topoisomerase II with decreased binding affinity to drug.
- Increased expression of glutathione and glutathione-associated enzymes.

Absorption

Not orally bioavailable.

Distribution

Rapid and extensive distribution to formed blood elements and to body tissues. Does not cross the blood-brain barrier. Epirubicin is extensively bound (about 80%) to plasma proteins. Peak plasma levels are achieved immediately.

Metabolism

Extensive metabolism by the liver microsomal P450 system. Both active (epirubicinol) and inactive metabolites are formed. Elimination is mainly through the hepatobiliary route. Renal clearance accounts for only 20% of drug elimination. The half-life is approximately 30–38 hours for the parent compound and 20–31 hours for the epirubicinol metabolite.

Indications

1. Breast cancer—FDA-approved as a component of adjuvant therapy in women with axillary node involvement following resection of primary breast cancer.

2. Metastatic breast cancer.

3. Gastric cancer.

Dosage Range

1. Usual dose is 100–120 mg/m^2 IV every 3 weeks.

2. In heavily pretreated patients, consider starting at lower dose of 75–90 mg/m^2 IV every 3 weeks.

3. Alternative schedule is 12–25 mg/m^2 IV on a weekly basis.

Drug Interaction 1

Heparin—Epirubicin is incompatible with heparin as a precipitate will form.

Drug Interaction 2

5-FU, cyclophosphamide—Increased risk of myelosuppression when epirubicin is used in combination with 5-FU and cyclophosphamide.

Drug Interaction 3

Cimetidine—Cimetidine decreases the AUC of epirubicin by 50% and should be discontinued upon initiation of epirubicin therapy.

Special Considerations

1. Use with caution in patients with abnormal liver function. Dose modification should be considered in patients with liver dysfunction.

2. Use with caution in patients with severe renal impairment. Dose should be reduced by at least 50% when serum creatinine >5 mg/dL.

3. Use with caution in elderly patients as they are at increased risk for developing toxicity.

4. Careful monitoring of drug administration is necessary to avoid extravasation. If extravasation is suspected, stop infusion immediately, withdraw fluid, elevate arm, and apply ice to site. In severe cases, consult plastic surgeon.

5. Monitor cardiac function before (baseline) and periodically during therapy with either MUGA radionuclide scan or echocardiogram to assess LVEF. Risk of cardiotoxicity is higher in elderly patients >70 years of age, in patients with prior history of hypertension or pre-existing heart disease, in patients previously treated with anthracyclines, or in patients with prior radiation therapy to the chest. In patients with no prior history of anthracycline therapy, cumulative doses of 900 mg/m^2 are associated with increased risk for cardiotoxicity.

6. Epirubicin may be administered on a weekly schedule to decrease the risk of cardiotoxicity.

7. Monitor weekly CBC while on therapy.

8. Use with caution in patients previously treated with radiation therapy as epirubicin may induce a radiation recall reaction.

9. Patients may experience red-orange discoloration of urine for 24 hours after drug administration.

10. Pregnancy category D. Breast-feeding should be avoided.

Toxicity 1

Myelosuppression. Dose-limiting toxicity with leukopenia more common than thrombocytopenia. Nadir typically occurs at 8–14 days after treatment, with recovery of counts by day 21. Risk of myelosuppression greater in elderly patients and in those previously treated with chemotherapy and/or radiation therapy.

Toxicity 2

Mild nausea and vomiting. Occur less frequently than with doxorubicin.

Toxicity 3

Mucositis and diarrhea. Dose-dependent, common, and generally mild.

Toxicity 4

Cardiotoxicity. Cardiac effects are similar to but less severe than those of doxorubicin. Acute toxicity presents as rhythm or conduction disturbances, chest pain, and myopericarditis syndrome that typically occurs within the first 24–48 hours of drug administration. Transient and mostly asymptomatic, not dose-related.

Chronic form of cardiotoxicity presents as a dilated cardiomyopathy with congestive heart failure. Risk of congestive heart failure increases significantly with cumulative doses >900 mg/m^2. Continuous infusion and weekly schedules are associated with decreased risk of cardiotoxicity. Dexrazoxane may be helpful in preventing epirubicin-mediated cardiotoxicity.

Toxicity 5

Alopecia. Onset within 10 days of initiation of therapy and regrowth of hair upon termination of treatment. Occurs much less commonly than with doxorubicin, being observed in only 25%–50% of patients.

Toxicity 6

Potent vesicant. Extravasation can lead to tissue injury, inflammation, and chemical thrombophlebitis at the site of injection.

Toxicity 7

Skin rash, flushing, hyperpigmentation of skin and nails, and photosensitivity. Radiation recall skin reaction can occur at previous sites of irradiation.

Toxicity 8

Red-orange discoloration of urine for 24 hours after drug administration.

Erlotinib

• HCl

Trade Names

Tarceva, OSI-774

Classification

Signal transduction inhibitor

Category

Chemotherapy drug

Drug Manufacturer

OSI, Genentech

Mechanism of Action

- Potent and selective small molecule inhibitor of the EGFR tyrosine kinase, resulting in inhibition of EGFR autophosphorylation and inhibition of EGFR signaling.
- Inhibition of the EGFR tyrosine kinase results in inhibition of critical mitogenic and anti-apoptotic signals involved in proliferation, growth, metastasis, angiogenesis, and response to chemotherapy and/or radiation therapy.

Mechanism of Resistance

- Mutations in the EGFR tyrosine kinase leading to decreased binding affinity to erlotinib.
- Presence of KRAS mutations.
- Activation/induction of alternative cellular signaling pathways, such as PI3K/Akt and IGF-1R.

Absorption

Oral bioavailability is approximately 60% and is increased by food to almost 100%.

Distribution

Extensive binding (90%) to plasma proteins, including albumin and α1-acid glycoprotein, and extensive tissue distribution. Peak plasma levels are achieved 4 hours after ingestion. Steady-state drug concentrations are reached in 7–8 days.

Metabolism

Metabolism in the liver primarily by the CYP3A4 microsomal enzyme and by CYP1A2 to a lesser extent. Elimination is mainly hepatic with excretion in the feces, and renal elimination of parent drug and its metabolites account for only about 8% of an administered dose. The terminal half-life of the parent drug is 36 hours.

Indications

1. FDA-approved as monotherapy for the treatment of locally advanced or metastatic non-small cell lung cancer after failure of at least one prior chemotherapy regimen.

2. FDA-approved in combination with gemcitabine for the first-line treatment of patients with locally advanced unresectable or metastatic pancreatic cancer.

Dosage Range

1. Non-small cell lung cancer—Recommended dose is 150 mg/day PO.

2. Pancreatic cancer—Recommended dose is 100 mg/day PO in combination with gemcitabine.

Drug Interaction 1

Dilantin and other drugs that stimulate the liver microsomal CYP3A4 enzyme, including carbamazepine, rifampicin, phenobarbital, and St. John's wort—These drugs may increase the metabolism of erlotinib, resulting in its inactivation.

Drug Interaction 2

Drugs that inhibit the liver microsomal CYP3A4 enzyme, including ketoconazole, itraconazole, erythromycin, and clarithromycin—These drugs may decrease the metabolism of erlotinib, resulting in increased drug levels and potentially increased toxicity.

Drug Interaction 3

Warfarin—Patients receiving coumarin-derived anticoagulants should be closely monitored for alterations in their clotting parameters (PT and INR) and/or bleeding, as erlotinib may inhibit the metabolism of warfarin by the liver P450 system. Dose of warfarin may require careful adjustment in the presence of erlotinib therapy.

Special Considerations

1. Use with caution in patients with hepatic impairment, and dose reduction and/or interruption should be considered.

2. Non-smokers and patients with EGFR-positive tumors are more sensitive to erlotinib therapy.

3. Erlotinib should not be used in combination with platinum-based chemotherapy as there is no evidence of clinical benefit.

4. Closely monitor patients for new or progressive pulmonary symptoms, including cough, dyspnea, and fever. Erlotinib therapy should be interrupted pending further diagnostic evaluation.

5. Consider increasing the dose of erlotinib to 300 mg in patients with NSCLC who are actively smoking, as the metabolism of erlotinib by CYP1A1/1A2 in the liver is induced.

6. Dose of erlotinib may need to be increased when used in patients with seizure disorders who are receiving phenytoin, as the metabolism of erlotinib by the liver P450 system is enhanced in the presence of phenytoin.

7. Coagulation parameters PT/INR should be closely monitored when patients are receiving both erlotinib and Coumadin, as erlotinib may inhibit the metabolism of Coumadin by the liver P450 system.

8. In patients who develop a skin rash, topical antibiotics such as Cleocin gel or either oral Cleocin and/or oral minocycline may help.

9. Patients should avoid contact lens use while on erlotinib therapy and for at least 14 days after termination of therapy.

10. Avoid grapefruit and grapefruit juice while on erlotinib therapy.

11. Pregnancy category D.

Toxicity 1

Pruritus, dry skin with mainly a pustular, acneiform skin rash occurring most often on face and upper trunk. Nail changes, paronychia, painful fissures or cracking of the skin on hands and feet, and hair growth abnormalities, including alopecia, thinning hair with increased fragility (trichorrhexis), darkening and increased thickness of eyelashes and eyebrows (trichomegaly), and hirsutism.

Toxicity 2

Diarrhea is most common GI toxicity. Mild nausea/vomiting and mucositis.

Toxicity 3

Pulmonary toxicity in the form of ILD manifested by increased cough, dyspnea, fever, and pulmonary infiltrates. Observed in less than 1% of patients and more frequent in patients with underlying pulmonary disease.

Toxicity 4

Mild to moderate elevations in serum transaminases. Usually transient and clinically asymptomatic.

E

Anorexia.

Conjunctivitis and keratitis. Rare cases of corneal perforation and ulceration.

Rare episodes of GI hemorrhage.

Erythropoietin

Trade Names

Procrit, Epogen, EPO, Epoetin alfa

Classification

Colony-stimulating growth factor, cytokine

Category

Biologic response modifier agent

Drug Manufacturer

Ortho Biotech, Amgen

Mechanism of Action

- Glycoprotein that is produced by recombinant DNA techniques. Has the same biologic effects as endogenous erythropoietin.
- Stimulates division and differentiation of red blood cells in the bone marrow.
- Does not possess antitumor activity.

Absorption

Administered either by the IV or SC route. Absorption is higher after SC injection in the thigh when compared to SC injection in the arm or abdomen. Plasma levels are detectable for 24 hours after injection.

Distribution

Distributes into total plasma volume. Binding to plasma proteins is not known.

Metabolism

Metabolism is not entirely clear, although catabolism in liver and bone marrow appears to play a role. About 10% of the drug is cleared in urine in unchanged form. The terminal half-life is 4–13 hours in patients with chronic renal failure.

Indications

1. Chemotherapy-induced anemia in patients with non-myeloid cancers.
2. Anemia in AZT-treated patients with HIV.
3. Anemia associated with chronic renal failure.
4. Anemia in patients scheduled to undergo elective, non-cardiac, non-vascular surgery to reduce the need for allogeneic blood transfusions.

Dosage Range

1. Chemotherapy-induced anemia: Usual starting dose is 40,000 units once a week, and if the hemoglobin is not increased >1 g/dL, the dose may be increased to 60,000 units once a week.

2. Anemia in AZT-treated HIV patients: 100 units/kg SC tiw.

3. Chronic renal failure: 50–100 units/kg SC tiw.

4. Surgery: 300 units/day for 10 days prior to surgery, on day of surgery, and for 4 days after surgery.

Drug Interaction 1

Heparin—Erythropoietin decreases the efficacy of heparin when given concurrently.

Drug Interaction 2

Aluminum-containing antacids—Efficacy of erythropoietin is decreased in the presence of aluminum-containing antacids.

Special Considerations

1. Contraindicated in patients with uncontrolled hypertension. Use with caution in patients with a history of hypertension and/or cardiovascular disease.

2. Contraindicated in patients with known hypersensitivity to mammalian-derived products.

3. Contraindicated in patients with known hypersensitivity to human albumin.

4. Use with caution in patients with known porphyria as exacerbation has been observed in patients treated with erythropoietin.

5. Obtain baseline erythropoietin levels before start of therapy. The optimal response is observed in cancer patients with endogenous levels ≤200 U/mL. A baseline serum ferritin level and transferrin saturation should also be obtained. Transferrin saturation should be at least 20%, and ferritin should be at least 100 mg/mL.

6. The lowest dose of erythropoietin should be used to increase gradually the need for hemoglobin concentrations to the lowest level sufficient to avoid the need for red blood cell transfusions. Blood counts should be monitored on a weekly basis during erythropoietin therapy. If the response is not satisfactory in terms of reducing transfusion requirements or increasing hematocrit after 4–8 weeks of therapy, the dose of erythropoietin can be doubled. If patients have not responded to this increase in dose, higher doses are unlikely to be beneficial. Increases in hemoglobin/hematocrit are usually seen after 7 days of therapy but may take up to 4–8 weeks.

7. Contraindicated in patients receiving myelosuppressive chemotherapy if the intent of treatment is cure. Remains indicated when myelosuppressive chemotherapy is intended for palliation.

8. Patients should be closely monitored to ensure that the hemoglobin levels are not greater than 12 g/dL. An increased risk of death and serious cardiovascular events, including myocardial infarction, heart failure, stroke, and thrombosis, has been observed in this setting (this represents a black-box warning).

9. Patients may benefit from concomitant treatment with iron supplementation, ferrous sulfate 1 tablet PO bid or tid, or with IV iron.

10. Pregnancy category C.

Toxicity 1

Diarrhea and occasional nausea and vomiting.

Toxicity 2

Hypertension is common but usually mild.

Toxicity 3

Local pain at injection site.

Toxicity 4

Fever, fatigue, asthenia, and headache.

Estramustine

Trade Names

Estracyte, Emcyt

Classification

Anti-microtubule agent

Category

Chemotherapy drug

Drug Manufacturer

Pfizer

Mechanism of Action

- Conjugate of nornitrogen mustard and estradiol phosphate.
- Cell cycle-specific agent with activity in the mitosis (M) phase.
- Initially designed to target cancer cells expressing estrogen receptors. However, active against estrogen receptor-negative tumor cells.
- Although this compound was initially designed as an alkylating agent, it has no alkylating activity.
- Inhibits microtubule structure and function and the process of microtubule assembly by binding to microtubule-associated proteins (MAPs).

Mechanism of Resistance

- Mechanisms of cellular resistance are different from those identified for other anti-microtubule agents.
- Estramustine-resistant cells do not express increased levels of P170 glycoprotein and are not cross-resistant to other anti-microtubule agents and/or natural products.
- Estramustine-resistant cells display increased efflux of drug with decreased drug accumulation. The underlying mechanism(s) remains ill-defined.

Absorption

Highly bioavailable via the oral route with 70%–75% of an oral dose absorbed.

Metabolism

Estramustine is supplied as the estramustine phosphate form, which renders it more water-soluble. Rapidly dephosphorylated in the GI tract so that the dephosphorylated form predominates about 4 hours after ingestion.

Metabolized primarily in the liver. About 15%–20% of the drug is excreted in urine. Only small amounts of unmetabolized drug are found. Biliary and fecal excretion of alkylating and estrogenic metabolites has also been demonstrated. Prolonged half-life of 20–24 hours.

Indications

Hormone-refractory, metastatic prostate cancer.

Dosage Range

1. Single agent: 14 mg/kg/day PO in three–four divided doses.

2. Combination: 600 mg/m^2/day PO days 1–42 every 8 weeks, as part of the estramustine/vinblastine regimen.

Drug Interactions

None known.

Special Considerations

1. Contraindicated in patients with active thrombophlebitis or thromboembolic disorders. Closely monitor patients with history of heart disease and/or stroke.

2. Contraindicated in patients with known hypersensitivity to estradiol or nitrogen mustard.

3. Contraindicated in patients with peptic ulcer disease, severe liver disease, or cardiac disease.

4. Instruct patients to take estramustine with water 1 hour before meals or 2 hours after meals to decrease the risk of GI upset.

5. Administer prophylactic antiemetics to avoid nausea and vomiting.

6. Instruct patients that milk, milk products, and calcium-rich foods may impair absorption of drug.

Toxicity 1

Nausea and vomiting. Occur within 2 hours of ingestion. Usually mild and respond to antiemetic therapy. However, intractable vomiting may occur after prolonged therapy (6–8 weeks).

Toxicity 2

Gynecomastia is reported in up to 50% of patients. Can be prevented by prophylactic breast irradiation.

Toxicity 3

Diarrhea occurs in about 15%–25% of patients.

Toxicity 4

Cardiovascular complications are rare and include congestive heart failure, cardiac ischemia, and thromboembolism.

Toxicity 5

Myelosuppression is rare.

Toxicity 6

Skin rash.

Etoposide

Trade Names
VePesid, VP-16

Classification
Epipodophyllotoxin, topoisomerase II inhibitor

Category
Chemotherapy drug

Drug Manufacturer
Bristol-Myers Squibb

Mechanism of Action

- Plant alkaloid extracted from the *Podophyllum peltatum* mandrake plant.
- Cell cycle-specific agent with activity in the late S- and G2-phase.
- Inhibits topoisomerase II by stabilizing the topoisomerase II-DNA complex and preventing the unwinding of DNA.

Mechanism of Resistance

1. Multidrug-resistant phenotype with increased expression of P170 glycoprotein. Results in enhanced drug efflux and decreased intracellular accumulation of drug. Cross-resistant to vinca alkaloids, anthracyclines, taxanes, and other natural products.

2. Decreased expression of topoisomerase II.

3. Mutations in topoisomerase II with decreased binding affinity to drug.

4. Enhanced activity of DNA repair enzymes.

Absorption

Bioavailability of oral capsules is approximately 50%, requiring an oral dose to be twice that of an IV dose. However, oral bioavailability is non-linear and decreases with higher doses of drug (>200 mg). Presence of food and/or other anticancer agents does not alter drug absorption.

Distribution

Rapidly distributed into all body fluids and tissues. Large fraction of etoposide (90%–95%) is protein-bound, mainly to albumin. Decreased albumin levels result in a higher fraction of free drug and a potentially higher incidence of host toxicity.

Metabolism

Metabolized primarily by the liver via glucuronidation to hydroxy acid metabolites, which are less active than the parent compound. About 30%–50% of etoposide is excreted in urine, and about 2%–6% is excreted in stool via biliary excretion. The elimination half-life ranges from 3 to 10 hours.

Indications

1. Germ cell tumors.

2. Small cell lung cancer.

3. Non-small cell lung cancer.

4. Non-Hodgkin's lymphoma.

5. Hodgkin's lymphoma.

6. Gastric cancer.

7. High-dose therapy in transplant setting for various malignancies, including breast cancer, lymphoma, and ovarian cancer.

Dosage Range

1. IV: Testicular cancer—As part of the PEB regimen, 100 mg/m^2 IV on days 1–5 with cycles repeated every 3 weeks.

2. IV: Small cell lung cancer—As part of cisplatin/VP-16 regimen, 100–120 mg/m^2 IV on days 1–3 with cycles repeated every 3 weeks.

3. Small cell lung cancer—50 mg/m^2/day PO for 21 days.

Drug Interactions

Warfarin—Etoposide may alter the anticoagulant effect of warfarin by prolonging the PT and INR. Coagulation parameters (PT and INR) need to be closely monitored and dose of warfarin may require adjustment.

Special Considerations

1. Use with caution in patients with abnormal renal function. Dose reduction is recommended in patients with renal dysfunction. Baseline creatinine clearance should be obtained, and renal status should be carefully monitored during therapy.

2. Use with caution in patients with abnormal liver function. Dose reduction is recommended in this setting.

3. Administer drug over a period of at least 30–60 minutes to avoid the risk of hypotension. Should the blood pressure drop, immediately discontinue the drug and administer IV fluids. Rate of administration must be reduced upon restarting therapy.

4. Carefully monitor for anaphylactic reactions. More commonly observed during the initial infusion of therapy and probably related to the polysorbate 80 vehicle in which the drug is formulated. In rare instances, such an allergic reaction can be fatal. The drug should be immediately stopped and treatment with antihistamines, steroids, H2 blockers such as cimetidine, and pressor agents should be administered.

5. Closely monitor injection site for signs of phlebitis and avoid extravasation.

6. Pregnancy category D.

Toxicity 1

Myelosuppression. Dose-limiting toxicity with leukopenia more common than thrombocytopenia. Nadir usually occurs 10–14 days after therapy with recovery by day 21.

Toxicity 2

Nausea and vomiting. Occur in about 30%–40% of patients and generally mild to moderate. More commonly observed with oral administration.

Toxicity 3

Anorexia.

Toxicity 4

Alopecia observed in nearly two-thirds of patients.

Toxicity 5

Mucositis and diarrhea are unusual with standard doses but more often observed with high doses in transplant setting.

Toxicity 6

Hypersensitivity reaction with chills, fever, bronchospasm, dyspnea, tachycardia, facial and tongue swelling, and hypotension. Occurs in less than 2% of patients.

Toxicity 7

Metallic taste during infusion of drug.

Toxicity 8

Local inflammatory reaction at injection site.

Toxicity 9

Radiation recall skin changes.

Toxicity 10

Increased risk of secondary malignancies, especially acute myelogenous leukemia. Associated with 11:23 translocation. Typically develops within 5–8 years of treatment and in the absence of preceding myelodysplastic syndrome.

Etoposide phosphate

Trade Names

Etopophos

Classification

Epipodophyllotoxin, topoisomerase II inhibitor

Category

Chemotherapy drug

Drug Manufacturer

Bristol-Myers Squibb

Mechanism of Action

- Water-soluble prodrug form of etoposide.
- Cell cycle-specific agent with activity in late S- and G2-phases.
- Must first be dephosphorylated for etoposide to be active.
- Once activated, it inhibits topoisomerase II by stabilizing the topoisomerase II-DNA complex and preventing the unwinding of DNA.

Mechanism of Resistance

- Multidrug-resistant phenotype with increased expression of P170 glycoprotein. Results in enhanced drug efflux and decreased intracellular accumulation of drug.
- Decreased expression of topoisomerase II.
- Mutations in topoisomerase II with decreased binding affinity to drug.
- Enhanced activity of DNA repair enzymes.

Absorption

Only administered via the IV route.

Distribution

Rapidly distributed into all body fluids and tissues. Large fraction of drug (90%–95%) is protein-bound, mainly to albumin. Decreased albumin levels result in a higher fraction of free drug and a potentially higher incidence of host toxicity.

Metabolism

Etoposide phosphate is rapidly and completely converted to etoposide in plasma, which is then metabolized primarily by the liver to hydroxyacid metabolites. These metabolites are less active than the parent compound. The elimination half-life of the drug ranges from 3 to 10 hours. About 15%–20% of the drug is excreted in urine and about 2%–6% is excreted in stool within 72 hours after IV administration.

Indications

1. Germ cell tumors.

2. Small cell lung cancer.

3. Non-small cell lung cancer.

Dosage Range

1. Testicular cancer: 100 mg/m² IV on days 1–5 with cycles repeated every 3 weeks.

2. Small cell lung cancer: 100 mg/m² IV on days 1–3 with cycles repeated every 3 weeks.

Drug Interactions

Warfarin—Etoposide may alter the anticoagulant effect of warfarin by prolonging the PT and INR. Coagulation parameters need to be closely monitored and dose of warfarin may require adjustment.

Special Considerations

1. Use with caution in patients with abnormal renal function. Dose reduction is recommended in this setting. Baseline creatinine clearance should be obtained and renal status should be closely monitored during therapy.

2. Use with caution in patients with abnormal liver function. Dose reduction is recommended in this setting.

3. Administer drug over a period of at least 30–60 minutes to avoid the risk of hypotension. Should the blood pressure drop, immediately discontinue the drug and administer IV fluids. The rate of administration must be reduced upon restarting therapy.

4. Carefully monitor for anaphylactic reactions. Occur more frequently during the initial infusion of therapy. In rare instances, such an allergic reaction can be fatal. The drug should be immediately stopped and treatment with antihistamines, steroids, H2 blockers such as cimetidine, and pressor agents should be administered.

5. Closely monitor injection site for signs of phlebitis. Carefully avoid extravasation.

6. Pregnancy category D.

Toxicity 1

Myelosuppression. Dose-limiting toxicity with leukopenia more common than thrombocytopenia. Nadir usually occurs 10–14 days after therapy with recovery by day 21.

Toxicity 2

Nausea and vomiting. Occur in about 30%–40% of patients and are generally mild to moderate.

Toxicity 3

Anorexia.

Toxicity 4

Alopecia.

Toxicity 5

Mucositis and diarrhea are only occasionally seen.

Toxicity 6

Hypersensitivity reaction with chills, fever, bronchospasm, dyspnea, tachycardia, facial and tongue swelling, and hypotension.

Toxicity 7

Metallic taste during infusion of drug.

Toxicity 8

Local inflammatory reaction at the injection site.

Toxicity 9

Radiation recall skin changes.

Toxicity 10

Increased risk of secondary malignancies, especially acute myelogenous leukemia. Associated with 11:23 translocation. Typically develops within 5–8 years of treatment and in the absence of preceding myelodysplastic syndrome.

Everolimus

Trade Names
Afinitor, RAD001

Classification
Signal transduction inhibitor

Category
Chemotherapy drug

Drug Manufacturer
Novartis

Mechanism of Action

- Potent inhibitor of the mammalian target of rapamycin (mTOR), a serine-threonine kinase that is a key component of cellular signaling pathways involved in the growth and proliferation of tumor cells.
- Inhibitor of expression of hypoxia-inducible factor (HIF-1), which leads to reduced expression of VEGF.
- Inhibition of mTOR signaling results in cell cycle arrest, induction of apoptosis, and inhibition of angiogenesis.

Mechanism of Resistance
None well characterized to date.

Absorption
Peak drug levels are achieved 1-2 hours after oral administration. Food with a high fat content reduces oral bioavailability by up to 20%.

Distribution

Steady-state drug concentrations are reached within two weeks after once-daily dosing. Significant binding (up to 75%) to plasma proteins.

Metabolism

Metabolism in the liver primarily by CYP3A4 microsomal enzymes. Six main metabolites have been identified, including 3 monohydroxylated metabolites, 2 hydrolytic ring-opened products, and a phosphatidylcholine conjugate of everolimus. In general, these metabolites are significantly less active than the parent compound. Elimination is mainly hepatic with excretion in feces, and renal elimination of parent drug and its metabolites accounts for only 5% of an administered dose. The terminal half-life of the parent drug is 30 hours.

Indications

FDA-approved for the treatment of advanced renal cell cancer after failure on sunitinib or sorafenib.

Dosage Range

Recommended dose is 10 mg PO once daily.

Drug Interaction 1

Dilantin and other drugs that induce liver microsomal CYP3A4, including carbamazepine, rifampin, phenobarbital, dexamethasone, and St. John's wort —These drugs may increase the rate of metabolism of everolimus, resulting in its inactivation.

Drug Interaction 2

Drugs that inhibit liver microsomal CYP3A4, including ketoconazole, itraconazole, fluconazole, verapamil or diltiazem, erythromycin, and clarithromycin—These drugs may decrease the rate of metabolism of everolimus, resulting in increased drug levels and potentially increased toxicity.

Special Considerations

1. Everolimus should be taken once daily at the same time with or without food. The tablets should be swallowed whole with a glass of water and never chewed or crushed.

2. Use with caution in patients with moderate liver impairment (Child-Pugh class B), and dose should be reduced to 5 mg daily. Should not be used in patients with severe liver impairment (Child-Pugh class C).

3. Consider increasing dose in 5 mg increments up to a maximum of 20 mg once daily if used in combination with drugs that are strong inducers of CYP3A4.

4. Closely monitor patients for new or progressive pulmonary symptoms, including cough, dyspnea, and fever. Non-infectious pneumonitis is a class effect of rapamycin analogs, and everolimus therapy should be interrupted pending further diagnostic evaluation.

5. Patients are at increased risk for developing opportunistic infections, such as pneumonia, other bacterial infections, and invasive fungal infections, while on everolimus.

6. Closely monitor serum glucose levels in all patients, especially those with diabetes mellitus.

7. Closely monitor serum triglyceride and cholesterol levels while on therapy.

8. Avoid alcohol or mouthwashes containing peroxide in the setting of oral ulcerations as they may worsen the condition.

9. Avoid grapefruit products while on everolimus, as they can result in a significant increase in drug levels.

10. Avoid the use of live vaccines and/or close contact with those who have received live vaccines while on everolimus.

11. Pregnancy category D.

Toxicity 1
Asthenia and fatigue.

Toxicity 2
Mucositis, oral ulcerations, and diarrhea.

Toxicity 3
Nausea/vomiting and anorexia.

Toxicity 4
Increased risk of opportunistic infections, such as pneumonia, other bacterial infections, and invasive fungal infections.

Toxicity 5
Pulmonary toxicity in the form of increased cough, dyspnea, fever, and pulmonary infiltrates.

Toxicity 6
Skin rash.

Toxicity 7
Myelosuppression with anemia, thrombocytopenia, and neutropenia.

Toxicity 8
Hyperlipidemia with increased serum triglycerides and/or cholesterol in up to 70-75% of patients.

Toxicity 9

Hyperglycemia in up to 50% of patients.

Toxicity 10

Mild liver toxicity with elevation in serum transaminases and alkaline phosphatase.

E

Exemestane

Trade Names

Aromasin

Classification

Steroidal aromatase inactivator

Category

Hormonal agent

Drug Manufacturer

Pfizer

Mechanism of Action

- Permanently binds to and irreversibly inactivates aromatase.
- Inhibits the synthesis of estrogens by inhibiting the conversion of adrenal androgens (androstenedione and testosterone) to estrogens (estrone, estrone sulfate, and estradiol).
- No inhibitory effect on adrenal corticosteroid or aldosterone biosynthesis.

Mechanism of Resistance

- None characterized.
- Lack of cross-resistance between exemestane and nonsteroidal aromatase inhibitors.

Absorption

Excellent bioavailability via the oral route with 85% of a dose absorbed within 2 hours of ingestion. Absorption is not affected by food.

Distribution

Widely distributed throughout the body. About 90% of drug is bound to plasma proteins.

Metabolism

Extensively metabolized in the liver by the cytochrome P450 3A4 enzyme (up to 85%) to inactive forms. Half-life of drug is about 24 hours. Steady-state levels of drug are achieved after 7 days of a once-daily administration. The major route of elimination is fecal with renal excretion accounting for only 10% of drug clearance.

Indications

Treatment of advanced breast cancer in postmenopausal women whose disease has progressed following tamoxifen therapy.

Dosage Range

Usual dose is 25 mg PO once daily after a meal.

Drug Interactions

None known.

Special Considerations

1. No dose adjustments are required for patients with either hepatic or renal dysfunction.
2. Should not be administered to premenopausal women.
3. Should not be administered with estrogen-containing agents as they may interfere with antitumor activity.
4. Caution patients about the risk of hot flashes.
5. No need for glucocorticoid and/or mineralocorticoid replacement.
6. Pregnancy category D.

Toxicity 1

Hot flashes.

Toxicity 2

Mild nausea.

Toxicity 3

Fatigue.

Toxicity 4

Headache.

Filgrastim

F

Filgrastim

Trade Names

Neupogen, G-CSF

Classification

Colony-stimulating growth factor, cytokine

Category

Biologic response modifier agent

Drug Manufacturer

Amgen

Mechanism of Action

- Pleiotropic cytokine that binds to specific surface receptors of hematopoietic progenitor cells.
- Stimulates the proliferation, differentiation, and activation of granulocyte progenitor cells and the activity of mature granulocytes.
- Enhances neutrophil chemotaxis and phagocytosis.
- Does not possess antitumor activity.

Absorption

Filgrastim is rapidly and completely absorbed into the circulation after a SC dose, with peak plasma concentration achieved in 2–8 hours after administration.

Distribution

Distributes into blood and bone marrow. Binding to plasma proteins is not known.

Metabolism

Metabolized in both the liver and the kidney. However, drug clearance is unaffected by hepatic and/or renal dysfunction. The terminal half-life is on the order of 3.5 hours.

Indications

1. Adjunct to myelosuppressive chemotherapy—Prophylactic use in patients receiving chemotherapy with either previous history of drug-related neutropenia and/or fever or in patients receiving drugs associated with a significant incidence of severe neutropenia and fever.

2. High-dose chemotherapy in bone marrow or peripheral stem cell transplant setting—Used to reduce the duration of neutropenia.

3. Mobilization of peripheral blood progenitor cells for collection by leukapheresis.

4. Chronic neutropenia such as congenital neutropenia, cyclic neutropenia, or idiopathic neutropenia.

5. Adjunct to induction or consolidation therapy for acute myelogenous leukemia.

Dosage Range

1. Prevention of chemotherapy-induced neutropenia: 5 µg/kg/day SC or IV, administered at least 24 hours after the completion of chemotherapy.

2. High-dose chemotherapy and stem cell transplant: 10 µg/kg/day IV infusion of 4 or 24 hours, administered 24 hours after infusion of stem cells. The dose can be reduced to 5 µg/kg when neutrophil count reaches >1,000/mm^3 and discontinued when absolute neutrophil count (ANC) remains >1,000/mm^3 for 3 consecutive days.

3. Stem cell mobilization: 10–20 µg/kg/day given at least 4 days before the first apheresis and continued until the last apheresis.

Drug Interactions

Steroids, lithium—Caution should be exercised when using these drugs concurrently with filgrastim as they may potentiate the release of neutrophils during filgrastim therapy.

Special Considerations

1. Contraindicated in patients with known hypersensitivity to *E. coli*–derived products.

2. Concurrent administration with chemotherapy or radiation therapy is contraindicated as an increased incidence of serious adverse events has been observed. Filgrastim must be given at least 24 hours after the last dose of chemotherapy and 12 hours after radiation therapy as the stimulatory effects of filgrastim on the hematopoietic precursors render them more susceptible to chemotherapy.

3. Instruct patients to rotate the SC injection sites.

4. Blood counts should be monitored at least twice a week during filgrastim therapy. The dose should be adjusted to prevent both persistent neutropenia and excessive leukocytosis. Therapy should be terminated once WBC >10,000/mm^3 or when ANC >1,000/mm^3 for 3 consecutive days.

5. Filgrastim is incompatible with saline-containing solutions.

6. Use with caution in patients on steroids or lithium as these drugs may potentiate the release of neutrophils.

7. Premedication with acetaminophen helps to relieve the bone pain that arises due to bone marrow expansion in response to treatment.

8. Pregnancy category C.

Toxicity 1

Transient bone pain occurs in up to 25% of patients. Usually mild to moderate and well-controlled with non-narcotic medications.

Toxicity 2

Hypersensitivity reaction is uncommon.

Toxicity 3

Neutrophilia with WBC counts >40,000/mm^3 is common with ongoing therapy after normal counts are achieved.

Toxicity 4

Transient elevations in serum lactate dehydrogenase and alkaline phosphatase.

Floxuridine

Trade Names

5-Fluoro-2'-deoxyuridine, FUDR

Classification

Antimetabolite

Category

Chemotherapy drug

Drug Manufacturer

Roche

Mechanism of Action

- Fluoropyrimidine deoxynucleoside analog.
- Cell cycle-specific with activity in the S-phase.
- Requires activation to cytotoxic metabolite forms. Metabolized to 5-FU metabolite FdUMP, which inhibits thymidylate synthase. This results in inhibition of DNA synthesis, function, and repair.
- Incorporation of 5-FU metabolite FUTP into RNA resulting in alterations in RNA processing and/or translation.
- Incorporation of 5-FU metabolite FdUTP into DNA resulting in inhibition of DNA synthesis and function.
- Inhibition of TS leads to accumulation of dUMP, which becomes misincorporated into DNA in the form of dUTP, resulting in inhibition of DNA synthesis and function.

Mechanism of Resistance

- Increased expression of thymidylate synthase.
- Decreased levels of reduced folate substrate 5, 10-methylenetetrahydrofolate for thymidylate synthase reaction.
- Decreased incorporation of 5-FU into RNA.
- Decreased incorporation of 5-FU into DNA.

- Increased activity of DNA repair enzymes, uracil glycosylase and dUTPase.
- Increased salvage of physiologic nucleosides including thymidine.
- Increased expression of dihydropyrimidine dehydrogenase.
- Decreased expression of mismatch repair enzymes (hMLH1, hMSH2).
- Alterations in thymidylate synthase with decreased binding affinity of enzyme for FdUMP.

Absorption

Poorly absorbed by the GI tract.

Distribution

After IV administration, floxuridine is rapidly extracted by the liver via first-pass metabolism. After hepatic intra-arterial administration, greater than 90% of drug is extracted by hepatocytes. Binding to plasma proteins has not been well characterized.

Metabolism

Undergoes extensive enzymatic metabolism to 5-FU and 5-FU metabolites. Catabolism accounts for >85% of drug metabolism. Dihydropyrimidine dehydrogenase is the main enzyme responsible for 5-FU catabolism, and it is present in liver and extrahepatic tissues, including GI mucosa, WBCs, and kidney. About 30% of an administered dose of drug is cleared in urine mainly as inactive metabolites. The terminal elimination half-life is 20 hours.

Indications

1. Metastatic colorectal cancer—Intrahepatic arterial treatment of colorectal cancer metastatic to the liver.
2. Metastatic GI adenocarcinoma—Patients with metastatic disease confined to the liver.

Dosage Range

Recommended dose is 0.1–0.6 mg/kg/day IA for 7–14 days via hepatic artery.

Drug Interaction 1

Leucovorin—Leucovorin enhances the toxicity and antitumor activity of floxuridine. Stabilizes the TS-FdUMP-reduced folate ternary complex resulting in maximal inhibition of TS.

Drug Interaction 2

Thymidine—Rescues against the toxic effects of floxuridine.

Drug Interaction 3

Vistonuridine (PN401)—Rescues against the toxic effects of floxuridine.

Special Considerations

1. Contraindicated in patients with poor nutritional status, depressed bone marrow function, or potentially serious infection.

2. No dose adjustments are necessary in patients with mild to moderate liver dysfunction or abnormal renal function. However, patients should be closely monitored as they may be at increased risk of toxicity.

3. Patients should be placed on an H2 blocker, such as ranitidine 150 mg PO bid, to prevent the onset of peptic ulcer disease while on therapy. Onset of ulcer-like pain is an indication to stop therapy as hemorrhage and/or perforation may occur.

4. Patients who experience unexpected, severe grade 3 or 4 host toxicities with initiation of therapy may have an underlying deficiency in dihydropyrimidine dehydrogenase. Therapy must be discontinued immediately. Further testing to identify the presence of this pharmacogenetic syndrome should be considered.

5. Pregnancy category D. Breast-feeding should be avoided.

Toxicity 1

Hepatotoxicity is dose-limiting. Presents as abdominal pain, elevated alkaline phosphatase, liver transaminases, and bilirubin. Sclerosing cholangitis is a rare event. Other GI toxicities include duodenitis, duodenal ulcer, and gastritis.

Toxicity 2

Nausea and vomiting are mild. Mucositis and diarrhea also observed.

Toxicity 3

Hand-foot syndrome (palmar-plantar erythrodysesthesia). Characterized by tingling, numbness, pain, erythema, dryness, rash, swelling, increased pigmentation, and/or pruritus of the hands and feet.

Toxicity 4

Myelosuppression. Nadir occurs at 7–10 days with full recovery by 14–17 days.

Toxicity 5

Neurologic toxicity manifested by somnolence, confusion, seizures, cerebellar ataxia, and rarely encephalopathy.

Toxicity 6

Cardiac symptoms of chest pain, EKG changes, and serum enzyme elevation. Rare event but increased risk in patients with prior history of ischemic heart disease.

Toxicity 7

Blepharitis, tear-duct stenosis, acute and chronic conjunctivitis.

Toxicity 8

Catheter-related complications include leakage, catheter occlusion, perforation, dislodgement, infection, bleeding at catheter site, and thrombosis and/or embolism of hepatic artery.

Fludarabine

2-Fluoro-ara-AMP, Fludara

Antimetabolite

Chemotherapy drug

Bayer Schering Pharma AG and Antisoma (oral form)

- 5-Monophosphate analog of arabinofuranosyladenosine (ara-A) with high specificity for lymphoid cells. Presence of the 2-fluoro group on adenine ring renders fludarabine resistant to breakdown by adenosine deaminase.

- Considered a prodrug. Following administration, it is rapidly dephosphorylated to 2-fluoro-ara-adenosine (F-ara-A). F-ara-A enters cells and is then re-phosphorylated first to its monophosphate form and eventually to the active 5-triphosphate metabolite (F-ara-ATP).

- Antitumor activity against both dividing and resting cells.

- Triphosphate metabolite incorporates into DNA resulting in inhibition of DNA chain extension.

- Inhibition of ribonucleotide reductase by the triphosphate metabolite.

- Inhibition of DNA polymerase-α and DNA polymerase-β by the triphosphate metabolite resulting in inhibition of DNA synthesis and DNA repair.

- Induction of apoptosis (programmed cell death).

Mechanism of Resistance

- Decreased expression of the activating enzyme, deoxycytidine kinase.
- Decreased nucleoside transport of drug.

Absorption

Fludarabine is orally bioavailable, in the range of 50-65%, and a tablet form is now available. Absorption is not affected by food.

Distribution

Widely distributed throughout the body. Concentrates in high levels in liver, kidney, and spleen. Binding to plasma proteins has not been well characterized.

Metabolism

Rapidly converted to 2-fluoro-ara-A, which enters cells via the nucleoside transport system and is re-phosphorylated by deoxycytidine kinase to fludarabine monophosphate. This metabolite undergoes two subsequent phosphorylation steps to yield fludarabine triphosphate, the active species. Major route of elimination is via the kidneys, and approximately 25% of 2-fluoro-ara-A is excreted unchanged in urine. The terminal half-life is on the order of 10–20 hours.

Indications

1. Chronic lymphocytic leukemia (CLL).
2. Non-Hodgkin's lymphoma (low-grade).
3. Cutaneous T-cell lymphoma.

Dosage Range

Usual dose is 25 mg/m² IV on days 1–5 every 28 days. For oral usage, the recommended dose is 40 mg/m² PO on days 1–5 every 28 days.

Drug Interaction 1

Cytarabine—Fludarabine may enhance the antitumor activity of cytarabine by inducing the expression of deoxycytidine kinase.

Drug Interaction 2

Cyclophosphamide, cisplatin, mitoxantrone—Fludarabine may enhance the antitumor activity of cyclophosphamide, cisplatin, and mitoxantrone by inhibiting nucleotide excision repair mechanisms.

Drug Interaction 3

Pentostatin—Increased incidence of fatal pulmonary toxicity when fludarabine is used in combination with pentostatin. Use of this combination is absolutely contraindicated.

Special Considerations

1. Use with caution in patients with abnormal renal function. Dose should be reduced in proportion to the creatinine clearance.

2. Use with caution in elderly patients and in those with bone marrow impairment as they are at increased risk of toxicity.

3. Monitor for signs of infection. Patients are at increased risk for opportunistic infections, including herpes, fungus, and *Pneumocystis carinii*. Patients should be empirically placed on Bactrim prophylaxis, 1 DS tablet PO bid three times/week.

4. Monitor for signs of tumor lysis syndrome, especially in patients with a high tumor cell burden. May occur as early as within the first week of treatment.

5. Allopurinol may be given prior to initiation of fludarabine therapy to prevent hyperuricemia.

6. Use irradiated blood products in patients requiring transfusions as transfusion-associated graft-versus-disease can occur rarely after transfusion of non-irradiated products in patients treated with fludarabine.

7. Pregnancy category D. Breast-feeding is not recommended.

Toxicity 1

Myelosuppression. Dose-limiting toxicity. Leukocyte nadir occurs in 10–13 days, with recovery by day 14–21. Autoimmune hemolytic anemia and drug-induced aplastic anemia also occur.

Toxicity 2

Immunosuppression. Decrease in CD4+ and CD8+ T cells occurs in most patients. Increased risk of opportunistic infections, including fungus, herpes, and *Pneumocystis carinii*. Recovery of CD4+ count is slow and may take over a year to return to normal.

Toxicity 3

Nausea and vomiting are usually mild.

Toxicity 4

Fever occurs in 20%–30% of patients. Most likely due to release of pyrogens and/or cytokines from tumor cells. Associated with fatigue, malaise, myalgias, arthralgias, and chills.

Toxicity 5

Hypersensitivity reaction with maculopapular skin rash, erythema, and pruritus.

Toxicity 6

Tumor lysis syndrome. Rarely seen (in less than 1%–2% of patients), and most often in the setting of high tumor-cell burden. However, it can be fatal upon presentation.

Toxicity 7

Transient elevation in serum transaminases. Clinically asymptomatic.

5-Fluorouracil

Trade Names

5-FU, Efudex

Classification

Antimetabolite

Category

Chemotherapy drug

Drug Manufacturer

Roche

Mechanism of Action

- Fluoropyrimidine analog.
- Cell cycle–specific with activity in the S-phase.
- Requires activation to cytotoxic metabolite forms. Complex process as outlined in Figure 1.
- Inhibition of the target enzyme thymidylate synthase by the 5-FU metabolite, FdUMP (Figure 2).
- Incorporation of the 5-FU metabolite FUTP into RNA resulting in alterations in RNA processing and/or translation.
- Incorporation of the 5-FU metabolite FdUTP into DNA resulting in inhibition of DNA synthesis and function.
- Inhibition of TS leads to accumulation of dUMP, which then gets misincorporated into DNA in the form of dUTP resulting in inhibition of DNA synthesis and function.

Mechanism of Resistance

- Increased expression of thymidylate synthase.
- Decreased levels of reduced folate substrate 5, 10-methylenetetrahydrofolate for thymidylate synthase reaction.

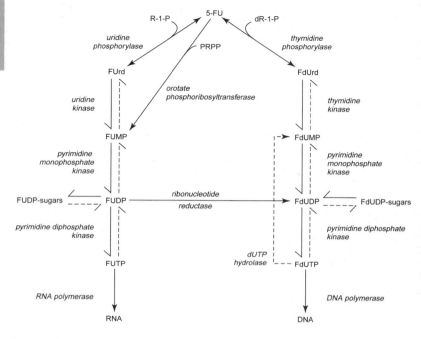

Figure 1 *Metabolic activation of 5-FU.*

- Decreased incorporation of 5-FU into RNA.
- Decreased incorporation of 5-FU into DNA.
- Increased activity of DNA repair enzymes, uracil glycosylase and dUTPase.
- Increased salvage of physiologic nucleosides including thymidine.
- Increased expression of dihydropyrimidine dehydrogenase.
- Decreased expression of mismatch repair enzymes (hMLH1, hMSH2).
- Alterations in thymidylate synthase with decreased binding affinity of enzyme for FdUMP.

Absorption

Oral absorption is variable and erratic with a bioavailability that ranges from 40% to 70%.

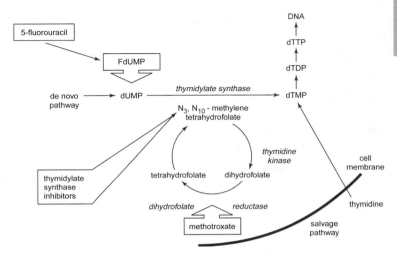

Figure 2 *Inhibition of thymidylate synthase by the 5-FU metabolite FdUMP.*

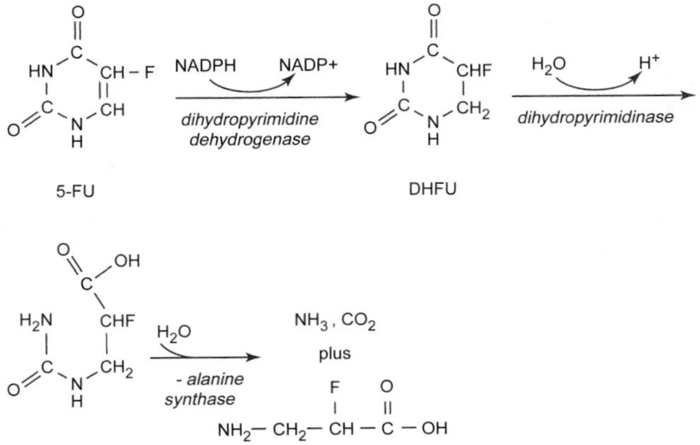

Figure 3 *Catabolic breakdown of 5-FU.*

Distribution

After IV administration, 5-FU is widely distributed to tissues with highest concentration in GI mucosa, bone marrow, and liver. Penetrates into third-space fluid collections such as ascites and pleural effusions. Crosses the blood-brain barrier and distributes into CSF and brain tissue. Binding to plasma proteins has not been well characterized.

Metabolism

Undergoes extensive enzymatic metabolism intracellularly to cytotoxic metabolites. Catabolism accounts for >85% of drug metabolism (see Figure 3). Dihydropyrimidine dehydrogenase is the main enzyme responsible for 5-FU catabolism, and it is highly expressed in liver and extrahepatic tissues such as GI mucosa, WBCs, and kidney. Greater than 90% of an administered dose of drug is cleared in urine and lungs. The terminal elimination half-life is short, ranging from 10 to 20 min.

Indications

1. Colorectal cancer—Adjuvant setting and advanced disease.
2. Breast cancer—Adjuvant setting and advanced disease.
3. GI malignancies, including anal, esophageal, gastric, and pancreatic cancer.
4. Head and neck cancer.
5. Hepatoma.
6. Ovarian cancer.
7. Topical use in basal cell cancer of skin and actinic keratoses.

Dosage Range

1. Bolus monthly schedule: 425–450 mg/m² IV on days 1–5 every 28 days.
2. Bolus weekly schedule: 500–600 mg/m² IV every week for 6 weeks every 8 weeks.
3. 24-hour infusion: 2,400–2,600 mg/m² IV every week.
4. 96-hour infusion: 800–1,000 mg/m²/day IV.
5. 120-hour infusion: 1,000 mg/m²/day IV on days 1–5 every 21–28 days.
6. Protracted continuous infusion: 200–400 mg/m²/day IV.

Drug Interaction 1

Leucovorin—Leucovorin enhances the antitumor activity and toxicity of 5-FU. Stabilizes the TS-FdUMP-reduced folate ternary complex resulting in maximal inhibition of TS.

Drug Interaction 2

Methotrexate, trimetrexate—Antifolate analogs increase the formation of 5-FU nucleotide metabolites when given 24 hours before 5-FU.

Drug Interaction 3

Thymidine—Rescues against the TS- and DNA-mediated toxic effects of 5-FU.

Drug Interaction 4

Vistonuridine—Rescues against the toxic effects of 5-FU.

Special Considerations

1. No dose adjustments are necessary in patients with mild to moderate liver or renal dysfunction. However, patients should be closely monitored as they may be at increased risk for host toxicity.

2. Contraindicated in patients with bone marrow depression, poor nutritional status, infection, active ischemic heart disease, or history of myocardial infarction within previous 6 months.

3. Patients should be monitored closely for mucositis and/or diarrhea as there is increased potential for dehydration, fluid imbalance, and infection. Elderly patients are at especially high risk for GI toxicity.

4. Patients who experience unexpected, severe grade 3 or 4 myelosuppression, GI toxicity, and/or neurologic toxicity with initiation of therapy may have an underlying deficiency in dihydropyrimidine dehydrogenase. Therapy must be discontinued immediately. Further testing to identify the presence of this pharmacogenetic syndrome should be considered.

5. Vistonuridine, at a dose of 10 gm PO every 6 hr, may be used in patients overdosed with 5-FU or in those who experience severe toxicity. For further information, call Wellstat Therapeutics.

6. Vitamin B6 (pyridoxine 50 mg PO bid) may be used to prevent and/ or reduce the incidence and severity of hand-foot syndrome.

7. Use of ice chips in mouth 10–15 minutes pre- and 10–15 minutes post-IV bolus injections of 5-FU may reduce the incidence and severity of mucositis.

8. Pregnancy category D. Breast-feeding should be avoided.

Toxicity 1

Myelosuppression. Dose-limiting for the qd × 5 or weekly schedules, less frequently observed with infusional therapy. Neutropenia and thrombocytopenia more common than anemia.

Toxicity 2

Mucositis and/or diarrhea. May be severe and dose-limiting for infusional schedules. Nausea and vomiting are mild and rare.

Toxicity 3

Hand-foot syndrome (palmar-plantar erythrodysesthesia). Characterized by tingling, numbness, pain, erythema, dryness, rash, swelling, increased pigmentation, nail changes, pruritus of the hands and feet, and/or desquamation. Most often observed with infusional therapy and can be dose-limiting.

Toxicity 4

Neurologic toxicity manifested by somnolence, confusion, seizures, cerebellar ataxia, and rarely encephalopathy.

Toxicity 5

Cardiac symptoms of chest pain, EKG changes, and serum enzyme elevation. Rare event but increased risk in patients with prior history of ischemic heart disease.

Toxicity 6

Blepharitis, tear-duct stenosis, acute and chronic conjunctivitis.

Toxicity 7

Dry skin, photosensitivity, and pigmentation of the infused vein are common.

Toxicity 8

Metallic taste in mouth during IV bolus injection.

Flutamide

Trade Names

Eulexin

Classification

Antiandrogen

Category

Hormonal agent

Drug Manufacturer

Schering

Mechanism of Action

Nonsteroidal, antiandrogen agent binds to androgen receptor and inhibits androgen uptake as well as inhibits androgen binding in nucleus in androgen-sensitive prostate cancer cells.

Mechanism of Resistance

- Decreased expression of androgen receptor.
- Mutation in androgen receptor leading to decreased binding affinity to flutamide.

Absorption

Rapidly and completely absorbed by the GI tract. Peak plasma levels observed 1–2 hours after oral administration.

Distribution

Distribution is not well characterized. Flutamide and its metabolites are extensively bound to plasma proteins (92%–96%).

Metabolism

Extensive metabolism by the liver cytochrome P450 system to both active and inactive metabolites. The main metabolite, α-hydroxyflutamide, is biologically active. Flutamide and its metabolites are cleared primarily in urine, and only 4% of drug is eliminated in feces. The elimination half-life of flutamide is about 8 hours, whereas the half-life of the hydroxyflutamide metabolite is 8–10 hours.

Indications

1. Locally confined stage B2–C prostate cancer.
2. Stage D2 metastatic prostate cancer.

Dosage Range

Recommended dose is 250 mg PO tid at 8-hour intervals.

Drug Interactions

Warfarin—Flutamide can inhibit metabolism of warfarin by the liver $P450$ system leading to increased anticoagulant effect. Coagulation parameters (PT and INR) must be followed closely when warfarin and flutamide are taken concurrently, and dose adjustments may be needed.

Special Considerations

1. Monitor LFTs at baseline and during therapy. In the presence of elevated serum transaminases to 2–3 times the upper limit of normal (ULN), therapy should be terminated.
2. Caution patients about the risk of diarrhea and, if severe, flutamide may need to be stopped.
3. Caution patients about the potential for hot flashes. Consider the use of clonidine 0.1–0.2 mg PO daily, Megace 20 mg PO bid, or soy tablets, one tablet PO tid for prevention and/or treatment.
4. Instruct patients on the potential risk of altered sexual function and impotence.
5. Pregnancy category D.

Toxicity 1

Hot flashes occur in 60% of patients, decreased libido (35%), impotence (30%), gynecomastia (10%), nipple pain, and galactorrhea.

Toxicity 2

Nausea, vomiting, and diarrhea.

Toxicity 3

Transient elevations in serum transaminases are rare but may necessitate discontinuation of therapy.

Toxicity 4

Amber-green discoloration of urine secondary to flutamide and/or its metabolites.

Fulvestrant

HO …''(CH$_2$)$_9$SO(CH$_2$)$_3$CF$_2$CF$_3$

OH

Trade Names
Faslodex

Classification
Estrogen receptor antagonist

Category
Hormonal agent

Drug Manufacturer
AstraZeneca

Mechanism of Action
- Potent and selective antagonist of the estrogen receptor (ER) with no known agonist effects. Affinity to the ER is comparable to that of estradiol.
- Downregulates the expression of the ER, presumably through enhanced degradation.

Mechanism of Resistance
None characterized.

Absorption
Not absorbed orally. After IM injection, peak plasma levels are achieved in approximately 7 days and are maintained for at least 1 month.

Distribution
Rapidly and widely distributed throughout the body. Approximately 99% of drug is bound to plasma proteins, and VLDL, LDL, and HDL are the main binding proteins.

Metabolism
Extensively metabolized in the liver by microsomal P450 3A4 enzymes to both active and inactive forms. Steady-state levels of drug are achieved after 7 days of a once-monthly administration and are maintained for at least up to 1 month. The major route of elimination is fecal (approximately 90%), with renal excretion accounting for only 1% of drug clearance.

Indications

Metastatic breast cancer—Treatment of ER+ postmenopausal women with advanced disease and disease progression following antiestrogen therapy.

Dosage Range

Recommended dose is 250 mg IM once every month.

Drug Interactions

None known.

Special Considerations

1. No dose adjustments are required for patients with either renal or mild hepatic dysfunction. The safety and efficacy have not been carefully studied in patients with moderate to severe hepatic impairment.

2. Use with caution in patients with bleeding diatheses, thrombocytopenia, and/or receiving anticoagulation therapy.

3. Pregnancy category D. Women of child-bearing potential should be strongly advised to avoid becoming pregnant. Breast-feeding should be avoided as it is not known whether fulvestrant is excreted in human milk.

Toxicity 1

Asthenia occurs in up to 25% of patients.

Toxicity 2

Mild nausea and vomiting. Constipation and/or diarrhea can also occur.

Toxicity 3

Hot flashes seen in 20% of patients.

Toxicity 4

Mild headache.

Toxicity 5

Injection site reactions with mild pain and inflammation that are usually transient in nature.

Toxicity 6

Back pain and arthralgias.

Toxicity 7

Flu-like syndrome in the form of fever, malaise, and myalgias. Occurs in 10% of patients.

Toxicity 8

Dry, scaling skin rash.

Gefitinib

Trade Names

Iressa, ZD1839

Classification

Signal transduction inhibitor

Category

Chemotherapy drug

Drug Manufacturer

AstraZeneca

Mechanism of Action

- Potent and selective small molecule inhibitor of the EGFR tyrosine kinase, resulting in inhibition of EGFR autophosphorylation and inhibition of EGFR signaling.
- Inhibition of the EGFR tyrosine kinase results in inhibition of critical mitogenic and anti-apoptotic signals involved in proliferation, growth, metastasis, angiogenesis, and response to chemotherapy and/or radiation therapy.

Mechanism of Resistance

- Mutations in the EGFR tyrosine kinase leading to decreased binding affinity to gefitinib.
- Presence of KRAS mutations.
- Activation/induction of alternative cellular signaling pathways, such as PI3K/Akt and IGF-1R.

Absorption

Oral absorption is relatively slow, and the oral bioavailability is approximately 60%. Food does not affect drug absorption.

Distribution

Extensive binding (90%) to plasma proteins, including albumin and α1-acid glycoprotein, and extensive tissue distribution. Steady-state drug concentrations are reached in 7–10 days.

Metabolism

Metabolism in the liver primarily by CYP3A4 microsomal enzymes. Other cytochrome P450 enzymes play a minor role in its metabolism. The main metabolite is the O-desmethyl piperazine derivative, and this metabolite is significantly less potent than the parent drug. Elimination is mainly hepatic with excretion in the feces, and renal elimination of the parent drug and its metabolites accounts for less than 4% of an administered dose. The terminal half-life of the parent drug is 48 hours.

Indications

Treatment of non-small cell lung cancer that is refractory to platinum-based chemotherapy and/or second-line docetaxel therapy. FDA-approved for patients who are currently receiving and benefiting or who have previously received and benefited from gefitinib treatment.

Dosage Range

Recommended dose is 250 mg/day PO.

Drug Interaction 1

Dilantin and other drugs that stimulate the liver microsomal CYP3A4 enzyme, including carbamazepine, rifampicin, phenobarbital, and St. John's wort—These drugs increase the rate of metabolism of gefitinib, resulting in its inactivation.

Drug Interaction 2

Drugs that inhibit the liver microsomal CYP3A4 enzyme, including ketoconazole, itraconazole, erythromycin, and clarithromycin—These drugs decrease the rate of metabolism of gefitinib, resulting in increased drug levels and potentially increased toxicity.

Drug Interaction 3

Warfarin—Patients receiving coumarin-derived anticoagulants should be closely monitored for alterations in their clotting parameters (PT and INR) and/or bleeding as gefitinib inhibits the metabolism of warfarin by the liver P450 system. Dose of warfarin may require careful adjustment in the presence of gefitinib therapy.

Special Considerations

1. Clinical responses may be observed within the first week of initiation of therapy.

2. Patients with bronchoalveolar non–small cell lung cancer may be more sensitive to gefitinib therapy than other histologic subtypes. Females and non-smokers also show increased sensitivity to gefitinib therapy.

3. Closely monitor patients with central lesions as they may be at increased risk for complications of hemoptysis.

4. Dose of gefitinib may need to be increased when used in patients with seizure disorders who are receiving phenytoin, as the metabolism of gefitinib by the liver P450 system is enhanced in the presence of phenytoin.

5. Coagulation parameters (PT/INR) should be closely monitored when patients are receiving both gefitinib and Coumadin, as gefitinib inhibits the metabolism of Coumadin by the liver P450 system.

6. In patients who develop a skin rash, topical antibiotics such as Cleocin gel or either oral Cleocin and/or oral minocycline may help.

7. Avoid grapefruit and grapefruit juice while on gefinitib.

8. Pregnancy category D.

Toxicity 1
Elevations in blood pressure, especially in those with underlying hypertension.

Toxicity 2
Pruritus, dry skin with mainly a pustular, acneiform skin rash.

Toxicity 3
Mild to moderate elevations in serum transaminases. Usually transient and clinically asymptomatic.

Toxicity 4
Asthenia and anorexia.

Toxicity 5
Mild nausea/vomiting and mucositis.

Toxicity 6
Conjunctivitis, blepharitis, and corneal erosions. Abnormal eyelash growth may occur in some patients.

Toxicity 7
Rare episodes of hemoptysis and GI hemorrhage.

Gemcitabine

Trade Names

Gemzar

Classification

Antimetabolite

Category

Chemotherapy drug

Drug Manufacturer

Eli Lilly

Mechanism of Action

- Fluorine-substituted deoxycytidine analog.
- Cell cycle-specific with activity in the S-phase.
- Requires intracellular activation by deoxycytidine kinase to the monophosphate form with eventual metabolism to the cytotoxic triphosphate nucleotide metabolite (dFdCTP). Antitumor activity of gemcitabine is determined by a balance between intracellular activation and degradation and the formation of cytotoxic triphosphate metabolites.
- Incorporation of dFdCTP triphosphate metabolite into DNA resulting in chain termination and inhibition of DNA synthesis and function.
- Triphosphate metabolite inhibits DNA polymerases α, β, and δ, which, in turn, interferes with DNA synthesis, DNA repair, and DNA chain elongation.
- Difluorodeoxycytidine diphosphate (dFdCDP) metabolite inhibits the enzyme ribonucleotide reductase, resulting in decreased levels of essential deoxyribonucleotides for DNA synthesis and function.
- Incorporation into RNA resulting in alterations in RNA processing and mRNA translation.

Mechanism of Resistance

- Decreased activation of drug through decreased expression of the anabolic enzyme deoxycytidine kinase.
- Increased breakdown of drug by the catabolic enzymes cytidine deaminase and dCMP deaminase.
- Decreased nucleoside transport of drug into cells.
- Increased concentration of the competing physiologic nucleotide dCTP, through increased expression of CTP synthetase.

Absorption

Poor oral bioavailability as a result of extensive deamination within the GI tract. Administered by the IV route.

Distribution

With infusions <70 minutes, drug is not extensively distributed. In contrast, with longer infusions, drug is slowly and widely distributed into body tissues. Does not cross the blood-brain barrier. Binding to plasma proteins is negligible.

Metabolism

Undergoes extensive metabolism by deamination to the difluorouridine (dFdU) metabolite with approximately >90% of drug being recovered in urine in this form. Deamination occurs in liver, plasma, and peripheral tissues. The principal enzyme involved in drug catabolism is cytidine deaminase. The terminal elimination half-life is dependent on the infusion time. With short infusions <70 minutes, the half-life ranges from 30 to 90 minutes, while for infusions >70 minutes, the half-life is 4–10 hours. Plasma clearance is also dependent on gender and age. Clearance is 30% lower in women and in elderly patients.

Indications

1. Pancreatic cancer—FDA-approved as monotherapy or in combination with erlotonib for first-line treatment of locally advanced or metastatic disease.

2. Non–small cell lung cancer—FDA-approved in combination with cisplatin for first-line treatment of inoperable, locally advanced or metastatic disease.

3. Breast cancer—FDA-approved in combination with paclitaxel for first-line treatment of metastatic breast cancer after failure of prior anthracycline-containing adjuvant chemotherapy.

4. Ovarian cancer—FDA-approved in combination with carboplatin for patients with advanced ovarian cancer that has relapsed at least 6 months after completion of platinum-based therapy.

5. Bladder cancer.

6. Soft tissue sarcoma.

Dosage Range

1. Pancreatic cancer: 1,000 mg/m^2 IV every week for 7 weeks with 1 week rest. Treatment then continues weekly for 3 weeks followed by 1 week off.

2. Bladder cancer: 1,000 mg/m^2 IV on days 1, 8, and 15 every 28 days.

3. Non–small cell lung cancer: 1,200 mg/m^2 IV on days 1, 8, and 15 every 28 days.

Drug Interaction 1

Cisplatin—Gemcitabine enhances the cytotoxicity of cisplatin by increasing the formation of cytotoxic platinum-DNA adducts.

Drug Interaction 2

Radiation therapy—Gemcitabine is a potent radiosensitizer.

Special Considerations

1. Monitor complete blood counts on a regular basis during therapy. Dose reduction is recommended based on the degree of hematologic toxicity.

2. Use with caution in patients with abnormal liver and/or renal function. Dose modification should be considered in this setting as there is an increased risk for toxicity.

3. Use with caution in women and in elderly patients as gemcitabine clearance is decreased.

4. Pregnancy category D.

Toxicity 1

Myelosuppression is dose-limiting. Leukopenia more common than thrombocytopenia. Nadir occurs by days 10–14, with recovery by day 21.

Toxicity 2

Nausea and vomiting. Usually mild to moderate, occur in 70% of patients. Diarrhea and/or mucositis observed in 15%–20% of patients.

Toxicity 3

Flu-like syndrome manifested by fever, malaise, chills, headache, and myalgias. Seen in 20% of patients. Fever, in the absence of infection, develops in 40% of patients within the first 6–12 hours after treatment but generally is mild.

Toxicity 4

Transient hepatic dysfunction with elevation of serum transaminases and bilirubin.

Toxicity 5

Pulmonary toxicity in the form of mild dyspnea and drug-induced pneumonitis. ARDS has been reported rarely.

Toxicity 6

Infusion reaction presents as flushing, facial swelling, headache, dyspnea, and/or hypotension. Usually related to the rate of infusion and resolves with slowing or discontinuation of infusion.

Toxicity 7

Mild proteinuria and hematuria. In rare cases, renal microangiopathy syndromes, including hemolytic-uremic syndrome (HUS) and thrombotic thrombocytopenic purpura (TTP), have been reported.

Toxicity 8

Maculopapular skin rash generally involving the trunk and extremities and pruritus. Alopecia is rarely observed.

G

G

Gemtuzumab ozogamicin

Trade Names

Mylotarg, CMA-676

Classification

Monoclonal antibody

Category

Biologic response modifier agent

Drug Manufacturer

Wyeth

Mechanism of Action

- Gemtuzumab ozogamicin is composed of a semisynthetic derivative of calicheamicin covalently linked to a recombinant humanized monoclonal antibody directed against the 67 kDa cell surface glycoprotein CD33. Calicheamicin is a potent cytotoxic antibiotic that binds to DNA in the minor groove resulting in double-strand breaks, inhibition of DNA synthesis and function, and cell death.

- CD33 antigen is expressed on myeloid leukemia cells from more than 90% of patients with acute myelogenous leukemia (AML) and on normal myeloid cells.

- CD33 antigen is not expressed on the surface of pluripotent hematopoietic stem cells nor on non-myeloid tissues.

- The antibody conjugate is internalized upon binding to the CD33 antigen, and calicheamicin is then released via hydrolysis.

Mechanism of Resistance

Not well characterized to date.

Absorption

Gemtuzumab is given only by the IV route.

Distribution

Within 30 minutes after infusion of gemtuzumab, nearly all of the CD33 sites on peripheral blood leukemic blast cells are bound by the drug conjugate. The AUC increases by nearly 2-fold from the first dose to the second dose of the drug conjugate.

Metabolism

Metabolism of gemtuzumab has not been extensively characterized in humans. In vitro studies suggest that the liver microsomal system plays an important role in the formation of various metabolites. While animal studies suggest that gemtuzumab undergoes hepatobiliary elimination, the clearance mechanism(s) in humans remains to be defined. Elimination half-lives of total and unconjugated calicheamicin are 39 and 100 hours, respectively, after the first dose. The half-life of total calicheamicin increases significantly to 63 hours with the second dose.

Indications

Relapsed CD33+ AML—Indicated in patients in first relapse who are 60 years of age or older and who are not considered for cytotoxic chemotherapy.

Dosage Range

Recommended dose is 9 mg/m² IV administered over 2 hours. Usually administer two doses of drug with the second dose being given 14 days after the first dose.

Drug Interactions

None known.

Special Considerations

1. Contraindicated in patients with known type I hypersensitivity or anaphylactic reactions to gemtuzumab or to any of its components.

2. Gemtuzumab should **NOT** be given by IV push or bolus.

3. Patients should be premedicated with acetaminophen, 650–1,000 mg PO, and diphenhydramine, 50 mg PO, 30 minutes before drug infusion to reduce the incidence of infusion-related reactions.

4. Monitor closely for infusion-related events, which usually occur during the infusion or within 2 hours after infusion. However, grade 3/4 hypotension has been observed several hours after infusion; this is usually transient and reversible with IV fluid support. Pulse, blood pressure, and oral temperature should be measured every 15 to 30 minutes. Immediate institution of diphenhydramine (50 mg IV), acetaminophen (625 mg PO), hydrocortisone (200 mg IV), and/or

vasopressors may be required. Resuscitation equipment should be readily available at bedside.

5. Reduction of WBC count to below 30,000 with either hydroxyurea or leukapheresis is highly recommended to reduce the risk of tumor lysis syndrome and pulmonary complications, including acute respiratory distress syndrome (ARDS) in patients treated with gemtuzumab.

6. Monitor CBC and platelet counts on a weekly basis during gemtuzumab therapy.

7. Pregnancy category D. Breast-feeding should be avoided.

Toxicity 1

Infusion-related symptoms, including fever, chills, nausea and vomiting, urticaria, skin rash, fatigue, headache, diarrhea, dyspnea, and/or hypotension. Usually occur during the infusion or within 2 hours after infusion. Transient hypotension can sometimes be observed up to 6 hours after infusion. Incidence decreases with second dose.

Toxicity 2

Myelosuppression is most common dose-limiting toxicity with neutropenia and thrombocytopenia.

Toxicity 3

Hepatotoxicity in the form of increased serum bilirubin and LFTs observed in up to 20% of patients. Usually transient and reversible. Rare cases of veno-occlusive disease (VOD), which can be fatal, most commonly seen in patients previously treated with hematopoietic stem cell transplantation.

Toxicity 4

GI toxicity in the form of nausea, vomiting, and mucositis.

Goserelin

pyro Glu-His-Trp-Ser-Tyr-D-Ser (tert Butyl)-Leu-Arg-Pro-Azgly
1   2   3   4   5   6   7   8   9   10

Trade Names

Zoladex

Classification

LHRH agonist

Category

Hormonal agent

Drug Manufacturer

AstraZeneca

Mechanism of Action

Administration leads to initial release of follicle-stimulating hormone (FSH) and luteinizing hormone (LH) followed by suppression of gonadotropin secretion as a result of desensitization of the pituitary to gonadotropin-releasing hormone. This results in decreased secretion of LH and FSH from the pituitary.

Absorption

Not orally absorbed because of extensive proteolysis in the GI tract. Bioavailability of subcutaneously administered drug is 75%–90%.

Distribution

Distribution is not well characterized. Slowly released over a 28-day period. Peak serum concentrations are achieved 10–15 days after drug administration. About 30% of goserelin is bound to plasma proteins.

Metabolism

Metabolism of goserelin occurs mainly via hydrolysis of the C-terminal amino acids. Goserelin is nearly completely eliminated in urine. The elimination half-life is normally 4–5 hours but is prolonged in patients with impaired renal function (12 hours).

Indications

Advanced prostate cancer.

Dosage Range

Administer 3.6 mg SC every 28 days or 10.8 mg SC every 90 days.

Drug Interactions

None known.

Special Considerations

1. Initiation of treatment with goserelin may induce a transient tumor flare. Goserelin should not be given in patients with impending ureteral obstruction and/or spinal cord compression or in those with painful bone metastases.

2. Serum testosterone levels decrease to castrate levels within 2–4 weeks after initiation of therapy.

3. Use with caution in patients with abnormal renal function.

4. Caution patients about the potential for hot flashes. Consider the use of soy tablets, one tablet PO tid for prevention and/or treatment.

Toxicity 1

Hot flashes occur in 50% of patients, decreased libido (10%), impotence (10%), and gynecomastia (10%).

Toxicity 2

Tumor flare. May occur in up to 20% of patients, usually within the first 2 weeks of starting therapy. May observe increased bone pain, urinary retention, or back pain with spinal cord compression. May be prevented by pretreating with an antiandrogen agent such as flutamide, bicalutamide, or nilutamide.

Toxicity 3

Local discomfort at the site of injection.

Toxicity 4

Elevated serum cholesterol levels.

Toxicity 5

Hypersensitivity reaction.

Toxicity 6

Nausea and vomiting. Rarely observed.

Toxicity 7

Myelosuppression. Rarely observed.

Hydroxyurea

$$H_2N - \overset{\overset{\displaystyle O}{\|}}{C} - \overset{\overset{\displaystyle H}{|}}{N} - OH$$

Trade Names
Hydrea

Classification
Antimetabolite

Category
Chemotherapy drug

Drug Manufacturer
MGI Pharma

Mechanism of Action
- Cell cycle–specific analog of urea with activity in the S-phase.
- Inhibits the enzyme ribonucleotide reductase, which converts ribonucleotides to deoxyribonucleotides, critical precursors for de novo DNA biosynthesis and DNA repair.

Mechanism of Resistance
Increased expression of ribonucleotide reductase due to gene amplification, increased transcription, and post-transcriptional mechanisms.

Absorption
Oral absorption is rapid and nearly complete with a bioavailability ranging between 80% and 100%. Peak plasma concentrations are achieved in 1–1.5 hours.

Distribution
Widely distributed in all tissues. High concentrations are found in third-space collections, including pleural effusions and ascites. Crosses the blood-brain barrier and enters the CSF. Excreted in significant levels in human breast milk.

Metabolism
Approximately 50% of drug is metabolized in the liver. About 50% of drug is excreted unchanged in urine. The carbon dioxide that results from drug metabolism is released through the lungs. Plasma half-life on the order of 3–4.5 hours.

Indications

1. Chronic myelogenous leukemia.
2. Essential thrombocytosis.
3. Polycythemia vera.
4. Acute myelogenous leukemia, blast crisis.
5. Head and neck cancer (in combination with radiation therapy).
6. Refractory ovarian cancer.

Dosage Range

1. Continuous therapy: 20–30 mg/kg PO daily.
2. Intermittent therapy: 80 mg/kg PO every third day.
3. Combination therapy with irradiation of head and neck cancer: 80 mg/kg PO every third day. In this setting, hydroxyurea is used as a radiation sensitizer and initiated at least 7 days before radiation therapy.

Drug Interaction 1

5-FU—Hydroxyurea may enhance the risk of 5-FU host toxicity.

Drug Interaction 2

Antiretroviral agents—Hydroxyurea may enhance the anti-HIV activity of azidothymidine (AZT), dideoxycytidine (ddC), and dideoxyinosine (ddI).

Special Considerations

1. Contraindicated in patients with bone marrow suppression presenting as WBC <2,500/mm^3 or platelet count <100,000/mm^3.
2. Monitor CBC on a weekly basis during therapy. Treatment should be stopped if the WBC count falls to less than 2,500/mm^3 or the platelet count drops to less than 100,000/mm^3 and held until the counts rise above these values.
3. Use with caution in patients previously treated with chemotherapy and/or radiation therapy as there is an increased risk of myelosuppression.
4. Use with caution in patients with abnormal renal function. Doses should be reduced in the setting of renal dysfunction.
5. Pregnancy category D. Use with caution in women who are breast-feeding as the drug is excreted in human breast milk.

Toxicity 1

Myelosuppression with leukopenia is dose-limiting. Median onset 7–10 days with recovery of WBC counts 7–10 days after stopping the drug. Median onset of thrombocytopenia and anemia usually by day 10. Effect on bone marrow may be more severe in patients previously treated with chemotherapy and/or radiation therapy.

Toxicity 2

Nausea and vomiting. Generally mild. Incidence can be reduced by dividing the daily dose into two or three doses. Stomatitis also occurs.

Toxicity 3

Maculopapular rash, facial and acral erythema, hyperpigmentation, dry skin with atrophy, and pruritus.

Toxicity 4

Radiation recall skin reaction.

Toxicity 5

Headache, drowsiness, and confusion.

Toxicity 6

Transient elevations of serum transaminases and bilirubin.

Toxicity 7

Teratogenic. Carcinogenic potential is not known.

Ibritumomab

Trade Names
Zevalin, IDEC-Y2B8

Classification
Monoclonal antibody

Category
Biologic response modifier agent

Drug Manufacturer
Cell Therapeutics

Mechanism of Action

- Immunoconjugate consisting of a stable thiourea covalent bond between the monoclonal antibody ibritumomab and the linker-chelator tiuxetan. This linker-chelator provides a high-affinity conformationally restricted site for indium-111 and/or yttrium-90.

- The antibody moiety is ibritumomab, which targets the CD20 antigen, a 35 kDa cell surface non-glycosylated phosphoprotein expressed during early pre–B cell development until the plasma cell stage. Binding of antibodies to CD20 induces a transmembrane signal that blocks cell activation and cell cycle progression.

- CD20 is expressed on more than 90% of all B-cell non-Hodgkin's lymphomas and leukemias. CD20 is not expressed on early pre–B cells, plasma cells, normal bone marrow stem cells, antigen-presenting dendritic reticulum cells, or other normal tissues.

- The beta emission from yttrium-90 induces cellular damage by the formation of free radicals in the target and neighboring cells.

Absorption
Ibritumomab is given only by the IV route.

Distribution
Peak and trough levels of rituximab correlate inversely with the number of circulating CD20-positive B cells. When In-111-ibritumomab is administered without unlabeled ibritumomab, only 18% of known sites of disease are imaged. In contrast, when In-111-ibritumomab administration is preceded by unlabeled ibritumomab, up to 90% of known sites of disease can be imaged.

Metabolism
The mean effective half-life of yttrium-90 in blood is 30 hours, and the mean area under the fraction of injected activity (FIA) versus time curve in

blood is 39 hours. Over a period of 7 days, a median of 7.2% of the injected activity is excreted in urine.

Indications

Relapsed and/or refractory low-grade, follicular, or transformed B-cell non-Hodgkin's lymphoma, including patients refractory to rituximab therapy.

Dosage Range

The regimen consists of two low doses of rituximab, an imaging dose, two or three whole body scans, and a therapeutic dose, all of which are delivered on an outpatient basis over a period of 8 days. The recommended dose is 0.4 mCi/kg for patients with platelet counts greater than 150,000 and 0.3 mCi/kg for patients with platelet counts between 100,000 and 149,000. In either case, the maximum dose is 32 mCi.

Drug Interactions

None characterized to date.

Special Considerations

1. Contraindicated in patients with known type I hypersensitivity, anaphylactic reactions to murine proteins or to any component of the product, including rituximab, yttrium chloride, and indium chloride.

2. Should not be administered to patients with an altered biodistribution of In-111 ibritumomab.

3. The prescribed and administered dose of yttrium-90 should not exceed the absolute maximum allowable dose of 32 mCi.

4. This therapy should be used only by physicians and health care professionals who are qualified and experienced in the safe use and handling of radioisotopes.

5. Patients should be premedicated with acetaminophen and diphenhydramine before each infusion of rituximab to reduce the incidence of infusion-related reactions.

6. Rituximab infusion should be started at an initial rate of 50 mg/hour. If no toxicity is observed during the first hour, the infusion rate can be escalated by increments of 50 mg/hour every 30 minutes to a maximum of 400 mg/hour. If the first treatment is well tolerated, the starting infusion rate for the second infusion can be administered at 100 mg/hour with 100 mg/hour increments at 30-minute intervals up to 400 mg/hour. Rituximab should NOT be given by IV push.

7. Monitor for infusion-related events resulting from rituximab infusion, which usually occur 30–120 minutes after the start of the first infusion. Infusion should be immediately stopped if signs or symptoms of an allergic reaction are observed. Immediate institution of diphenhydramine, acetaminophen, corticosteroids, IV fluids, and/or vasopressors may be necessary. In most instances, the infusion can

be restarted at a reduced rate (50%) once symptoms have completely resolved. Resuscitation equipment should be readily available at bedside.

8. Infusion-related deaths within 24 hours of rituximab infusions have been reported.

9. Ibritumomab therapy should not be given to patients with >25% involvement of the bone marrow by lymphoma and/or impaired bone marrow reserve.

10. Ibritumomab therapy should not be given to patients with platelet counts below 100,000.

11. Complete blood counts and platelet counts should be monitored weekly following ibritumomab therapy and should continue until levels recover.

12. The ibritumomab regimen should be given only as a single-course treatment.

13. The ibritumomab regimen may have direct toxic effects on the male and female reproductive organs, and effective contraception should be used during therapy and for up to 12 months following the completion of therapy.

14. Pregnancy category D. Breast-feeding should be avoided as it is not known whether ibritumomab is excreted in human milk.

Toxicity 1

Infusion-related symptoms, including fever, chills, urticaria, flushing, fatigue, headache, bronchospasm, rhinitis, dyspnea, angioedema, nausea, and/or hypotension. Severe symptoms include pulmonary infiltrates, acute respiratory distress syndrome, myocardial infarction, ventricular fibrillation, and/or cardiogenic shock. Usually occur within 30 minutes to 2 hours after the start of the first infusion. Usually resolve upon slowing or interrupting the infusion and with supportive care.

Toxicity 2

Myelosuppression is most common side effect. Thrombocytopenia observed more frequently than neutropenia. The median duration of cytopenias ranges from 22 to 35 days, and the median time to nadir is 7–9 weeks. In <5% of patients, severe cytopenias were extended beyond 12 weeks after therapy.

Toxicity 3

Mild asthenia occurs in up to 40% of patients.

Toxicity 4

Infections develop in nearly 30% of patients during the first 3 months after therapy.

Toxicity 5

Mild nausea and vomiting.

Toxicity 6

Cough, rhinitis, dyspnea, and sinusitis are observed in up to 35% of patients.

Toxicity 7

Secondary malignancies occur in about 2% of patients. Acute myelogenous leukemia and myelodysplastic syndrome have been reported at a range of 8–34 months following therapy.

Toxicity 8

Development of human anti-mouse (HAMA) and human anti-chimeric antibodies (HACA). Rare event in less than 1%–2% of patients.

Idarubicin

Trade Names

Idamycin, 4-Demethoxydaunorubicin

Classification

Antitumor antibiotic

Category

Chemotherapy drug

Drug Manufacturer

Pfizer

Mechanism of Action

- Semisynthetic anthracycline glycoside analog of daunorubicin.
- Intercalates into DNA, which results in inhibition of DNA synthesis and function.
- Inhibits topoisomerase II by forming a cleavable complex with topoisomerase II and DNA.
- In the presence of iron, drug forms oxygen free radicals, which cause single- and double-stranded DNA breaks.
- Specificity, in part, for the late S- and G2-phases of the cell cycle.

Mechanism of Resistance

- Increased expression of the multidrug-resistant gene with enhanced drug efflux. This results in decreased intracellular drug accumulation.
- Decreased expression of topoisomerase II.
- Mutation in topoisomerase II with decreased binding affinity to drug.
- Increased expression of sulfhydryl proteins, including glutathione and glutathione-associated enzymes.

Absorption

Administered only by the IV route.

Distribution

Rapid and extensive tissue distribution. Peak concentrations in nucleated blood and bone marrow cells are achieved within minutes of administration and are 100-fold greater than those in plasma. Drug and its major metabolite, idarubicinol, are extensively bound (>90%) to plasma proteins.

Metabolism

Significant metabolism in liver and in extrahepatic tissues. Metabolism by the liver microsomal system yields the active metabolite, idarubicinol, which may be responsible for the cardiotoxic effects. Idarubicin is eliminated mainly by biliary excretion into feces, with renal clearance accounting for only about 15% of drug elimination. The half-life of the parent drug is on the order of 20 hours, while the half-life of drug metabolites may exceed 45 hours.

Indications

1. Acute myelogenous leukemia.
2. Acute lymphoblastic leukemia.
3. Chronic myelogenous leukemia in blast crisis.
4. Myelodysplastic syndromes.

Dosage Range

Acute myelogenous leukemia, induction therapy: 12 mg/m^2 IV on days 1–3 in combination with cytarabine, 100 mg/m^2/day IV continuous infusion for 7 days.

Drug Interaction 1

Probenecid and sulfinpyrazone—Avoid concomitant use of probenecid and sulfinpyrazone as these are uricosuric agents and may lead to uric acid nephropathy.

Drug Interaction 2

Heparin—Idarubicin is incompatible with heparin as it forms a precipitate.

Special Considerations

1. Use with caution in patients with abnormal liver function. Dose modification should be considered in patients with liver dysfunction. Dose reduction by 50% is recommended for serum bilirubin in the range of 2.6–5.0 mg/dL. Absolutely contraindicated in patients with bilirubin >5.0 mg/dL.
2. Careful administration of drug, usually through a central venous catheter, is necessary as it is a strong vesicant. If peripheral venous access is used, careful monitoring of drug administration is necessary

to avoid extravasation. If extravasation is suspected, stop infusion immediately, withdraw fluid, elevate arm, and apply ice to site. In severe cases, consult a plastic surgeon.

3. Alkalinization of the urine, allopurinol, and vigorous IV hydration are recommended to prevent tumor lysis syndrome in patients with acute myelogenous leukemia.

4. Monitor cardiac function before (baseline) and periodically during therapy with either MUGA radionuclide scan or echocardiogram to assess LVEF. Risk of cardiotoxicity is higher in elderly patients >70 years of age, in patients with prior history of hypertension or pre-existing heart disease, in patients previously treated with anthracyclines, or in patients with prior radiation therapy to the chest. While maximum dose of idarubicin that may be administered safely is not known, cumulative doses of >150 mg/m^2 have been associated with decreased LVEF.

5. Caution patients against sun exposure and to wear sun protection when outside.

6. Caution patients about the potential for red discoloration of urine for 1–2 days after drug administration.

7. Pregnancy category D. Breast-feeding should be avoided.

Toxicity 1

Myelosuppression. Dose-limiting toxicity with neutropenia and thrombocytopenia. Nadir typically occurs at 10–14 days after treatment, with recovery of counts by day 21. Risk of myelosuppression is greater in elderly patients and in those previously treated with chemotherapy and/or radiation therapy.

Toxicity 2

Nausea and vomiting. Usually mild and occurs in up to 80%–90% of patients.

Toxicity 3

Cardiotoxicity. Cardiac effects are similar to but less severe than those of doxorubicin. Acute toxicity presents as atrial arrhythmias, chest pain, and myopericarditis syndrome that typically occur within the first 24–48 hours of drug administration. Dilated cardiomyopathy with congestive heart failure can occur, usually with higher cumulative doses above 150 mg/m^2.

Toxicity 4

Alopecia. Nearly universal but reversible.

Toxicity 5

Generalized skin rash, increased sensitivity to sunlight, hyperpigmentation of nails and at the injection site. Rarely, radiation recall skin reaction.

Toxicity 6

Strong vesicant. Extravasation can lead to extensive tissue damage.

Toxicity 7

Mucositis and diarrhea. Common but usually not severe.

Toxicity 8

Reversible effects on liver enzymes, including SGOT and SGPT.

Toxicity 9

Red discoloration of urine. Usually within the first 1–2 days after drug administration.

Ifosfamide

$$
\begin{array}{c}
\text{Cl} \\
| \\
\text{CH}_2 \\
| \\
\text{CH}_2 \\
| \\
\text{Cl}-\text{CH}_2-\text{CH}_2 \quad \text{O} \quad \text{N}-\text{CH}_2 \\
\diagdown \qquad \| / \qquad \diagdown \\
\text{N}-\text{P} \qquad \text{CH}_2 \\
/ \qquad \diagdown \qquad / \\
\text{H} \qquad \text{O}-\text{CH}_2
\end{array}
$$

Trade Names

Ifex, Isophosphamide

Classification

Alkylating agent

Category

Chemotherapy drug

Drug Manufacturer

Bristol-Myers Squibb

Mechanism of Action

- Inactive in its parent form.
- Activated by the liver cytochrome P450 microsomal system to various cytotoxic metabolites, including ifosfamide mustard and acrolein.
- Cytotoxic metabolites form cross-links with DNA resulting in inhibition of DNA synthesis and function.
- Cell cycle-nonspecific agent, active in all phases of the cell cycle.

Mechanism of Resistance

- Decreased cellular uptake of drug.
- Decreased expression of liver P450 activating enzymes.
- Increased expression of sulfhydryl proteins, including glutathione and glutathione-associated enzymes.
- Increased expression of aldehyde dehydrogenase resulting in enhanced inactivation of drug.
- Enhanced activity of DNA repair enzymes.

Absorption

Well-absorbed by the GI tract with a bioavailability of nearly 100%. However, only IV form is available commercially because oral form is highly neurotoxic.

Distribution

Widely distributed into body tissues. About 20% of drug is bound to plasma protein.

Metabolism

Extensively metabolized in the liver by the cytochrome P450 system. Activated at a 4-fold slower rate than cyclophosphamide because of lower affinity to the liver P450 system. For this reason, about 4-fold more drug is required to produce equitoxic antitumor effects with cyclophosphamide. The half-life of the drug is 3–10 hours for standard therapy and up to 14 hours for high-dose therapy. Approximately 50%–70% of the drug and its metabolites are excreted in urine.

Indications

1. Recurrent germ cell tumors.
2. Soft tissue sarcoma, osteogenic sarcoma.
3. Non-Hodgkin's lymphoma.
4. Hodgkin's lymphoma.
5. Non–small cell and small cell lung cancer.
6. Bladder cancer.
7. Head and neck cancer.
8. Cervical cancer.
9. Ewing's sarcoma.

Dosage Range

1. Testicular cancer: 1,200 mg/m^2 IV on days 1–5 every 21 days, as part of the VeIP salvage regimen.
2. Soft tissue sarcoma: 2,000 mg/m^2 IV continuous infusion on days 1–3 every 21 days, as part of the MAID regimen.
3. Non-Hodgkin's lymphoma: 1,000 mg/m^2 on days 1 and 2 every 28 days, as part of the ICE regimen.
4. Head and neck cancer: 1,000 mg/m^2 on days 1–3 every 21–28 days, as part of the TIC regimen.

Drug Interaction 1

Phenobarbital, phenytoin, and other drugs that stimulate the liver P450 system—Increase the rate of metabolic activation of ifosfamide to its toxic metabolites resulting in enhanced toxicity.

Drug Interaction 2

Cimetidine and allopurinol—Increase the formation of ifosfamide metabolites resulting in increased toxicity.

Drug Interaction 3

Cisplatin—Increases ifosfamide-associated renal toxicity.

Drug Interaction 4

Warfarin—Ifosfamide may enhance the anticoagulant effects of warfarin. Need to closely monitor coagulation parameters, PT and INR.

Special Considerations

1. Administer prophylactic antiemetics to avoid nausea and vomiting.

2. Contraindicated in patients with a history of thrombophlebitis or thromboembolic disorders.

3. Use with caution in patients with abnormal renal function. Dose reduction is necessary in this setting. Baseline creatinine clearance must be obtained, and renal function should be monitored during therapy.

4. Uroprotection with mesna and hydration must be used to prevent bladder toxicity. Pre- and post-hydration (1,500–2,000 mL/day) or continuous bladder irrigations are recommended to prevent hemorrhagic cystitis. Important to monitor urine for presence of gross and/or microscopic hematuria before each cycle of therapy.

5. Monitor coagulation parameters, including PT and INR, when ifosfamide is used concurrently with warfarin, as ifosfamide may enhance its anticoagulant effects.

6. Contraindicated in patients with peptic ulcer disease, severe liver disease, and/or cardiac disease.

7. Pregnancy category D.

Toxicity 1

Myelosuppression is dose-limiting. Mainly leukopenia and to a lesser extent thrombocytopenia. Nadir occurs at 10–14 days with recovery in 21 days.

Toxicity 2

Bladder toxicity can be dose-limiting and manifested by hemorrhagic cystitis, dysuria, and increased urinary frequency. Chronic fibrosis of bladder leads to an increased risk of secondary bladder cancer. Uroprotection with mesna and hydration must be used to prevent bladder toxicity.

Toxicity 3

Nausea and vomiting. Usually occurs within 3–6 hours of therapy and may last up to 3 days. Anorexia is fairly common.

Toxicity 4

Neurotoxicity in the form of lethargy, confusion, seizure, cerebellar ataxia, weakness, hallucinations, cranial nerve dysfunction, and rarely stupor and coma. Incidence may be higher in patients receiving high-dose therapy and in those with impaired renal function.

Toxicity 5

Alopecia is common (>80%). Skin rash, hyperpigmentation, and nail changes are occasionally seen.

Toxicity 6

Syndrome of inappropriate secretion of antidiuretic hormone (SIADH).

Toxicity 7

Amenorrhea, oligospermia, and infertility.

Toxicity 8

Mutagenic, teratogenic, and carcinogenic.

Imatinib

Trade Names
STI571, Gleevec

Classification
Signal transduction inhibitor

Category
Chemotherapy drug

Drug Manufacturer
Novartis

Mechanism of Action
- Phenylaminopyrimidine methanesulfonate compound that occupies the ATP binding site of the BCR-ABL protein and a very limited number of other tyrosine kinases. Binding in this ATP pocket results in subsequent inhibition of substrate phosphorylation.
- Potent and selective inhibitor of the P210 BCR-ABL tyrosine kinase resulting in inhibition of clonogenicity and tumorigenicity of BCR-ABL and Ph+ cells.
- Induces apoptosis in BCR-ABL positive cells without causing cell differentiation.
- Inhibits other activated ABL tyrosine kinases, including P185 BCR-ABL, and inhibits other receptor tyrosine kinases for platelet-derived growth factor receptor (PDGFR), stem cell factor (SCF), and c-kit.

Mechanism of Resistance
- Increased expression of BCR-ABL tyrosine kinase through amplification of the BCR-ABL gene.
- Alterations in the binding affinity of the BCR-ABL tyrosine kinase to the drug as a result of mutations in the protein.
- Increased expression of P170 glycoprotein resulting in enhanced drug efflux and decreased intracellular drug accumulation.

- Increased degradation and/or metabolism of the drug through as yet undefined mechanisms.

Absorption

Oral bioavailability is nearly 100%.

Distribution

Extensive binding (95%) to plasma proteins, including albumin and α_1-acid glycoprotein. Steady-state drug concentrations are reached in 2–3 days.

Metabolism

Metabolism in the liver primarily by the CYP3A4 microsomal enzyme. Other cytochrome P450 enzymes play a minor role in its metabolism. The main metabolite is the N-desmethylated piperazine derivative, and this metabolite shows in vitro potency similar to that of the parent drug. Elimination is mainly in the feces, predominantly as metabolites. The terminal half-life of the parent drug is 18 hours, while that of its main metabolite, the N-desmethyl derivative, is on the order of 40 hours.

Indications

1. Chronic phase of CML—First-line therapy in adult patients, FDA-approved.

2. Chronic phase of CML after failure on interferon-α therapy—FDA-approved.

3. CML in accelerated phase and/or in blast crisis—FDA-approved.

4. Chronic phase Ph+ CML in pediatric patients whose disease has recurred after stem cell transplant or is resistant to interferon-α.

5. Myelodysplastic/myeloproliferative diseases (MDS/MPD) associated with PDGFR gene rearrangements.

6. Hypereosinophilic syndrome/chronic eosinophilic leukemia (HES/CEL).

7. Relapsed/refractory Ph+ acute lymphocytic leukemia (PH+ ALL).

8. Gastrointestinal stromal tumors (GIST) expressing c-kit (CD117)—unresectable and/or metastatic disease.

9. Gastrointestinal stromal tumors (GIST) expressing c-kit (CD117)—adjuvant therapy following resection of localized disease.

Dosage Range

1. Recommended starting dose is 400 mg/day for patients in chronic phase CML and 600 mg/day for patients in accelerated phase or blast crisis. Dose increases from 400 mg to 600 mg or 800 mg in patients with chronic phase disease, or from 600 mg to a maximum of 800 mg (given as 400 mg twice daily) in patients with accelerated phase or blast crisis may be considered in the absence of severe adverse drug reaction and severe nonleukemia-related

neutropenia or thrombocytopenia in the following circumstances: disease progression (at any time); failure to achieve a satisfactory hematological response after at least 3 months of treatment; failure to achieve a cytogenetic response after 12 months of treatment; or loss of a previously achieved hematological and/or cytogenetic response. Patients should be monitored closely following dose escalation given the potential for an increased incidence of adverse reactions at higher dosages.

2. Recommended starting dose is 400 mg/day for patients with unresectable and/or metastatic GIST. Limited data exist on the effect of dose increases from 400 mg to 600 mg or 800 mg in patients progressing at the lower dose.

3. Recommended dose is 400 mg/day for adjuvant therapy of patients with early-stage GIST.

4. Recommended starting dose is 400 mg/day for patients with MDS/MPD.

5. Recommended starting dose is 400 mg/day for patients with HES/CEL.

6. Recommended starting dose is 600 mg/day for patients with Ph+ ALL.

Drug Interaction 1

Dilantin and other drugs that stimulate the liver microsomal CYP3A4 enzyme, including carbamazepine, rifampin, phenobarbital, and St. John's wort—These drugs increase the rate of metabolism of imatinib resulting in its inactivation.

Drug Interaction 2

Drugs that inhibit the liver microsomal CYP3A4 enzyme, including ketoconazole, itraconazole, erythromycin, and clarithromycin—These drugs decrease the rate of metabolism of imatinib resulting in increased drug levels and potentially increased toxicity.

Drug Interaction 3

Warfarin—Patients on coumarin-derived anticoagulants should be closely monitored for alterations in their clotting parameters (PT and INR) and/or bleeding as imatinib inhibits the metabolism of warfarin by the liver P450 system. Dose of warfarin may require careful adjustment in the presence of imatinib therapy.

Special Considerations

1. Patients should be weighed and monitored regularly for signs and symptoms of fluid retention. The risk of fluid retention and edema is increased with higher drug doses and in patients whose age >65 years.

2. Use with caution in patients with underlying hepatic impairment. Dose adjustment is not required in patients with mild to moderate hepatic impairment. Patients with severe hepatic impairment should have a 25% reduction in the recommended dose.

3. Use with caution in patients with underlying renal impairment. For patients with moderate renal impairment (CrCL 20-39 mL/min), doses greater than 400 mg are not recommended, and patients should have a 50% reduction in the recommended starting dose. For patients with mild renal impairment, CrCL 40-59 mL/min, doses greater than 600 mg are not recommended.

4. Monitor CBC on a weekly basis for the first month, biweekly for the second month, and periodically thereafter.

5. Imatinib should be taken with food and a large glass of water to decrease the risk of GI irritation. Imatinib tablets can be dissolved in water or apple juice for patients having difficulty swallowing.

6. Hematologic responses typically occur within 2 weeks after initiation of therapy while complete hematologic responses are observed within 4 weeks after starting therapy.

7. Cytogenetic responses are observed as early as 2 months and up to 10 months after starting therapy. The median time to best cytogenetic response is about 5 months.

8. Carefully monitor dose of drug when used in patients with seizure disorders on phenytoin. Dose of drug may need to be increased as the metabolism of imatinib by the CYP3A4 enzyme is enhanced in the presence of phenytoin.

9. Patients who require anticoagulation should receive low-molecular weight or standard heparin as imatinib inhibits the metabolism of warfarin.

10. Monitor cardiac function before (baseline) and periodically during therapy with either MUGA radionuclide scan or echocardiogram to assess LVEF. The diagnosis of CHF should be considered in patients who experience edema while on imatinib.

11. Avoid grapefruit products while on imatinib therapy.

12. Pregnancy category D.

Toxicity 1

Nausea and vomiting occur in 40%–50% of patients. Usually related to the swallowing of capsules and relieved when the drug is taken with food.

Toxicity 2

Transient ankle and periorbital edema. Usually mild to moderate in nature.

Toxicity 3

Occasional myalgias.

Toxicity 4

Fluid retention with pleural effusion, ascites, pulmonary edema, and weight gain. Usually dose-related and more common in elderly patients and in those in blast crisis and the accelerated phase of CML. CHF is a rare but serious adverse event.

Toxicity 5

Diarrhea is observed in 25%–30% of patients.

Toxicity 6

Myelosuppression with neutropenia and thrombocytopenia.

Toxicity 7

Mild, transient elevation in serum transaminases. Clinically asymptomatic in most cases.

Toxicity 8

Skin toxicity in the form of bullous reactions, including erythema multiforme and Stevens-Johnson syndrome.

Interferon-α

Trade Names

α-interferon, IFN-α, Interferon-α 2a, Roferon Interferon-α 2b, Intron A

Classification

Immunotherapy

Category

Biologic response modifier agent

Drug Manufacturer

Roche (Roferon), Schering (Intron A)

Mechanism of Action

- Precise mechanism of antitumor action remains unknown.
- Direct antiproliferative effects on tumor cell mediated by: induction of 2'5'-oligoadenylate synthetase and protein kinase leading to decreased translation and inhibition of tumor cell protein synthesis; induction of differentiation; prolongation of the cell cycle; modulation of oncogene expression.
- Indirect induction of host antitumor mechanisms mediated by: induced activity of at least four immune effector cells, including cytotoxic T cells, helper T cells, NK cells, and macrophages; enhancement of tumor surface expression of critical antigens that are recognized by the immune system; inhibition of angiogenesis through decreased expression of various angiogenic factors.

Mechanism of Resistance

- Development of neutralizing antibodies to interferon-α.
- Decreased expression of cell surface receptors to interferon-α.

Absorption

Not available for oral use and is administered only via the parenteral route. Approximately 80%–90% of interferon-α is absorbed into the systemic circulation after IM or SC injection. Peak plasma levels are achieved in 4 hours after intramuscular injection and 7 hours after subcutaneous administration.

Distribution

Does not cross the blood-brain barrier. Binding to plasma proteins has not been well characterized.

Metabolism

Interferon-α is catabolized by renal tubule cells to various breakdown products. The major route of elimination is through the kidneys by both glomerular filtration and tubular secretion. Hepatic metabolism and biliary excretion play only a minor role in drug clearance. The elimination half-life is approximately 2–7 hours and depends on the specific route of drug administration.

Indications

1. Malignant melanoma—Adjuvant therapy.
2. Chronic myelogenous leukemia—Chronic phase.
3. Hairy cell leukemia.
4. AIDS-related Kaposi's sarcoma.
5. Cutaneous T-cell lymphoma.
6. Multiple myeloma.
7. Low-grade, non-Hodgkin's lymphoma.
8. Renal cell cancer.
9. Hemangioma.

Dosage Range

1. Chronic myelogenous leukemia: 9 million IU SC or IM daily.
2. Hairy cell leukemia: 3 million IU SC or IM daily for 16–24 weeks.
3. Malignant melanoma: 20 million IU/m^2 IV, five times weekly for 4 weeks, then 10 million IU/m^2 SC, three times weekly for 48 weeks.
4. Kaposi's sarcoma: 36 million IU SC or IM daily for 12 weeks.

Drug Interaction 1

Phenytoin, phenobarbital—Effects of phenytoin and phenobarbital may be increased as interferon-α inhibits the liver P450 system. Drug levels must be monitored closely and dose adjustments made accordingly.

Drug Interaction 2

Live vaccines—Vaccination with live vaccines is contraindicated during and for at least 3 months after completion of interferon therapy.

Special Considerations

1. Use with caution in patients with pre-existing cardiac, pulmonary, CNS, hepatic, and/or renal impairment as they are at increased risk for developing serious and sometimes fatal reactions.
2. Contraindicated in patients with history of autoimmune disease, autoimmune hepatitis, or in those who have received immunosuppressive therapy for organ transplants.

3. Contraindicated in patients with a known allergy to benzyl alcohol as the injectable solution form contains benzyl alcohol.

4. Use with caution in patients with myelosuppression or those who are receiving concurrent agents known to cause myelosuppression.

5. Use with caution in patients with a history of depression and/or other psychological disorders. Routine neuropsychiatric monitoring of all patients on interferon-α is recommended.

6. Use with caution in older patients (>65 years of age) as they are at increased risk for developing fatigue and neurologic toxicities secondary to interferon-α.

7. Premedicate patient with acetaminophen to reduce the risk and/or severity of flu-like symptoms, including fever and chills. In the event that acetaminophen is unsuccessful, indomethacin can be used.

8. Pregnancy category C.

Toxicity 1

Flu-like symptoms with fever, chills, headache, myalgias, and arthralgias. Occur in 80%–90% of patients, usually beginning a few hours after the first injection and lasting for up to 8–9 hours. Incidence decreases with subsequent injections. Can be controlled with acetaminophen and/or indomethacin.

Toxicity 2

Fatigue and anorexia are dose-limiting with chronic administration.

Toxicity 3

Somnolence, confusion, or depression. Patients >65 years of age are more susceptible to the neurologic sequelae of interferon-α.

Toxicity 4

Myelosuppression with mild leukopenia and thrombocytopenia. Reversible upon discontinuation of therapy.

Toxicity 5

Mild, transient elevations in serum transaminases. Dose-dependent toxicity observed more frequently in the presence of pre-existing liver abnormalities.

Toxicity 6

Renal toxicity is uncommon and is manifested by mild proteinuria and hypocalcemia. Acute renal failure and nephrotic syndrome have been reported in rare instances.

Toxicity 7

Alopecia, skin rash, pruritus with dry skin, and irritation at the injection site.

Toxicity 8

Cardiotoxicity in the form of chest pain, arrhythmias, and congestive heart failure. Uncommon and almost always reversible.

Toxicity 9

Impotence, decreased libido, menstrual irregularities, and an increased incidence of spontaneous abortions.

Toxicity 10

Rare cases of autoimmune disorders, including thrombocytopenia, vasculitis, Raynaud's disease, lupus, rheumatoid arthritis, and rhabdomyolysis.

Toxicity 11

Retinopathy with cotton-wool spots and small hemorrhages. Usually asymptomatic and resolves upon termination of therapy.

Irinotecan

CPT-11 lactone

CPT-11 converting enzyme

SN-38 lactone

CPT-11 carboxylate

SN-38 carboxylate

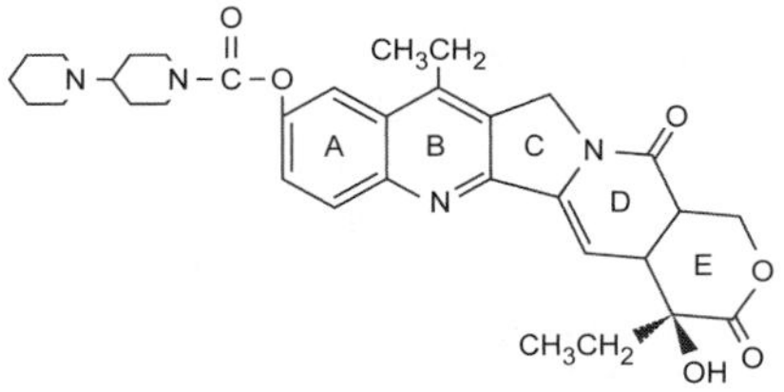

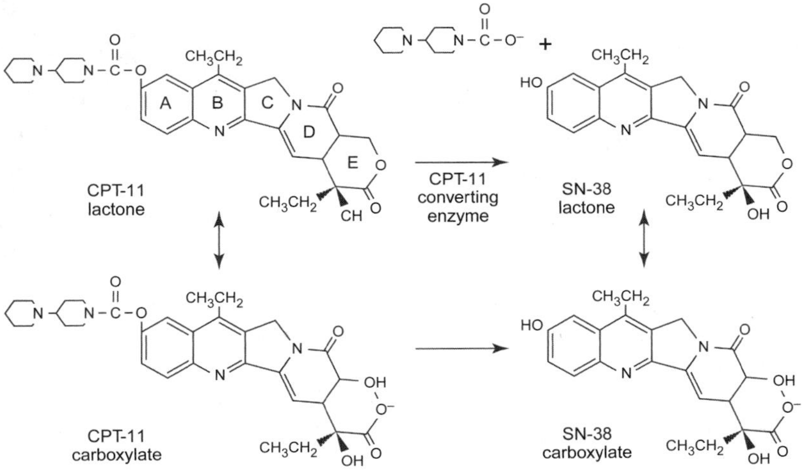

Trade Names

Camptosar, CPT-11

Classification

Topoisomerase I inhibitor

Category

Chemotherapy drug

Drug Manufacturer

Pfizer

Mechanism of Action

- Semisynthetic derivative of camptothecin, an alkaloid extract from the *Camptotheca acuminata* tree.

- Inactive in its parent form. Converted by the carboxylesterase enzyme to its active metabolite form, SN-38.

- SN-38 binds to and stabilizes the topoisomerase I-DNA complex and prevents the religation of DNA after it has been cleaved by topoisomerase I. The collision between this stable cleavable complex and the advancing replication fork results in double-strand DNA breaks and cellular death.

- Antitumor activity of drug requires the presence of ongoing DNA synthesis.

- Cell cycle–nonspecific agent with activity in all phases of the cell cycle.

- Colorectal tumors express higher levels of topoisomerase I than normal colonic mucosa, making this an attractive target for chemotherapy.

Mechanism of Resistance

- Decreased expression of topoisomerase I.

- Mutations in topoisomerase I enzyme with decreased affinity for the drug.

- Increased expression of the multidrug-resistant phenotype with overexpression of P170 glycoprotein. Results in enhanced efflux of drug and decreased intracellular accumulation of drug.

- Decreased formation of the cytotoxic metabolite SN-38 through decreased activity and/or expression of the carboxylesterase enzyme.

- Decreased accumulation of drug into cells by mechanisms not well identified.

Absorption

Irinotecan is not given by the oral route.

Distribution

Widely distributed in body tissues. Irinotecan exhibits moderate binding to plasma proteins (30%–60%). In contrast, SN-38 shows extensive plasma protein binding (95%). Peak levels of SN-38 are achieved within 1 hour after drug administration.

Metabolism

The conversion of irinotecan to the active metabolite SN-38 occurs primarily in the liver. However, this conversion can also take place in plasma and in intestinal mucosa. SN-38 subsequently undergoes conjugation in the liver to the glucuronide metabolite, which is essentially inactive. In aqueous solution, the lactone ring undergoes rapid hydrolysis to the carboxylate form. Only about 34%–44% of CPT-11 and 45%–64% of the active metabolite SN-38 are present in the active lactone form at 1 hour after drug administration. The major route of elimination of both irinotecan and SN-38 is in bile and feces, accounting for 50%–70% of drug clearance. Only 10%–14% of CPT-11 and <1% of SN-38 is cleared in urine. The half-lives of irinotecan and SN-38 are 6–12 and 10–20 hours, respectively.

Indications

1. Colorectal cancer—Irinotecan is FDA-approved in combination with 5-FU and leucovorin as first-line treatment of patients with metastatic colorectal cancer.

2. Colorectal cancer—Irinotecan is FDA-approved as a single agent for second-line treatment of patients with metastatic colorectal cancer after failure of 5-FU–based chemotherapy.

3. Non–small cell lung cancer.

4. Small cell lung cancer.

Dosage Range

1. In the United States, irinotecan can be administered at 180 mg/m^2 IV as monotherapy or in combination with infusional 5-FU/LV on an every-2-week schedule.

2. An alternative regimen is 300–350 mg/m^2 IV on an every-3-week schedule.

Drug Interaction 1

Dilantin and other drugs that stimulate the liver microsomal CYP3A4 enzyme, including carbamazepine, rifampin, phenobarbital, and St. John's wort—These drugs increase the rate of metabolism of irinotecan and SN-38, resulting in its inactivation.

Drug Interaction 2

Drugs that inhibit the liver microsomal CYP3A4 enzyme, including ketoconazole, itraconazole, erythromycin, and clarithromycin—These drugs decrease the rate of metabolism of irinotecan and SN-38, resulting in increased drug levels and potentially increased toxicity.

Special Considerations

1. Irinotecan is an emetogenic drug. Patients should routinely receive antiemetic prophylaxis with a 5-HT3 antagonist, such as ondansetron or granisetron, in combination with dexamethasone.

2. Treatment with irinotecan is complicated by a syndrome of "early diarrhea," which consists of diarrhea, diaphoresis, and abdominal cramping during the infusion or within 24 hours of drug administration. This complication is thought to be due to a cholinergic effect. The recommended treatment is atropine (0.25–1.0

mg) administered IV unless clinically contraindicated. The routine use of atropine for prophylaxis is not recommended. However, atropine prophylaxis should be administered if a cholinergic event has been experienced.

3. Instruct patients about the possibility of late diarrhea (starting after 24 hours of drug administration), which can lead to serious dehydration and/or electrolyte imbalances if not managed promptly. This side effect is thought to be due to a direct irritation of the gastrointestinal mucosa by SN-38, although other as yet unidentified mechanisms may be involved. Loperamide should be taken immediately after the first loose bowel movement. The recommended dose is 4 mg PO as a loading dose, followed by 2 mg every 2 hours around the clock (4 mg every 4 hours during the night). Loperamide can be discontinued once the patient is diarrhea-free for 12 hours. If diarrhea should continue without improvement in the first 24 hours, an oral fluoroquinolone should be added. Hospitalization with IV antibiotics and IV hydration should be considered with continued diarrhea.

4. Irinotecan should be held for grade 3 (7–9 stools/day, incontinence, or severe cramping) and/or grade 4 (<10 stools/day, grossly bloody stool, or need for parenteral support) diarrhea. Dose of drug must be reduced upon recovery by the patient.

5. Patients should be warned against taking laxatives while on therapy.

6. Carefully monitor administration of drug as it is a moderate vesicant. The site of infusion should be carefully inspected for extravasation, in which case flushing with sterile water, elevation of the extremity, and local application of ice are recommended.

7. Use with caution in patients >65 years of age, in patients with poor performance status, and in those previously treated with pelvic and/or abdominal irradiation as they are at increased risk for myelosuppression and diarrhea.

8. Careful monitoring of patients on a weekly basis, especially during the first treatment cycle. Monitor complete blood cell count and platelet count on a weekly basis.

9. Patients with the UGT1A1 7/7 genotype may be at increased risk for developing GI toxicity and myelosuppression. Approximately 10% of the North American population is homozygous for this genotype. Dose reduction should be considered in this setting.

10. Patients should be warned to be off St. John's wort for at least 2 weeks before starting irinotecan therapy and should remain off until after the completion of irinotecan therapy. St. John's wort has been shown to reduce the efficacy of irinotecan chemotherapy by inhibiting metabolism of irinotecan to the active SN-38 metabolite.

11. Pregnancy category D. Breast-feeding should be avoided.

Toxicity 1

Myelosuppression. Dose-limiting with neutropenia being most commonly observed. Patients with prior history of abdominal/pelvic irradiation are particularly prone to developing myelosuppression after treatment with irinotecan. Typical nadir occurs at days 7–10 with full recovery by days 21–28.

Toxicity 2

Diarrhea. Dose-limiting with two different forms, early and late. Early form occurs within 24 hours of drug treatment and is thought to be a cholinergic event. Characterized by flushing, diaphoresis, abdominal pain, and diarrhea.

Late-form diarrhea occurs after 24 hours, typically at 3–10 days after treatment, can be severe and prolonged, and can lead to dehydration and electrolyte imbalance. Up to 80%–90% of patients may experience some aspect of late diarrhea, although only 10%–20% of patients will experience grade 3 or 4 diarrhea. Anorexia, nausea, and vomiting are usually mild and dose-related.

Toxicity 3

Mild alopecia.

Toxicity 4

Transient elevation in serum transaminases, alkaline phosphatase, and bilirubin.

Toxicity 5

Asthenia and fever.

Ixabepilone

Trade Names
Ixempra, BMS-247550

Classification
Epothilone, anti-microtubule agent

Category
Chemotherapy drug

Drug Manufacturer
Bristol-Myers Squibb

Mechanism of Action
- Semisynthetic analog of epothilone B.
- Cell cycle–specific, active in the mitosis (M) phase of the cell cycle.
- Binds directly to β-tubulin subunits on microtubules, leading to inhibition of normal microtubule dynamics.
- Exhibits activity in drug-resistant tumors that overexpress P-glycoprotein, MRP-1, βIII tubulin isoforms, and tubulin mutations.

Mechanism of Resistance
None well characterized to date.

Absorption
Not orally bioavailable. Administered only by the IV route.

Distribution
Distributes widely to all body tissues. Moderate binding (60%–70%) to plasma proteins.

Metabolism

Metabolized extensively by the hepatic P450 microsomal system via oxidation by CYP3A4. About 85% of drug is excreted via fecal elimination. Less than 10% is eliminated as the parent form with the majority being eliminated as metabolites. Renal clearance is relatively minor with less than 10% of drug cleared via the kidneys. The terminal elimination half-life is on the order of 52 hours. Gender, race, and age do not impact drug pharmacokinetics.

Indications

FDA-approved in combination with capecitabine for metastatic or locally advanced breast cancer resistant to treatment with an anthracycline and a taxane, or whose cancer is taxane-resistant and for whom further anthracycline therapy is contraindicated.

FDA-approved as monotherapy for metastatic or locally advanced breast cancer in patients whose tumors are resistant or refractory to anthracyclines, taxanes, and capecitabine.

Dosage Range

Recommended dose is 40 mg/m^2 IV every 3 weeks.

Drug Interaction 1

Drugs such as ketoconazole, fluconazole, itraconazole, erythromycin, clarithromycin, and verapamil may decrease the rate of metabolism of ixabepilone, resulting in increased drug levels and potentially increased toxicity.

Drug Interaction 2

Drugs such as rifampin, dilantin, phenobarbital, and carbamazepine may increase the rate of metabolism of ixabepilone, resulting in its inactivation.

Drug Interaction 3

St. John's wort may alter the metabolism of ixabepilone and should be avoided while on therapy.

Drug Interaction 4

Ixabepilone does not appear to affect the metabolism of drugs that are substrates of liver CYP enzymes.

Special Considerations

1. Contraindicated in patients with history of severe hypersensitivity reaction to paclitaxel or to other drugs formulated in Cremophor EL.
2. Use with caution in patients with abnormal liver function. When used as monotherapy, dose reduction is required in the setting of mild to moderate hepatic impairment. Contraindicated when used in

combination with capecitabine in patients with SGOT or SGPT >2.5 × ULN or bilirubin >1 × ULN.

3. Contraindicated in patients with a neutrophil count <1,500 cells/mm³ or a platelet count <100,000 cells/mm³.

4. Use with caution in patients with prior history of diabetes mellitus and chronic alcoholism or prior therapy with known neurotoxic agents such as cisplatin.

5. Patients should receive premedication prior to treatment to prevent the incidence of hypersensitivity reactions (HSR). Give an H1 antagonist (diphenhydramine 50 mg PO) and an H2 antagonist (cimetidine 300 mg) 1 hour prior to drug administration. Patients experiencing an HSR require premedication with dexamethasone 20 mg IV 30 minutes before drug treatment, along with diphenhydramine 50 mg IV and cimetidine 300 mg IV.

6. Medical personnel should be available at the time of drug administration. Emergency equipment, including Ambu bag, EKG machine, IV fluids, pressors, and other drugs for resuscitation, must be at bedside before initiation of treatment.

7. Pregnancy category D. Breast-feeding should be avoided.

Toxicity 1

Myelosuppression with neutropenia and thrombocytopenia. The onset of neutropenia occurs on days 10–14 with recovery usually by day 21.

Toxicity 2

HSR characterized by generalized skin rash, flushing, erythema, hypotension, dyspnea, and/or bronchospasm. Premedication regimen, as outlined in Special Considerations, has significantly decreased incidence.

Toxicity 3

Neurotoxicity mainly in the form of peripheral sensory neuropathy with numbness and paresthesias. Occurs in up to 20% of patients.

Toxicity 4

Fatigue and asthenia.

Toxicity 5

GI toxicity in the form of nausea/vomiting, mucositis, and/or diarrhea.

Toxicity 6

Myalgias, arthralgias, and musculoskeletal pain.

Lapatinib

Trade Names

Tykerb, GW572016

Classification

Signal transduction inhibitor

Category

Chemotherapy drug

Drug Manufacturer

GlaxoSmithKline

Mechanism of Action

- Potent small molecule inhibitor of the tyrosine kinases associated with epidermal growth factor receptor (ErbB1;EGFR) and HER2 (ErbB2), resulting in inhibition of phosphorylation and downstream signaling.
- Inhibition of the EGFR and HER2 tyrosine kinases results in inhibition of critical mitogenic and anti-apoptotic signals involved in proliferation, growth, invasion/metastasis, angiogenesis, and response to chemotherapy and/or radiation therapy.

Mechanism of Resistance

None well characterized to date.

Absorption

Oral absorption is incomplete and variable and is increased when administered with food.

Distribution

Extensive binding (99%) to plasma proteins, including albumin and α1-acid glycoprotein, and extensive tissue distribution. Peak plasma levels are achieved 4 hours after ingestion. Steady-state drug concentrations are reached in 6 to 7 days.

Metabolism

Metabolism in the liver primarily by the CYP3A4 and CYP3A5 microsomal enzymes and by CYP2C19 and CYP2C8 to a lesser extent. Elimination is mainly hepatic with excretion in the feces, and renal elimination of parent drug and its metabolites accounts for less than 2% of an administered dose. The terminal half-life of the parent drug is 14 hours, and with repeat dosing, the effective half-life is 24 hours.

Indications

FDA-approved in combination with capecitabine for the treatment of patients with advanced or metastatic breast cancer whose tumors overexpress HER2 and who have received prior therapy, including an anthracycline, a taxane, and trastuzumab.

Dosage Range

Recommended dose is 1,250 mg PO daily on days 1 to 21 continuously in combination with capecitabine 1,000 mg/m^2 PO bid on days 1 to 14, with each cycle repeated every 21 days.

Drug Interaction 1

Dilantin and other drugs that stimulate the liver microsomal CYP3A4 enzyme, including carbamazepine, rifampicin, phenobarbital, and St. John's wort. These drugs may increase the rate of metabolism of lapatinib, resulting in its inactivation.

Drug Interaction 2

Drugs that inhibit the liver microsomal CYP3A4 enzyme, including ketoconazole, itraconazole, erythromycin, and clarithromycin. These drugs may decrease the rate of metabolism of lapatinib, resulting in increased drug levels and potentially increased toxicity.

Drug Interaction 3

Warfarin—Patients receiving coumarin-derived anticoagulants should be closely monitored for alterations in their clotting parameters (PT and INR) and/or bleeding, as lapatinib may inhibit the metabolism of warfarin by the liver P450 system. The dose of warfarin may require careful adjustment in the presence of lapatinib therapy.

Special Considerations

1. Use with caution in patients with hepatic impairment, and dose reduction and/or interruption should be considered.

2. Monitor cardiac function at baseline and periodically during therapy with either MUGA or echocardiogram to assess LVEF. The majority of LVEF decreases occur within the first 9 weeks of therapy. Use with caution in patients with pre-existing conditions that could impair LVEF.

3. Monitor EKG with QT measurement at baseline and periodically during therapy, as QT prolongation has been observed. Use with caution in patients at risk of developing QT prolongation, including hypokalemia, hypomagnesemia, congenital long QT syndrome, patients taking antiarrhythmic medications or any other products that may cause QT prolongation, and cumulative high-dose anthracycline therapy.

4. Lapatinib should be taken 1 hour before or after a meal, and the daily dose should not be divided. When capecitabine is co-administered, capecitabine should be taken with a glass of water within 30 minutes after a meal.

5. Avoid grapefruit products while on therapy.

6. Closely monitor patients for diarrhea, as severe diarrhea may develop while on therapy. Aggressive management with anti-diarrheal agents as well as replacement of fluids. Electrolyte status should be closely followed.

7. Pregnancy category D.

Toxicity 1

Diarrhea is the most common dose-limiting toxicity and occurs in 65% of patients. Mild nausea/vomiting may also occur.

Toxicity 2

Cardiac toxicity with reduction in LVEF. QT prolongation observed in <1% of patients.

Toxicity 3

Myelosuppression with anemia more common than thrombocytopenia or neutropenia.

Toxicity 4

Fatigue and anorexia.

Toxicity 5

Mild to moderate elevation of serum transaminases and serum bilirubin.

Toxicity 6

Hand-foot syndrome (palmar-plantar erythrodysesthesia) and skin rash.

Lenalidomide

Trade Name

Revlimid, CC-5013

Classification

Immunomodulatory analog of thalidomide, anti-angiogenic agent

Category

Unclassified therapeutic agent, biologic response modifier agent

Drug Manufacturer

Celgene

Mechanism of Action

- Mechanism of action is not fully characterized.
- Immunomodulatory drug (IMid) that stimulates T-cell proliferation as well as IL-2 and IFN-γ production.
- Inhibition of TNF-α and IL-6 synthesis and down-modulation of cell surface adhesion molecules similar to thalidomide.
- May exert anti-angiogenic effect by inhibition of basic fibroblast growth (bFBG) and vascular endothelial growth factor (VEGF) and through as yet undefined mechanisms.
- Overcomes cellular drug resistance to thalidomide.

Mechanism of Resistance

None characterized to date.

Absorption

Lenalidomide is rapidly absorbed following oral administration with peak plasma concentrations at 60–90 minutes post ingestion. Co-administration with food does not alter the extent of absorption (AUC) but does reduce maximal plasma concentration (C_{max}) by 36%.

Distribution

Not well characterized.

Metabolism

Lenalidomide does not appear to be metabolized or induced by the cytochrome P450 pathway. Approximately 66% of an administered dose is excreted unchanged in the urine. The elimination half-life of the drug is approximately 3 hours.

Indications

1. FDA-approved for the treatment of low- or intermediate-1-risk myelodysplastic syndromes (MDS) associated with the deletion 5q (del 5q) cytogenetic abnormality with or without additional cytogenetic abnormalities.

2. FDA-approved for the treatment of multiple myeloma in combination with dexamethasone for patients who have received at least one prior therapy.

Dosage Range

1. Myelodysplastic syndrome: 10 mg PO daily.

2. Multiple myeloma: 25 mg PO daily on days 1–21 and 40 mg Decadron PO on days 1–4, 9–12, and 17–20 of a 28-day cycle.

Drug Interactions

None well characterized to date.

Special Considerations

1. Pregnancy category X. Lenalidomide is a thalidomide analog, a known human teratogen that causes severe or life-threatening birth defects. As such, women who are pregnant or who wish to become pregnant should not take lenalidomide. Severe fetal malformations can occur if even one capsule is taken by a pregnant woman. All women should have a baseline β-human chorionic gonadotropin (β-HCG) before starting lenalidomide therapy. Women of reproductive age must have two negative pregnancy tests before starting therapy: one should be 10 to 14 days before therapy is begun, and the second should be 24 hours before therapy.

2. All women of childbearing potential should practice two forms of birth control throughout therapy with lenalidomide: one highly effective form (intrauterine device, hormonal contraception [patch, implant, pill, injection], partner's vasectomy, or tubal ligation) and one additional barrier method (latex condom, diaphragm, or cervical cap). It is strongly recommended that these precautionary measures be taken 1 month before initiation of therapy, continue while on therapy, and continue at least 1 month after therapy is discontinued.

3. Lenalidomide is only available under a special restricted distribution program called "RevAssist^{SM}." Only prescribers and pharmacists registered with the RevAssist^{SM} program are able to prescribe

and dispense the drug. Lenalidomide should only be dispensed to those patients who are registered and meet all the conditions of the RevAssist[SM] program.

4. Breast-feeding while on therapy should be avoided, as it remains unknown if lenalidomide is excreted in breast milk.

5. Men taking lenalidomide must use latex condoms for every sexual encounter with a woman of childbearing potential, as the drug may be present in semen.

6. Patients taking lenalidomide should not donate blood or semen while receiving treatment, and for at least 1 month after stopping this drug.

7. Monitor complete blood counts while on therapy as lenalidomide is toxic to the bone marrow.

8. Use with caution in patients with impaired renal function, as the risk of toxicity may be greater.

9. There is a significantly increased risk of thromboembolic complications, including deep venous thrombosis (DVT) and pulmonary embolism (PE), especially in myeloma patients treated with lenalidomide and Decadron. Prophylaxis with low molecular weight heparin or aspirin [325 mg PO qd) can help prevent and/or reduce this risk.

Toxicity 1

Potentially severe or fatal teratogenic effects.

Toxicity 2

Myelosuppression with neutropenia and thrombocytopenia that is usually reversible.

Toxicity 3

Increased risk of thromboembolic complications, such as DVT and PE.

Toxicity 4

Nausea/vomiting, diarrhea, and constipation are most common GI side effects.

Toxicity 5

Neurotoxic side effects are rare with almost no sedation.

Letrozole

Trade Names
Femara

Classification
Aromatase inhibitor

Category
Hormonal agent

Drug Manufacturer
Novartis

Mechanism of Action
- Nonsteroidal, competitive inhibitor of aromatase. Nearly 200-fold more potent than aminoglutethimide.
- Inhibits synthesis of estrogens by inhibiting the conversion of adrenal androgens (androstenedione and testosterone) to estrogens (estrone, estrone sulfate, and estradiol). Serum estradiol levels are suppressed by 90% within 14 days, and nearly completely suppressed after 6 weeks of therapy.
- No inhibitory effect on adrenal corticosteroid biosynthesis.

Absorption
Rapidly and completely absorbed after oral administration. Food does not interfere with oral absorption.

Distribution
Significant uptake in peripheral tissues and in breast cancer cells. Minimal binding to plasma proteins.

Metabolism
Metabolism occurs in the liver by the cytochrome P450 system. Process of glucuronidation leads to inactive metabolites. Parent drug and metabolites are excreted via the kidneys with over 75%–90% cleared in urine.

Indications

1. First-line treatment of postmenopausal women with hormone-receptor positive or hormone-receptor unknown locally advanced or metastatic breast cancer.

2. Second-line treatment of postmenopausal women with advanced breast cancer after progression on antiestrogen therapy.

3. Adjuvant treatment of postmenopausal women with hormone-receptor positive early-stage breast cancer.

4. Extended adjuvant treatment of early-stage breast cancer in postmenopausal women who have received 5 years of adjuvant tamoxifen therapy.

Dosage Range

Metastatic disease: 2.5 mg PO qd until disease progression.

Adjuvant setting: 2.5 mg PO qd until disease relapse.

Drug Interactions

None known.

Special Considerations

1. Letrozole is indicated only for postmenopausal women. Efficacy in premenopausal women has not been established, and there may be an increased risk of benign ovarian tumors and cystic ovarian disease in this population.

2. Use with caution in patients with abnormal liver function. Monitor liver function at baseline and periodically during therapy. The dose should be reduced by 50% in patients with cirrhosis and severe hepatic dysfunction. In this setting, the recommended dose is 2.5 mg PO every other day.

3. No need for glucocorticoid and/or mineralocorticoid replacement.

4. Closely monitor women with osteoporosis or at risk of osteoporosis by performing bone densitometry at the start of therapy and at regular intervals. Treatment or prophylaxis for osteoporosis should be initiated when appropriate.

5. Letrozole can be taken with or without food.

6. Pregnancy category D.

Toxicity 1

Mild musculoskeletal pains and arthralgias are the most common adverse events.

Toxicity 2

Headache and fatigue.

Toxicity 3

Mild nausea with less frequent vomiting and anorexia. Thromboembolic events are rare, and less common than with megestrol acetate.

Toxicity 4

Hot flashes occur in less than 10% of patients.

Toxicity 5

Mild elevation in serum transaminases and serum bilirubin. Most often seen in patients with established metastatic disease in the liver.

Toxicity 6

Thromboembolic events are rarely observed.

Leuprolide

pyro Glu-His-Trp-Ser-Tyr-D-Leu-Leu-Arg-Pro-ethylamide
 1   2   3   4   5   6   7   8   9   10

Trade Names
Lupron

Classification
LHRH agonist

Category
Hormonal agent

Drug Manufacturer
TAP Pharmaceuticals

Mechanism of Action
Administration of this LHRH agonist leads to initial release of FSH and LH followed by suppression of gonadotropin secretion as a result of desensitization of the pituitary to gonadotropin-releasing hormone. This eventually leads to decreased secretion of LH and FSH from the pituitary, resulting in castration levels of testosterone. Plasma levels of testosterone fall to castrate levels after 2–4 weeks of therapy.

Absorption
Leuprolide is not orally absorbed. After SC injection, approximately 90% of a dose is absorbed into the systemic circulation.

Distribution
Distribution is not well characterized. Leuprolide is slowly released over a 28-day period. Peak serum concentrations are achieved 10–15 days after drug administration. About 45%–50% of drug is bound to plasma proteins.

Metabolism
Metabolism of leuprolide occurs mainly via hydrolysis of the C-terminal amino acids. Leuprolide is nearly completely eliminated in its parent form in urine (>90%) with an elimination half-life of 3–4 hours. The half-life is prolonged in patients with impaired renal function.

Indications
1. Advanced prostate cancer.
2. Neoadjuvant therapy of early-stage prostate cancer.

Dosage Range

Administer 22.5 mg SC every 3 months. Can also be given as 30 mg SC every 4 months.

Drug Interactions

None known.

Special Considerations

1. Initiation of treatment with leuprolide may induce a transient tumor flare due to the initial release of LH and FSH. Patients with impending ureteral obstruction and/or spinal cord compression or those with painful bone metastases are at especially high risk. To prevent tumor flare, patients should be started on antiandrogen therapy at least 2 weeks before starting leuprolide.

2. Serum testosterone levels decrease to castrate levels within 2–4 weeks after initiation of therapy.

3. Use with caution in patients with abnormal renal function.

4. Caution patients about the possibility of hot flashes. Consider the use of clonidine 0.1–0.2 mg PO daily, Megace 20 mg PO bid, or soy tablets, one tablet PO tid for prevention and/or treatment.

Toxicity 1

Hot flashes, impotence, and gynecomastia. Decreased libido occurs less commonly.

Toxicity 2

Tumor flare. May occur in up to 20% of patients, usually within the first 2 weeks of starting therapy. May observe increased bone pain, urinary retention, or back pain with spinal cord compression. May be prevented by pretreating with an anti-androgen agent such as flutamide, bicalutamide, or nilutamide.

Toxicity 3

Local discomfort at the site of injection.

Toxicity 4

Elevated serum cholesterol levels.

Toxicity 5

Nausea and vomiting. Rarely observed.

Toxicity 6

Hypersensitivity reaction.

Toxicity 7

Myelosuppression. Rarely observed.

Toxicity 8

Peripheral edema. Results from sodium retention.

Toxicity 9

Asthenia.

Lomustine

$$Cl - CH_2 - CH_2 - \underset{\underset{NO}{|}}{N} - \overset{\overset{O}{\|}}{C} - NH - \bigcirc$$

Trade Names

CCNU

Classification

Alkylating agent

Category

Chemotherapy drug

Drug Manufacturer

Bristol-Myers Squibb

Mechanism of Action

- Cell cycle–nonspecific nitrosourea analog.
- Alkylation and carbamoylation by lomustine metabolites interfere with the synthesis and function of DNA, RNA, and proteins.
- Antitumor activity appears to correlate best with formation of intrastrand cross-linking of DNA.

Mechanism of Resistance

- Decreased cellular uptake of drug.
- Increased intracellular thiol content due to glutathione and/or glutathione-related enzymes.
- Enhanced activity of DNA repair enzymes.

Absorption

Readily and completely absorbed orally. Peak plasma concentrations are observed within 3 hours after oral administration.

Distribution

Lipid-soluble drug with broad tissue distribution. Well-absorbed after oral administration and crosses the blood-brain barrier. CNS levels approach 15%–30% of plasma levels.

Metabolism

Metabolized by the liver microsomal P450 system to active metabolites. The elimination half-life of the drug is about 72 hours, and excretion mainly occurs via the kidneys. Approximately 50% of a dose is excreted in urine within the first 12–24 hours, while 60% of a dose is excreted after 48 hours.

Indications

1. Brain tumors—primary or metastatic.
2. Hodgkin's lymphoma.
3. Non-Hodgkin's lymphoma.

Dosage Range

As a single agent, the recommended dose in previously untreated patients is 130 mg/m² PO every 6 weeks. In patients with compromised bone marrow function, the dose should be reduced to 100 mg/m² PO every 6 weeks.

Drug Interaction 1

Cimetidine—Cimetidine enhances the toxicity of lomustine.

Drug Interaction 2

Alcohol—Ingestion of alcohol should be avoided for at least 1 hour before and after administration of lomustine.

Special Considerations

1. Monitor CBC while on therapy. Subsequent cycles should not be given before 6 weeks, given the delayed and potentially cumulative effects of the drug. Platelet and leukocyte counts must return to normal before starting the next course of therapy.
2. PFTs should be obtained at baseline and monitored periodically during therapy. There is an increased risk of pulmonary toxicity in patients with a prior history of lung disease and a baseline FVC or DLCO below 70% of predicted.
3. Administer drug on an empty stomach as food may inhibit absorption.
4. Pregnancy category D.

Toxicity 1

Myelosuppression. Dose-limiting toxicity. In contrast to most other anticancer agents, myelosuppression involving all elements is delayed and cumulative. Nadirs typically occur 4–6 weeks after therapy and may persist for 1–3 weeks.

Toxicity 2

Nausea and vomiting may occur within 2–6 hours after a dose of drug and can last for up to 24 hours.

Toxicity 3

Anorexia may be present but short-lived. Mucositis is unusual.

Toxicity 4

Impotence, male sterility, amenorrhea, ovarian suppression, menopause, and infertility. Gynecomastia is occasionally observed.

Toxicity 5

Pulmonary toxicity is uncommon at doses lower than 1,100 mg/m².

Toxicity 6

Interstitial lung disease and pulmonary fibrosis in the form of an insidious cough, dyspnea, pulmonary infiltrates, and/or respiratory failure may be observed.

Toxicity 7

Renal toxicity is uncommon at total cumulative doses of lower than 1,000 mg/m². Usually manifested by progressive azotemia and decrease in kidney size, which can progress to renal failure.

Toxicity 8

Neurotoxicity in the form of confusion, lethargy, dysarthria, and ataxia.

Toxicity 9

Increased risk of secondary malignancies with long-term use, especially acute myelogenous leukemia and myelodysplasia.

Toxicity 10

Alopecia is rarely seen.

Mechlorethamine

$$CICH_2CH_2 - \overset{\overset{\displaystyle CH_3}{|}}{\underset{\underset{\displaystyle H}{|}}{\overset{\oplus}{N}}} - CH_2CH_2CI$$

Trade Names

Mustargen, Nitrogen mustard

Classification

Alkylating agent

Category

Chemotherapy drug

Drug Manufacturer

Merck

Mechanism of Action

- Analog of mustard gas.
- Classic alkylating agent that forms interstrand and intrastrand cross-links with DNA resulting in inhibition of DNA synthesis and function.
- Cell cycle–nonspecific with activity in all phases of the cell cycle.

Mechanism of Resistance

- Decreased cellular uptake of drug.
- Increased inactivation of cytotoxic species through increased expression of sulfhydryl proteins, including glutathione and glutathione-associated enzymes.
- Enhanced activity of DNA repair enzymes.

Absorption

Not orally bioavailable.

Distribution

Distribution of drug is not well characterized.

Metabolism

Undergoes rapid hydrolysis in plasma to reactive metabolites. Extremely short plasma half-life on the order of 15–20 minutes. No significant organ metabolism. Greater than 50% of inactive drug metabolites are excreted in urine within 24 hours.

Indications

1. Hodgkin's lymphoma.
2. Non-Hodgkin's lymphoma.
3. Cutaneous T-cell lymphoma (topical use).
4. Intrapleural, intrapericardial, and intraperitoneal treatment of metastatic disease resulting in pleural effusion.

Dosage Range

1. Hodgkin's lymphoma: Administer 6 mg/m² IV on days 1 and 8 every 28 days, as part of the MOPP regimen.
2. Cutaneous T-cell lymphoma: Dilute 10 mg in 60 mL sterile water and apply topically to skin lesions.
3. Intracavitary use: Administer 0.2–0.4 mg/kg into the pleural and/or peritoneal cavity.

Drug Interactions

Sodium thiosulfate—Sodium thiosulfate inactivates the activity of mechlorethamine.

Special Considerations

1. Mechlorethamine is a potent vesicant, and caution should be exercised in preparing and administering the drug.
2. Administer drug into either a new IV site or one that is less than 24 hours old to decrease the risk of extravasation.
3. In the event of drug extravasation, inflammation and necrosis may be prevented by the immediate instillation of 2.6% sodium thiosulfate solution into the area to neutralize the active drug. Elevate arm and apply ice packs for 6–12 hours. May need to consult a plastic surgeon for further evaluation.
4. Pregnancy category D.

Toxicity 1

Myelosuppression. Dose-limiting toxicity with leukopenia and thrombocytopenia. Nadirs occur at day 7–10 and recover by day 21.

Toxicity 2

Nausea and vomiting. Usually occur within the first 3 hours after drug administration, lasting for 4–8 hours and up to 24 hours, and often severe. Can be dose limiting in some patients.

Toxicity 3

Potent vesicant. Pain, inflammation, erythema, induration, and necrosis can be observed at the injection site.

Toxicity 4

Alopecia.

Toxicity 5

Amenorrhea and azoospermia.

Toxicity 6

Hyperuricemia.

Toxicity 7

CNS toxicities, including weakness, sleepiness, and headache, are rare.

Toxicity 8

Hypersensitivity reactions. Rarely observed.

Toxicity 9

Increased risk of secondary malignancies including acute myelogenous leukemia with IV administration and basal cell and squamous cell cancers of the skin with topical application.

Megestrol acetate

Trade Names

Megace

Classification

Progestational agent

Category

Hormonal agent

Drug Manufacturer

Bristol-Myers Squibb

Mechanism of Action

- Synthetic derivative of the naturally occurring steroid hormone progesterone.
- Possesses antiestrogenic effects. Induces the activity of 17-hydroxysteroid dehydrogenase, which then oxidizes estradiol to the less active metabolite estrone. Also activates estrogen sulfatransferase, which metabolizes estrogen to less potent metabolites.
- Inhibits release of luteinizing hormone receptors resulting in a decrease in estrogen levels.
- Inhibits stability, availability, and turnover of estrogen receptors.

Mechanism of Resistance

None known.

Absorption

Rapidly and completely absorbed after an oral dose. Peak plasma concentration is reached within 1–3 hours after oral administration.

Distribution

Large fraction of megestrol is distributed into body fat.

Metabolism

About 70% of drug is metabolized in the liver to inactive steroid metabolites. The drug is primarily eliminated in urine in the form of parent drug and metabolites, and 60%–80% of the drug is renally excreted within 10 days after administration. Elimination half-life is quite variable and ranges from 15 to 105 hours with a mean of 34 hours.

Indications

1. Breast cancer.
2. Endometrial cancer.
3. Renal cell cancer.
4. Appetite stimulant in cancer and HIV patients.

Dosage Range

1. Breast cancer: 40 mg PO qid.
2. Endometrial cancer: 40 mg PO qid.
3. Appetite stimulant: 80–200 mg PO qid.

Drug Interactions

Aminoglutethimide—Aminoglutethimide enhances the hepatic metabolism of megestrol resulting in decreased serum levels.

Special Considerations

1. Use with caution in patients with either a history of thromboembolic or hypercoagulable disorders as megestrol acetate has been associated with an increased incidence of thromboembolic events.
2. Use with caution in patients with diabetes mellitus as megestrol may exacerbate this condition.
3. Use with caution in patients with abnormal liver function. Dose reduction is recommended in this setting.
4. Caution patients on the risk of weight gain and fluid retention. Patients should be advised to go on a low-salt diet.
5. Pregnancy category D.

Toxicity 1

Weight gain results from a combination of fluid retention and increased appetite.

Toxicity 2

Thromboembolic events are rarely observed.

Toxicity 3

Nausea and vomiting.

Toxicity 4

Breakthrough menstrual bleeding.

Toxicity 5

Tumor flare.

Toxicity 6

Hyperglycemia.

Toxicity 7

Hot flashes, sweating, and mood changes.

M

Melphalan

$$\text{Cl}\diagdown\text{N}\diagup\text{Cl} - \langle\text{C}_6\text{H}_4\rangle - \text{CH}_2\overset{\text{NH}_2}{\underset{|}{\text{CHCO}_2\text{H}}}$$

Trade Names

Alkeran, Phenylalanine mustard, L-PAM

Classification

Alkylating agent

Category

Chemotherapy drug

Drug Manufacturer

GlaxoSmithKline

Mechanism of Action

- Analog of nitrogen mustard.
- Classic bifunctional alkylating agent that forms interstrand and intrastrand cross-links with DNA resulting in inhibition of DNA synthesis and function.
- Cell cycle–nonspecific as it acts at all stages of the cell cycle.

Mechanism of Resistance

- Decreased cellular uptake of drug.
- Increased inactivation of cytotoxic species through increased expression of sulfhydryl proteins, including glutathione and glutathione-associated enzymes.
- Enhanced activity of DNA repair enzymes.

Absorption

Oral absorption is poor and incomplete. Oral bioavailability ranges between 25% and 90% with a mean of 60%, and oral absorption is decreased when taken with food.

Distribution

Widely distributed in all tissues. Approximately 80%–90% of drug is bound to plasma proteins.

Metabolism

Undergoes rapid hydrolysis in plasma to reactive metabolites. Short plasma half-life on the order of 60–90 minutes. No significant organ metabolism. About 25%–30% of drug is excreted in urine within 24 hours after administration, with the majority of the drug being excreted in feces (up to 50%) over 6 days.

Indications

1. Multiple myeloma.
2. Breast cancer.
3. Ovarian cancer.
4. High-dose chemotherapy and transplant setting.
5. Polycythemia vera.

Dosage Range

1. Multiple myeloma: Administer 9 mg/m² IV on days 1–4 every 4 weeks as part of the melphalan-prednisone regimen.
2. Transplant setting: Administer 140 mg/m² as a single agent in bone marrow/stem cell transplant setting.

Drug Interaction 1

Cimetidine—Cimetidine decreases the oral bioavailability of melphalan by up to 30%.

Drug Interaction 2

Steroids—Steroids enhance the antitumor effects of melphalan.

Drug Interaction 3

Cyclosporine—Cyclosporine enhances the risk of renal toxicity secondary to melphalan.

Special Considerations

1. Use with caution in patients with abnormal renal function. Although the drug has been used in high doses in the transplant setting in the face of renal dysfunction without increased toxicity, dose reduction should be considered in the setting of renal dysfunction.
2. When administered orally, drug should be taken on an empty stomach to maximize absorption.
3. IV administration may cause hypersensitivity reaction.
4. Monitor complete blood cell count as melphalan therapy is associated with delayed and prolonged nadir.
5. Monitor injection site for erythema, pain, and/or burning.
6. Pregnancy category D.

Toxicity 1

Myelosuppression. Dose-limiting toxicity with leukopenia and thrombocytopenia equally affected. Effect may be prolonged and cumulative with a nadir 4–6 weeks after therapy.

Toxicity 2

Nausea and vomiting, mucositis, and diarrhea. Generally mild with conventional doses, but severe with high-dose therapy.

Toxicity 3

Hypersensitivity reactions are rare with oral form. Observed in about 10% of patients treated with IV form of drug, and manifested as diaphoresis, urticaria, skin rashes, bronchospasm, dyspnea, tachycardia, and hypotension.

Toxicity 4

Alopecia is uncommon.

Toxicity 5

Skin ulcerations and other skin reactions at the injection site are uncommon.

Toxicity 6

Increased risk of secondary malignancies including acute myelogenous leukemia and myelodysplasia with prolonged use. Mutagenic and teratogenic.

Mercaptopurine

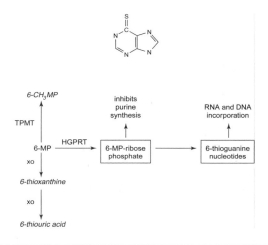

Trade Names

6-MP, Purinethol

Classification

Antimetabolite

Category

Chemotherapy drug

Drug Manufacturer

GlaxoSmithKline

Mechanism of Action

- Cell cycle–specific purine analog with activity in the S-phase.
- Parent drug is inactive. Requires intracellular phosphorylation by the enzyme hypoxanthine-guanine phosphoribosyltransferase (HGPRT) to the cytotoxic monophosphate form, which is then metabolized to the eventual triphosphate metabolite.
- Inhibits de novo purine synthesis by inhibiting 5-phosphoribosyl-1 pyrophosphate (PRPP) amidotransferase.
- Incorporation of thiopurine triphosphate nucleotides into DNA resulting in inhibition of DNA synthesis and function.
- Incorporation of thiopurine triphosphate nucleotides into RNA resulting in alterations in RNA processing and/or translation.

Mechanism of Resistance

- Decreased expression of the activating enzyme HGPRT.
- Increased expression of the catabolic enzyme alkaline phosphatase or the conjugating enzyme thiopurine methyltransferase (TPMT).
- Decreased transmembrane transport of drug.
- Decreased expression of mismatch repair enzymes (e.g., hMLH1, hMSH2).
- Cross-resistance observed between mercaptopurine and thioguanine.

Absorption

Oral absorption is erratic and incomplete. Only 50% of an oral dose is absorbed.

Distribution

Widely distributed in total body water. Does not cross the blood brain barrier. About 20%–30% of drug is bound to plasma proteins.

Metabolism

Metabolized in the liver by methylation to inactive metabolites and via oxidation by xanthine oxidase to inactive metabolites. About 50% of parent drug and metabolites are eliminated in urine within the first 24 hours. Plasma half-life after oral administration is 1.5 hours in contrast to the plasma half-life after IV administration, which ranges between 20 and 50 minutes.

Indications

Acute lymphoblastic leukemia.

Dosage Range

1. Induction therapy: 2.5 mg/kg PO daily.
2. Maintenance therapy: 1.5–2.5 mg/kg PO daily.

Drug Interaction 1

Coumadin—Anticoagulant effects of Coumadin are inhibited by mercaptopurine through an unknown mechanism. Monitor coagulation parameters (PT and INR), and adjust dose accordingly.

Drug Interaction 2

Allopurinol—Allopurinol inhibits xanthine oxidase and the catabolic breakdown of mercaptopurine, resulting in enhanced toxicity. Dose of mercaptopurine must be reduced by 50%–75% when given concurrently with allopurinol.

Drug Interaction 3

Bactrim DS may enhance the myelosuppressive effects of mercaptopurine when given concurrently.

Special Considerations

1. Dose reduction of 50%–75% is required when mercaptopurine is given concurrently with allopurinol. This is because allopurinol inhibits the catabolic breakdown of mercaptopurine by xanthine oxidase.

2. Use with caution in patients with abnormal liver and/or renal function. Dose reduction should be considered in this setting.

3. Use with caution in the presence of other hepatotoxic drugs as risk of mercaptopurine-associated hepatic toxicity is increased.

4. Patients with a deficiency in the metabolizing enzyme 6-thiopurine methyltransferase (TPMT) are at increased risk for developing severe toxicities. This enzyme deficiency is a pharmacogenetic syndrome.

5. Administer on an empty stomach to facilitate oral absorption. Advise patient to take mercaptopurine at bedtime.

6. Pregnancy category D.

Toxicity 1

Myelosuppression. Mild to moderate with leukopenia more common than thrombocytopenia. Leukopenia nadir at days 10–14 with recovery by day 21.

Toxicity 2

Mucositis and/or diarrhea. Usually seen with higher doses.

Toxicity 3

Hepatotoxicity in the form of elevated serum bilirubin and transaminases, presenting as jaundice. Usually occurs 2–3 months after therapy.

Toxicity 4

Mild nausea and vomiting.

Toxicity 5

Dry skin, urticaria, and photosensitivity.

Toxicity 6

Immunosuppression. Increased risk of bacterial, fungal, and parasitic infections.

Toxicity 7

Mutagenic, teratogenic, and carcinogenic.

Mesna

Mesnex, 2-Mercaptoethanesulfonic acid

Classification

Sulfhydryl compound

Category

Chemoprotective drug

Drug Manufacturer

Bristol-Myers Squibb

Mechanism of Action

- Synthetic sulfhydryl compound with no intrinsic antitumor activity.
- Used to prevent ifosfamide- and cyclophosphamide-induced hemorrhagic cystitis.
- Mesna is initially metabolized to the dimesna form (mesna disulfide). In the kidneys, dimesna is reduced back to mesna, which then binds to and detoxifies the urotoxic ifosfamide metabolites, acrolein and 4-hydroxy ifosfamide.
- Identical mode of action to detoxify urotoxic cyclophosphamide metabolites.

Absorption

About 75% of mesna is bioavailable after an oral dose.

Distribution

Distributed in total body water and in the intravascular compartment.

Metabolism

Rapidly metabolized in plasma via oxidation to its sole metabolite, dimesna. Rapidly eliminated in the kidneys, where it is reduced to mesna, the free thiol compound. Mesna then binds to acrolein and other urotoxic metabolites, and the soluble complexes are excreted in urine. Most of given dose is eliminated within 4 hours of administration, and approximately 32% of the drug is eliminated as mesna and 33% as dimesna. The half-lives of mesna and dimesna are 0.36 and 1.1 hours, respectively.

Indications

1. Prevention of ifosfamide-induced hemorrhagic cystitis.
2. Prevention of high-dose cyclophosphamide-induced hemorrhagic cystitis.

Dosage Range

1. Dose of mesna is based on the administered dose of ifosfamide and/ or cyclophosphamide.

2. Usually given as IV bolus three times daily at a total dose that is 60% of the administered dose of ifosfamide and/or cyclophosphamide. The first dose of mesna is given 15 minutes before ifosfamide, the second dose is given 4 hours after ifosfamide, and the third dose is given 8 hours after ifosfamide.

3. Alternative regimen is to combine equivalent doses of ifosfamide and mesna in same IV bag.

4. Mesna can be administered via a combination of intravenous and oral dosing. Mesna is given as IV bolus at a dose equal to 20% of the ifosfamide dose at the time of ifosfamide administration. Mesna tablets are given orally at a dose equal to 40% of the ifosfamide dose at 2 and 6 hours after each dose of ifosfamide. The total daily dose of mesna is 100% of the ifosfamide dose.

Drug Interaction 1

Cisplatin, carboplatin—Mesna is incompatible with cisplatin and carboplatin.

Drug Interaction 2

Epirubicin—Mesna is incompatible with epirubicin.

Drug Interaction 3

Ifosfamide, cyclophosphamide—Mesna decreases the risk of bladder toxicity associated with ifosfamide and cyclophosphamide but does not alter their antitumor activity.

Special Considerations

1. Use with caution in patients with diabetes mellitus as treatment with mesna can cause false-positive results on urinalysis for ketones.

2. Monitoring of urine for hematuria is recommended for early detection of hemorrhagic cystitis. Urinalysis should be checked for gross and/or microscopic hematuria before each dose of ifosfamide. Mesna does not prevent drug-induced hemorrhagic cystitis in all patients, especially in those receiving high doses of ifosfamide (>2–4 mg/m^2).

3. Use with caution in patients with known allergies to thiol-containing compounds.

4. Patients who vomit within 2 hours of taking oral mesna should repeat the dose or receive IV mesna.

5. Mesna does not prevent and/or reduce any of the non-bladder adverse reactions associated with ifosfamide therapy.

6. Pregnancy category B.

Toxicity 1

Mild nausea and vomiting, diarrhea.

Toxicity 2

Allergic reaction in the form of skin rash or pruritus. Usually mild.

Toxicity 3

Flu-like symptoms, including fever, flushing, and sore throat.

Methotrexate

H_2N ... chemical structure ...

Trade Names

MTX, Amethopterin

Classification

Antimetabolite

Category

Chemotherapy drug

Drug Manufacturer

Lederle Laboratories and Immunex

Mechanism of Action

- Cell cycle–specific antifolate analog, active in S-phase of the cell cycle.
- Enters cells through specific transport systems mediated by the reduced folate carrier and the folate receptor protein.
- Requires polyglutamation by the enzyme folylpolyglutamate synthase (FPGS) for its cytotoxic activity.
- Inhibition of dihydrofolate reductase (DHFR) resulting in depletion of critical reduced folates.
- Inhibition of de novo thymidylate synthesis.
- Inhibition of de novo purine synthesis.
- Incorporation of dUTP into DNA resulting in inhibition of DNA synthesis and function.

Mechanism of Resistance

- Increased expression of the target enzyme DHFR through either gene amplification or increased transcription, translation, and/or post-translational events.
- Alterations in the binding affinity of DHFR for methotrexate.
- Decreased carrier-mediated transport of drug into cell through decreased expression and/or activity of reduced folate carrier (RFC) or folate-receptor protein.

- Decreased formation of cytotoxic MTX polyglutamates through either decreased expression of FPGS or increased expression of gamma-glutamyl hydrolase (GGH).
- Decreased expression of mismatch repair enzymes may contribute to drug resistance.

Absorption

Oral bioavailability is saturable and erratic at doses greater than 25 mg/m^2. Peak serum levels are achieved within 1–2 hours of oral administration. Methotrexate is completely absorbed from parenteral routes of administration, and peak serum concentrations are reached in 30–60 minutes after IM injection.

Distribution

Widely distributed throughout the body. At conventional doses, CSF levels are only about 5%–10% of those in plasma. High-dose MTX yields therapeutic concentrations in the CSF. Distributes into third-space fluid collections such as pleural effusion and ascites. Only about 50% of drug bound to plasma proteins, mainly to albumin.

Metabolism

Extensive metabolism in liver and in cells by FPGS to higher polyglutamate forms. About 10%–20% of parent drug and the 7-hydroxymetabolite are eliminated in bile and then reabsorbed via enterohepatic circulation. Renal excretion is the main route of elimination and is mediated by glomerular filtration and tubular secretion. About 80%–90% of an administered dose is eliminated unchanged in urine within 24 hours. Terminal half-life of drug is on the order of 8–10 hours.

Indications

1. Breast cancer.
2. Head and neck cancer.
3. Osteogenic sarcoma.
4. Acute lymphoblastic leukemia.
5. Non-Hodgkin's lymphoma.
6. Primary CNS lymphoma.
7. Meningeal leukemia and carcinomatous meningitis.
8. Bladder cancer.
9. Gestational trophoblastic cancer.

Dosage Range

1. Low dose: 10–50 mg/m^2 IV every 3–4 weeks.
2. Low dose weekly: 25 mg/m^2 IV weekly.
3. Moderate dose: 100–500 mg/m^2 IV every 2–3 weeks.

4. High dose: 1–12 gm/m² IV over a 3- to 24-hour period every 1–3 weeks.

5. Intrathecal: 10–15 mg IT two times weekly until CSF is clear, then weekly dose for 2–6 weeks, followed by monthly dose.

6. Intramuscular: 25 mg/m² IM every 3 weeks.

Drug Interaction 1

Aspirin, penicillins, probenecid, nonsteroidal anti-inflammatory agents, cephalosporins, and phenytoin—These drugs inhibit the renal excretion of methotrexate leading to enhanced drug effect and toxicity.

Drug Interaction 2

Warfarin—Methotrexate may enhance the anticoagulant effect of warfarin through competitive displacement from plasma proteins.

Drug Interaction 3

5-Fluorouracil—Methotrexate enhances the antitumor activity of 5-fluorouracil when given 24 hours before fluoropyrimidine treatment.

Drug Interaction 4

Leucovorin—Leucovorin rescues the toxic effects of methotrexate and may also impair the antitumor activity. The active form of leucovorin is the L-isomer.

Drug Interaction 5

Thymidine—Thymidine rescues the toxic effects of methotrexate and may also impair the antitumor activity.

Drug Interaction 6

Folic acid supplements—Folic acid supplements may counteract the antitumor effects of methotrexate and should be discontinued while on therapy.

Drug Interaction 7

Omeprazole—Omeprazole increases serum methotrexate levels, leading to enhanced antitumor activity and host toxicity.

Drug Interaction 8

L-Asparaginase—L-Asparaginase antagonizes the antitumor activity of methotrexate.

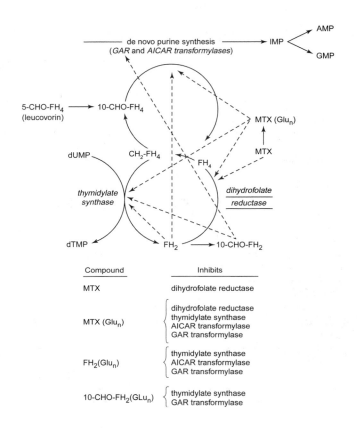

Compound	Inhibits
MTX	dihydrofolate reductase
MTX (Glu$_n$)	dihydrofolate reductase thymidylate synthase AICAR transformylase GAR transformylase
FH$_2$(Glu$_n$)	thymidylate synthase AICAR transformylase GAR transformylase
10-CHO-FH$_2$(GLu$_n$)	thymidylate synthase GAR transformylase

Special Considerations

1. Use with caution in patients with abnormal renal function. Dose should be reduced in proportion to the creatinine clearance. Important to obtain baseline creatinine clearance and to monitor renal status during therapy.

2. Instruct patients to stop folic acid supplements during therapy as they may counteract the effects of methotrexate.

3. Monitor complete blood counts on a weekly basis and more frequently with high-dose therapy.

4. Use with caution in patients with third-space fluid collections such as pleural effusion and ascites, as the half-life of methotrexate is prolonged, leading to enhanced clinical toxicity. Fluid collections should be drained before methotrexate therapy.

5. Use with caution in patients with bladder cancer status post cystectomy and ileal conduit diversion as they are at increased risk for delayed elimination of methotrexate and subsequent toxicity.

6. With high-dose therapy, methotrexate doses >1 gm/m², important to vigorously hydrate the patient with 2.5–3.5 liters/m²/day of IV 0.9% sodium chloride starting 12 hours before and for 24–48 hours after methotrexate infusion. Sodium bicarbonate (1–2 amps/L solution) should be included in the IV fluid to ensure that the urine pH is greater than 7.0 at the time of drug infusion and ideally for up to 48–72 hours after drug is given.

7. Methotrexate blood levels should be monitored in patients receiving high-dose therapy, patients with renal dysfunction (creatinine clearance <60 mL/min) regardless of dose, and patients who have experienced excessive toxicity with prior treatment with methotrexate.

8. With high-dose therapy, methotrexate blood levels should be monitored every 24 hours starting at 24 hours after methotrexate infusion. Rescue with leucovorin or L-leucovorin, the active isomer of leucovorin, should begin at 24 hours after drug infusion and should continue until the methotrexate drug level is <50 nM.

9. Patients should be instructed to lie on their side for at least 1 hour after intrathecal administration of methotrexate. This will ensure adequate delivery of drug throughout the CSF.

10. Intrathecal administration of methotrexate may lead to myelosuppression and/or mucositis as therapeutic blood levels can be achieved.

11. Methotrexate overdose can be treated with leucovorin, L-leucovorin and/or thymidine.

12. Instruct patients to avoid sun exposure for at least 1 month after therapy.

13. Pregnancy category D.

Toxicity 1

Myelosuppression. Dose-limiting toxicity with leukocyte nadir at days 4–7 and recovery usually by day 14.

Toxicity 2

Mucositis. Can be dose-limiting. Typical onset is 3–7 days after methotrexate therapy and precedes the decrease in leukocyte and platelet count. Nausea and vomiting are dose-dependent.

Toxicity 3

Acute renal failure, azotemia, urinary retention, and uric acid nephropathy. Renal toxicity results from the intratubular precipitation of methotrexate and its metabolites. Methotrexate itself may exert a direct toxic effect on the renal tubules.

Toxicity 4

Transient elevation in serum transaminases and bilirubin are often observed with high-dose therapy. May occur within the first 12–24 hours after start of infusion and returns to normal within 10 days.

Toxicity 5

Poorly defined pneumonitis characterized by fever, cough, and interstitial pulmonary infiltrates.

Toxicity 6

Acute chemical arachnoiditis with headaches, nuchal rigidity, seizures, vomiting, fever, and an inflammatory cell infiltrate in the CSF observed immediately after intrathecal administration. Chronic, demyelinating encephalopathy observed in children months to years after intrathecal methotrexate and presents as dementia, limb spasticity, and in advanced cases, coma.

Toxicity 7

Acute cerebral dysfunction with paresis, aphasia, behavioral abnormalities, and seizures observed in 5%–15% of patients receiving high-dose methotrexate. Usually occurs within 6 days of treatment and resolves within 48–72 hours. A chronic form of neurotoxicity manifested as an encephalopathy with dementia and motor paresis can develop 2–4 months after treatment.

Toxicity 8

Erythematous skin rash, pruritus, urticaria, photosensitivity, and hyperpigmentation. Radiation recall skin reaction is also observed.

Toxicity 9

Menstrual irregularities, abortion, and fetal deaths in women. Reversible oligospermia with testicular failure reported in men with high-dose therapy.

Mitomycin-C

Trade Names

Mutamycin, Mitomycin

Classification

Antitumor antibiotic

Category

Chemotherapy drug

Drug Manufacturer

Bristol-Myers Squibb

Mechanism of Action

- Isolated from the broth of *Streptomyces caespitosus* species.
- Acts as an alkylating agent to cross-link DNA resulting in inhibition of DNA synthesis and function.
- Inhibits transcription by targeting DNA-dependent RNA polymerase.
- Bioreductive activation by NADPH cytochrome P450 reductase, NADH cytochrome B450 reductase, and DT-diaphorase to oxygen free radical forms, semiquinone or hydroquinone species, which target DNA and inhibit DNA synthesis and function.
- Preferential activation of mitomycin-C in hypoxic tumor cells.

Mechanism of Resistance

- Increased expression of the multidrug-resistant gene with elevated P170 protein levels. This leads to increased drug efflux and decreased intracellular drug accumulation. Cross-resistance to anthracyclines, vinca alkaloids, and other natural products.
- Decreased bioactivation through decreased expression of DT-diaphorase.
- Increased activity of DNA excision repair enzymes.
- Increased expression of glutathione and glutathione-dependent detoxifying enzymes.

Absorption

Not available for oral use and is administered only by the IV route.

Distribution

Rapidly cleared from plasma after IV administration and widely distributed to tissues. Does not cross the blood-brain barrier.

Metabolism

Metabolism in the liver with formation of both active and inactive metabolites. Mediated by the liver cytochrome P450 system and DT-diaphorase. Bioactivation can also occur in spleen, kidney, and heart. Parent compound and its metabolites are excreted mainly through the hepatobiliary system into feces. Renal clearance accounts for only 8%–10% of drug elimination. Elimination half-life of about 50 minutes.

Indications

1. Gastric cancer.
2. Pancreatic cancer.
3. Breast cancer.
4. Non–small cell lung cancer.
5. Cervical cancer.
6. Head and neck cancer (in combination with radiation therapy).
7. Superficial bladder cancer.

Dosage Range

1. Gastric cancer: 10 mg/m^2 IV every 8 weeks, as part of the FAM regimen.
2. Breast cancer: Usual dose in various combination regimens is 10 mg/m^2 IV every 8 weeks.
3. Intravesicular therapy: Usual dose for intravesicular instillation is 40 mg administered in 20 mL of water.

Drug Interactions

None well characterized.

Special Considerations

1. Use with caution in patients with abnormal liver function. Dose reduction is required in the setting of liver dysfunction.
2. Because mitomycin-C is a potent vesicant, administer slowly over 30–60 minutes with a rapidly flowing IV. Administer drug carefully, usually through a central venous catheter. Careful monitoring is necessary to avoid extravasation. If extravasation is suspected, immediately stop infusion, withdraw fluid, elevate extremity, and apply ice to involved site. May administer local steroids. In severe cases, consult a plastic surgeon.
3. Monitor complete blood cell counts on a weekly basis. Mitomyin-C therapy results in delayed and cumulative myelosuppression.

4. Monitor patients for acute dyspnea and severe bronchospasm following drug administration. Bronchodilators, steroids, and/or oxygen may help to relieve symptoms. Risk of pulmonary toxicity increased with cumulative doses of mitomycin-C >50 mg/m².

5. FIO_2 concentrations in the perioperative period should be maintained below 50% as patients receiving mitomycin-C concurrently with other anticancer agents are at increased risk for developing ARDS. Careful attention to fluid status is important.

6. Monitor for signs of hemolytic-uremic syndrome (anemia with fragmented cells on peripheral blood smear, thrombocytopenia, and renal dysfunction), especially when total cumulative doses of mitomycin-C are >50 mg/m².

7. Monitor when used in combination with other myelosuppressive anticancer agents.

8. Pregnancy category D. Breast-feeding should be avoided.

Toxicity 1

Myelosuppression. Dose-limiting and cumulative toxicity with leukopenia being more common than thrombocytopenia. Nadir counts are delayed at about 4–6 weeks.

Toxicity 2

Nausea and vomiting. Usually mild and occurs within 1–2 hours of treatment, lasting for up to 3 days.

Toxicity 3

Mucositis is common but not dose-limiting. Observed within the first week of treatment.

Toxicity 4

Potent vesicant. Extravasation can lead to tissue necrosis and chemical thrombophlebitis at the site of injection.

Toxicity 5

Anorexia and fatigue are common.

Toxicity 6

Hemolytic-uremic syndrome. Consists of microangiopathic hemolytic anemia (hematocrit <25%), thrombocytopenia (<100,000/mm³), and renal failure (serum creatinine >1.6 mg/dL). Other complications include pulmonary edema, neurologic abnormalities, and hypertension. Rare event, seen in <2% of patients treated. Can occur at any time during treatment but usually occurs at total doses >50 mg/m². In rare cases, syndrome can be fatal.

Toxicity 7

Interstitial pneumonitis. Presents with dyspnea, non-productive cough, and interstitial infiltrates on chest x-ray. Occurs more frequently with total cumulative doses >50 mg/m².

Toxicity 8

Hepatic veno-occlusive disease. Presents with abdominal pain, hepatomegaly, and liver failure. Occurs only with high-dose therapy in transplant setting.

Toxicity 9

Chemical cystitis and bladder contraction. Observed only in setting of intravesicular therapy.

Mitotane

$$\text{(structure: benzene ring with Cl substituent)}-CH(-CHCl_2)-\text{(benzene ring)}-Cl$$

Trade Names

Lysodren

Classification

Adrenolytic agent

Category

Chemotherapy drug

Drug Manufacturer

Bristol-Myers Squibb

Mechanism of Action

- Dichloro derivative of the insecticide DDD.
- Direct toxic effect on mitochondria of adrenal cortical cells resulting in inhibition of adrenal steroid production.
- Alters the peripheral metabolism of steroids resulting in decreased levels of 17-OH corticosteroid.

Absorption

About 35%–45% of an oral dose is absorbed. Peak plasma levels are achieved in 3–5 hours.

Distribution

Widely distributed to tissues. Highly fat-soluble with large amounts of drug distributed in adipose tissues. Mitotane is slowly released with drug levels being detectable for up to 10 weeks. Does not cross the blood-brain barrier.

Metabolism

Metabolism in the liver with formation of both active and inactive metabolites. Parent compound and its metabolites are excreted mainly through the hepatobiliary system into feces (60%). Renal clearance accounts for only 10%–25% of drug elimination. Variable elimination half-life of up to 160 hours due to storage of drug in adipose tissue.

Indications

Adrenocortical cancer.

Dosage Range

Usual dose is 2–10 gm/day PO in three or four divided doses.

Drug Interaction 1

Warfarin—Mitotane alters the metabolism of warfarin, leading to an increased requirement for warfarin. Coagulation parameters, including PT and INR, should be monitored closely, and dose adjustments made accordingly.

Drug Interaction 2

Barbiturates, phenytoin, cyclophosphamide—Mitotane alters the metabolism of various drugs that are metabolized by the liver microsomal P450 system, including barbiturates, phenytoin, and cyclophosphamide.

Drug Interaction 3

Steroids—Mitotane interferes with steroid metabolism. If steroid replacement is required, doses higher than those for physiologic replacement may be needed.

Special Considerations

1. Use with caution in patients with abnormal liver function. Dose reduction is required in the setting of liver dysfunction.

2. Adrenal insufficiency may develop, and adrenal steroid replacement with glucocorticoid and/or mineralocorticoid therapy is indicated.

3. Stress-dose IV steroids are required in the event of infection, stress, trauma, and/or shock.

4. Patients should be cautioned about driving, operating complicated machinery, and/or other activities that require increased mental alertness as mitotane causes lethargy and somnolence.

5. Concurrent use of mitotane and warfarin requires careful monitoring of coagulation parameters, including PT and INR, as mitotane can alter warfarin metabolism.

6. Pregnancy category C.

Toxicity 1

Mild nausea and vomiting. Dose-limiting, occur in 80% of patients.

Toxicity 2

Lethargy, somnolence, vertigo, and dizziness. CNS side effects occur in 40% of patients.

Toxicity 3

Mucositis is common but not dose-limiting. Observed within the first week of treatment.

Toxicity 4

Transient skin rash and hyperpigmentation.

Toxicity 5

Adrenal insufficiency. Rarely occurs with steroid replacement therapy.

Mitoxantrone

$$\text{OH} \quad \text{O} \quad \text{NH}-\text{CH}_2\text{CH}_2-\text{NH}-\text{CH}_2\text{CH}_2-\text{OH}$$

$$\text{OH} \quad \text{O} \quad \text{NH}-\text{CH}_2\text{CH}_2-\text{NH}-\text{CH}_2\text{CH}_2-\text{OH}$$

Trade Names

Novantrone

Classification

Antitumor antibiotic

Category

Chemotherapy drug

Drug Manufacturer

OSI

Mechanism of Action

- Synthetic planar anthracenedione analog.
- Intercalates into DNA resulting in inhibition of DNA synthesis and function.
- Inhibits topoisomerase II by forming a cleavable complex with topoisomerase II and DNA.

Mechanism of Resistance

- Increased expression of the multidrug-resistant gene with enhanced drug efflux, resulting in decreased intracellular drug accumulation.
- Decreased expression of topoisomerase II.
- Mutation in topoisomerase II with decreased binding affinity to drug.
- Increased expression of sulfhydryl proteins, including glutathione and glutathione-associated enzymes.

Absorption

Not orally bioavailable.

Distribution

Rapid and extensive distribution to formed blood elements and to body tissues. Distributes in high concentrations in liver, bone marrow, heart, lung, and kidney. Does not cross the blood-brain barrier. Extensively bound (about 80%) to plasma proteins. Peak plasma levels are achieved immediately after IV injection.

Metabolism

Metabolism by the liver microsomal P450 system. Elimination is mainly through the hepatobiliary route with 25% of the drug excreted in feces. Renal clearance accounts for only 6%–10% of drug elimination, mainly as unchanged drug. The elimination half-life ranges from 23 to 215 hours with a median of 75 hours.

Indications

1. Advanced, hormone-refractory prostate cancer—Used in combination with prednisone as initial chemotherapy.
2. Acute myelogenous leukemia.
3. Breast cancer.
4. Non-Hodgkin's lymphoma.

Dosage Range

1. Acute myelogenous leukemia, induction therapy: 12 mg/m^2 IV on days 1–3, given in combination with ara-C, 100 mg/m^2/day IV continuous infusion for 5–7 days.
2. Prostate cancer: 12 mg/m^2 IV on day 1 every 21 days, given in combination with prednisone 5 mg PO bid.
3. Non-Hodgkin's lymphoma: 10 mg/m^2 IV on day 1 every 21 days, given as part of the CNOP or FND regimens.

Drug Interactions

Heparin—Mitoxantrone is incompatible with heparin as a precipitate will form.

Special Considerations

1. Use with caution in patients with abnormal liver function. Dose modification should be considered in patients with liver dysfunction.
2. Carefully monitor the IV injection site as mitoxantrone is a vesicant. Skin may turn blue at site of injection. Avoid extravasation, but ulceration and tissue injury are rare when drug is properly diluted.
3. Alkalinization of the urine, allopurinol, and vigorous IV hydration are recommended to prevent tumor lysis syndrome in patients with acute myelogenous leukemia.
4. Monitor cardiac function prior to (baseline) and periodically during therapy with either MUGA radionuclide scan or echocardiogram to assess LVEF. Risk of cardiac toxicity is higher in elderly patients >70 years of age, in patients with prior history of hypertension or pre-existing heart disease, in patients previously treated with anthracyclines, or in patients with prior radiation therapy to the chest. Cumulative doses of 140 mg/m^2 in patients with no prior history of anthracycline therapy and 120 mg/m^2 in patients with

prior anthracycline therapy are associated with increased risk for cardiotoxicity. A decrease in LVEF by 15%–20% is an indication to discontinue treatment.

5. Monitor complete blood counts while on therapy.

6. Patients may experience blue-green urine for up to 24 hours after drug administration.

7. Pregnancy category D. Breast-feeding should be avoided.

Toxicity 1

Myelosuppression. Dose-limiting toxicity with neutropenia more common than thrombocytopenia. Nadir typically occurs at 10–14 days after treatment but may occur earlier in acute leukemia, with recovery of counts by day 21. Risk of myelosuppression is greater in elderly patients and in those previously treated with chemotherapy and/or radiation therapy.

Toxicity 2

Nausea and vomiting are observed in 70% of patients. Usually mild, occurs less frequently than with doxorubicin.

Toxicity 3

Mucositis and diarrhea. Common but usually not severe.

Toxicity 4

Cardiotoxicity. Cardiac effects are similar to but less severe than those of doxorubicin. Acute toxicity presents as atrial arrhythmias, chest pain, and myopericarditis syndrome that typically occurs within the first 24–48 hours of drug administration. Transient and mostly asymptomatic.

Chronic toxicity is manifested in the form of a dilated cardiomyopathy with congestive heart failure. Cumulative doses of 140 mg/m^2 in patients with no prior history of anthracycline therapy and 120 mg/m^2 in patients with prior anthracycline therapy are associated with increased risk for developing congestive cardiomyopathy.

Toxicity 5

Alopecia. Observed in 40% of patients but less severe than with doxorubicin.

Toxicity 6

Transient and reversible effects on liver enzymes including SGOT and SGPT.

Toxicity 7

Blue discoloration of fingernails, sclera, and urine for 1–2 days after treatment.

Secondary acute myelogenous leukemia.

Nelarabine

Trade Names

Arranon, 9-β-D-Arabinofuranosylguanine, Ara-G

Classification

Antimetabolite

Category

Chemotherapy drug

Drug Manufacturer

GlaxoSmithKline

Mechanism of Action

- Prodrug of the deoxyguanosine analog 9-β-D-arabinofuranosylguanine (ara-G).
- Cell cycle–specific with activity in the S-phase.
- Requires intracellular activation to the nucleotide metabolite ara-GTP.
- Incorporation of ara-GTP into DNA resulting in chain termination and inhibition of DNA synthesis and function.

Mechanism of Resistance

- Decreased activation of drug through decreased expression of the anabolic enzyme deoxycytidine kinase.
- Decreased transport of drug into cells.

Absorption

Poor oral bioavailability. Administered by the IV route.

Distribution

Extensively distributed in the body. Binding to plasma proteins has not been well characterized.

Metabolism

Undergoes metabolism by adenosine deaminase to form ara-G, which undergoes subsequent hydrolysis to form guanine. A minor route of nelarabine metabolism is via hydrolysis to form methylguanine, which is then demethylated to form guanine. Nelarabine and ara-G are rapidly eliminated from plasma with a half-life in adults of approximately 30 minutes and 3 hours, respectively. Nelarabine (5-10%) and ara-G (20-30%) are eliminated, to a minor extent, by the kidneys. The mean clearance of nelarabine is approximately 30% higher in pediatric patients than adult patients, while the clearance of ara-G is similar in the two patient populations. Age and gender have no effects on nelarabine or ara-G pharmacokinetics.

Indications

1. FDA-approved for T-cell acute lymphoblastic leukemia (T-ALL) that has not responded to or has relapsed following treatment with at least 2 chemotherapy regimens.
2. FDA-approved for T-cell lymphoblastic lymphoma (T-LBL) that has not responded to or has relapsed following treatment with at least 2 chemotherapy regimens.

Dosage Range

1. Pediatric patients: 650 mg/m^2/day IV over 1 hour on days 1–5 every 21 days.
2. Adult patients: 1,500 mg/m^2/day IV over 2 hours on days 1, 3, and 5 every 28 days.

Drug Interactions

Pentostatin—Treatment with adenosine deaminase inhibitors, such as pentostatin, may reduce the conversion of nelarabine to its active form, thereby leading to a change in its efficacy and/or safety profile.

Special Considerations

1. Monitor CBCs on a regular basis during therapy.
2. Closely monitor for neurologic events, as this represents a black-box warning.
3. Patients treated previously or concurrently with intrathecal chemotherapy and/or previously with craniospinal radiation therapy may be at increased risk for developing neurotoxicity.
4. Patients should be advised against performing activities that require mental alertness, including operating hazardous machinery and driving.

5. Alkalinization of the urine (pH >7.0), allopurinol, and vigorous IV hydration are recommended to prevent tumor lysis syndrome.

6. Pregnancy category D.

Toxicity 1

Myelosuppression is the most common toxicity with neutropenia, thrombocytopenia, and anemia.

Toxicity 2

Nausea and vomiting. Mild to moderate emetogenic agent.

Toxicity 3

Neurotoxicity is dose-limiting with headache, altered mental status, seizures, and peripheral neuropathy with numbness, paresthesias, motor weakness, and paralysis. Rare events of demyelination and ascending peripheral neuropathies similar to Guillain-Barre syndrome have been reported.

Toxicity 4

Mild hepatic dysfunction with elevation of serum transaminases and bilirubin.

Toxicity 5

Fatigue and asthenia.

Nilotinib

N

HCl, H₂O

Trade Name	
	Tasigna, AMN107

Classification	
	Signal transduction inhibitor

Category	
	Chemotherapy drug

Drug Manufacturer	
	Novartis

Mechanism of Action

- Second-generation phenylaminopyrimidine inhibitor of the BCR-ABL, c-KIT, and PDGFR-β tyrosine kinases.
- Higher binding affinity (up to 20- to 50-fold) and selectivity for ABL kinase domain when compared to imatinib and overcomes imatinib resistance resulting from BCR-ABL mutations.

Mechanism of Resistance

Single-point mutation within the ATP-binding pocket of the ABL tyrosine kinase (T315I).

Absorption

Nilotinib has good oral bioavailability. Rapidly absorbed following oral administration. Peak plasma concentrations are observed within 3 hours of oral ingestion.

Distribution

Extensive binding of parent drug to plasma proteins in the range of 95%–98%.

Metabolism

Metabolized in the liver primarily by CYP3A4 microsomal enzymes. Other liver P450 enzymes, such as UGT, play a relatively minor role in metabolism. None of the metabolites are biologically active. Approximately 90% of an administered dose is eliminated in feces within 7 days. The terminal half-life of the parent drug is in the order of 15–17 hours.

Indications

FDA-approved for the treatment of adults with chronic phase (CP) and accelerated phase (AP) Philadelphia chromosome-positive CML with resistance or intolerance to prior therapy that included imatinib.

Dosage Range

Recommended dose is 400 mg PO bid.

Drug Interaction 1

Nilotinib is an inhibitor of CYP3A4 and may decrease the metabolic clearance of drugs that are metabolized by CYP3A4.

Drug Interaction 2

Drugs such as ketoconazole, itraconazole, erythromycin, and clarithromycin may decrease the rate of metabolism of nilotinib, resulting in increased drug levels and potentially increased toxicity.

Drug Interaction 3

Drugs such as rifampin, Dilantin, phenobarbital, carbamazepine, and St. John's wort may increase the rate of metabolism of nilotinib, resulting in its inactivation.

Drug Interaction 4

Nilotinib is a substrate of the P-glycoprotein (Pgp) transporter. Caution should be used in patients on drugs that inhibit Pgp (e.g., verapamil) as this may lead to increased concentrations of nilotinib.

Special Considerations

1. Nilotinib tablets should not be taken with food for at least 2 hours before a dose is taken and for at least 1 hour after a dose is taken.

2. Important to review patient's list of medications as nilotinib has several potential drug–drug interactions.

3. Monitor CBC every 2 weeks for the first 2 months, and monthly thereafter.

4. Use with caution in patients with a prior history of pancreatitis. Serum lipase levels should be checked periodically.

5. Nilotinib should not be used in patients with hypokalemia, hypomagnesemia, or long QT syndrome. Electrolyte abnormalities must be corrected prior to initiation of therapy, and electrolyte status should be monitored periodically during therapy.

6. ECGs should be performed at baseline, 7 days after initiation of therapy, and periodically thereafter.

7. Patients should be warned about not taking St. John's wort while on nilotinib therapy.

8. Avoid grapefruit and grapefruit juice while on therapy.

9. Pregnancy category D.

Toxicity 1

Myelosuppression with thrombocytopenia, neutropenia, and anemia.

Toxicity 2

Prolongation of QT interval, which on rare occasions, may lead to sudden death.

Toxicity 3

Elevations in serum lipase.

Toxicity 4

Electrolyte abnormalities with hypophosphatemia, hypokalemia, hypocalcemia, and hyponatremia.

Toxicity 5

Fatigue, asthenia, and anorexia.

Toxicity 6

Elevations in serum transaminases and/or bilirubin (usually indirect bilirubin).

Nilutamide

Trade Names
Nilandron

Classification
Antiandrogen

Category
Hormonal agent

Drug Manufacturer
Sanofi-Aventis

Mechanism of Action
Nonsteroidal, anti-androgen agent that binds to androgen receptor and inhibits androgen uptake. It also inhibits androgen binding in the nucleus of androgen-sensitive prostate cancer cells.

Mechanism of Resistance
- Decreased expression of androgen receptor.
- Mutation in androgen receptor leading to decreased binding affinity to nilutamide.

Absorption
Rapidly and completely absorbed by the GI tract. Absorption is not affected by food.

Distribution
Distribution is not well characterized. Moderate binding of nilutamide to plasma proteins.

Metabolism
Extensive metabolism occurs in the liver to both active and inactive metabolites. About 60% of the drug is excreted in urine, mainly in metabolite form, and only minimal clearance in feces. The elimination half-life is approximately 41–49 hours.

Indications

Stage D2 metastatic prostate cancer in combination with surgical castration.

Dosage Range

Recommended dose is 300 mg PO daily for 30 days, then 150 mg PO daily.

Drug Interaction 1

Warfarin—Nilutamide can inhibit metabolism of warfarin by the liver P450 system leading to increased anticoagulant effect. Coagulation parameters, PT and INR, must be followed routinely, and dose adjustments may be needed.

Drug Interaction 2

Drugs metabolized by the liver P450 system—Nilutamide inhibits the activity of liver cytochrome P450 enzymes and may therefore reduce the metabolism of various compounds, including phenytoin and theophylline. Enhanced toxicity of these agents may be observed, requiring dose adjustment.

Drug Interaction 3

Alcohol—Increased risk of alcohol intolerance following treatment with nilutamide.

Special Considerations

1. Should be given on the same day or on the day after surgical castration to achieve maximal benefit.

2. Nilutamide can be taken with or without food.

3. Should be used with caution in patients with abnormal liver function and is contraindicated in patients with severe liver impairment. Monitor liver function tests at baseline and during therapy.

4. Contraindicated in patients with severe respiratory insufficiency. Baseline PFTs and chest x-ray should be obtained in all patients and periodically during therapy. If findings of interstitial pneumonitis appear on chest x-ray or there is a significant decrease by 20%–25% in DLCO and FVC on PFTs, treatment with nilutamide should be terminated.

5. Caution patients about the potential for hot flashes. Consider the use of clonidine 0.1–0.2 mg PO daily, Megace 20 mg PO bid, or soy tablets one tablet PO tid for prevention and/or treatment.

6. Instruct patients on the potential risk of altered sexual function and impotence.

7. Patients should be advised to abstain from alcohol while on nilutamide as there is an increased risk of intolerance (facial flushes, malaise, hypotension) to alcohol.

8. Pregnancy category C.

Toxicity 1

Hot flashes, decreased libido, impotence, gynecomastia, nipple pain, and galactorrhea.

Toxicity 2

Visual disturbances in the form of impaired adaptation to dark, abnormal vision, and alterations in color vision. Occurs in up to 57% of patients and results in treatment discontinuation in 1%–2% of patients.

Toxicity 3

Anorexia, nausea, and constipation. Transient elevations in serum transaminases are uncommon.

Toxicity 4

Cough, dyspnea, and interstitial pneumonitis occur rarely in about 2% of patients. Usually observed within the first 3 months of treatment. Incidence may be higher in patients of Asian descent.

Oxaliplatin

Trade Names

Eloxatin, Diaminocyclohexane platinum, DACH-platinum

Classification

Platinum analog

Category

Chemotherapy drug

Drug Manufacturer

Sanofi-Aventis

Mechanism of Action

- Third-generation platinum compound.
- Cell cycle–nonspecific with activity in all phases of the cell cycle.
- Covalently binds to DNA with preferential binding to the N-7 position of guanine and adenine.
- Reacts with two different sites on DNA to produce cross-links, either intrastrand (>90%) or interstrand (<5%). Formation of DNA adducts results in inhibition of DNA synthesis and function as well as inhibition of transcription.
- DNA mismatch repair enzymes are unable to recognize oxaliplatin-DNA adducts in contrast with other platinum-DNA adducts as a result of their bulkier size.
- Binding to nuclear and cytoplasmic proteins may result in additional cytotoxic effects.

Mechanism of Resistance

- Decreased drug accumulation due to alterations in cellular transport.
- Increased inactivation by thiol-containing proteins such as glutathione and glutathione-related enzymes.
- Increased DNA repair enzyme activity (e.g., ERCC-1).
- Non–cross-resistant to cisplatin and carboplatin in tumor cells that are deficient in MMR enzymes (e.g., hMHL1, hMSH2).

O

Absorption

Not orally bioavailable.

Distribution

Widely distributed to all tissues with a 50-fold higher volume of distribution than cisplatin. About 40% of drug is sequestered in red blood cells within 2–5 hours of infusion. Extensively binds to plasma proteins in time-dependent manner (up to 98%).

Metabolism

Oxaliplatin undergoes extensive non-enzymatic conversion to its active cytotoxic species. As observed with cisplatin, oxaliplatin undergoes aquation reaction in the presence of low concentrations of chloride. The major species are monochloro-DACH, dichloro-DACH, and mono-diaquo-DACH platinum. Renal excretion accounts for >50% of oxaliplatin clearance. More than 20 different metabolites have been identified in the urine. Only 2% of drug is excreted in feces. Prolonged terminal half-life of up to 240 hours.

Indications

1. Metastatic colorectal cancer—FDA-approved in combination with infusional 5-FU/LV in patients with advanced, metastatic disease.

2. Early-stage colon cancer—FDA-approved as adjuvant therapy in combination with infusional 5-FU/LV in patients with stage III colon cancer. Also effective in patients with high-risk stage II disease.

3. Metastatic pancreatic cancer.

4. Metastatic gastro-esophageal cancer.

Dosage Range

Recommended dose is 85 mg/m² IV over 2 hours, on an every-2-week schedule. Can also administer 100–130 mg/m² IV on an every-3-week schedule.

Drug Interactions

None known.

Special Considerations

1. Use with caution in patients with abnormal renal function, especially when CrCl <20 mL/min. Baseline creatinine clearance should be obtained, and renal status should be closely monitored during treatment.

2. Oxaliplatin should not be administered with basic solutions (e.g., solutions containing 5-FU) as it may be partially degraded.

3. Careful neurologic evaluation should be performed before starting therapy and at the beginning of each cycle as the dose-limiting toxicity of oxaliplatin is neurotoxicity.

4. Caution patients to avoid exposure to cold following drug administration, which can trigger and/or worsen acute neurotoxicity.

5. Calcium/magnesium infusions (1 gm calcium gluconate/1 gm magnesium sulfate) prior to and at the completion of the oxaliplatin infusion can be used to reduce the incidence of acute neurotoxicity. There is no evidence that these infusions impair the clinical activity of oxaliplatin.

6. Anaphylactic reactions to oxaliplatin have been reported and may occur within minutes of drug administration. This represents a black-box warning.

7. Pregnancy category D.

Toxicity 1

Neurotoxicity with acute and chronic forms. Acute toxicity is seen in 80%–85% of patients and is characterized by a peripheral sensory neuropathy with distal paresthesias, visual and voice changes, often triggered or exacerbated by cold. Dysesthesias in the upper extremities and laryngopharyngeal region with episodes of difficulty breathing or swallowing are also observed usually within hours or 1–3 days after therapy. Risk increases upon exposure to cold and usually is spontaneously reversible. Chronic toxicity is dose-dependent with a 15% and >50% risk of impairment in proprioception and neurosensory function at cumulative doses of 850 and 1,200 mg/m^2, respectively. In contrast to cisplatin-induced neurotoxicity, oxaliplatin-induced neuropathy is reversible, and returns to normal usually within 3–4 months of discontinuation of oxaliplatin. Gait abnormalities and cognitive dysfunction can also occur.

Toxicity 2

Nausea and vomiting. Occur in 65% of patients treated with single-agent oxaliplatin and in 90% of patients treated with the combination of 5-FU/LV and oxaliplatin. Well-controlled with antiemetic therapy.

Toxicity 3

Diarrhea.

Toxicity 4

Myelosuppression. Relatively mild with thrombocytopenia and anemia more common than neutropenia.

Toxicity 5

Allergic reactions with facial flushing, rash, urticaria, and less frequently, bronchospasm and hypotension. In rare cases, anaphylactic-like reactions can occur.

Toxicity 6

Hepatotoxicity with sinusoidal injury resulting in portal hypertension, ascites, splenomegaly, thrombocytopenia, and varices.

Toxicity 7

RPLS has been observed with headache, lethargy, seizures, visual disturbances, and encephalopathy.

Paclitaxel

Trade Names

Taxol

Classification

Taxane, anti-microtubule agent

Category

Chemotherapy drug

Drug Manufacturer

Bristol-Myers Squibb

Mechanism of Action

- Isolated from the bark of the Pacific yew tree, *Taxus brevifolia*.
- Cell cycle–specific, active in the mitosis (M) phase of the cell cycle.
- High-affinity binding to microtubules enhances tubulin polymerization. Normal dynamic process of microtubule network is inhibited, leading to inhibition of mitosis and cell division.

Mechanism of Resistance

- Alterations in tubulin with decreased binding affinity for drug.
- Multidrug-resistant phenotype with increased expression of P170 glycoprotein. Results in enhanced drug efflux with decreased intracellular accumulation of drug. Cross-resistant to other natural products, including vinca alkaloids, anthracyclines, taxanes, and VP-16.

Absorption

Poorly soluble and not orally bioavailable.

Distribution

Distributes widely to all body tissues, including third-space fluid collections such as ascites. Negligible penetration into the CNS. Extensive binding (>90%) to plasma and cellular proteins.

Metabolism

Metabolized extensively by the hepatic P450 microsomal system. About 70%–80% of drug is excreted via fecal elimination. Less than 10% is eliminated as the parent form with the majority being eliminated as metabolites. Renal clearance is relatively minor with less than 10% of drug cleared via the kidneys. Terminal elimination half-life ranges from 9 to 50 hours depending on the schedule of administration.

Indications

1. Ovarian cancer.
2. Breast cancer.
3. Non–small cell and small cell lung cancer.
4. Head and neck cancer.
5. Esophageal cancer.
6. Prostate cancer.
7. Bladder cancer.
8. AIDS-related Kaposi's sarcoma.

Dosage Range

1. Ovarian cancer: 135–175 mg/m² IV as a 3-hour infusion every 3 weeks.
2. Breast cancer: 175 mg/m² IV as a 3-hour infusion every 3 weeks.
3. Bladder cancer, head and neck cancer: 250 mg/m² IV as a 24-hour infusion every 3 weeks.
4. Weekly schedule: 80–100 mg/m² IV each week for 3 weeks with 1 week rest.
5. Infusional schedule: 140 mg/m² as a 96-hour infusion.

Drug Interaction 1

Radiation therapy–Paclitaxel is a radiosensitizing agent.

Drug Interaction 2

Concomitant use of inhibitors and/or activators of the liver cytochrome P450 CYP3A4 enzyme system may affect paclitaxel metabolism and its subsequent antitumor and host toxic effects.

Drug Interaction 3

Phenytoin, phenobarbital—Accelerate the metabolism of paclitaxel resulting in lower plasma levels of drug.

Drug Interaction 4

Cisplatin, carboplatin—Myelosuppression is greater when platinum compound is administered before paclitaxel. Platinum compounds inhibit plasma clearance of paclitaxel. When a platinum analog is used in combination, paclitaxel must be given first.

Drug Interaction 5

Cyclophosphamide—Myelosuppression is greater when cyclophosphamide is administered before paclitaxel.

Drug Interaction 6

Doxorubicin—Paclitaxel reduces the plasma clearance of doxorubicin by 30%–35%, resulting in increased severity of myelosuppression.

Special Considerations

1. Contraindicated in patients with history of severe hypersensitivity reaction to paclitaxel or to other drugs formulated in Cremophor EL, including cyclosporine, etoposide, or teniposide.

2. Use with caution in patients with abnormal liver function. Dose reduction is required in this setting. Patients with abnormal liver function are at significantly higher risk for host toxicity. Contraindicated in patients with severe hepatic dysfunction.

3. Use with caution in patients with prior history of diabetes mellitus and chronic alcoholism or prior therapy with known neurotoxic agents such as cisplatin.

4. Use with caution in patients with previous history of ischemic heart disease, with myocardial infarction within the preceding 6 months, conduction system abnormalities, or on medications known to alter cardiac conduction (beta blockers, calcium channel blockers, and digoxin).

5. Patients should receive premedication to prevent the incidence of hypersensitivity reactions (HSR). Give dexamethasone 20 mg PO at 12 and 6 hours before drug administration, diphenhydramine 50 mg IV, and cimetidine 300 mg IV at 30 minutes before drug administration. Patients experiencing major HSR may be rechallenged after receiving multiple high doses of steroids, dexamethasone 20 mg IV every 6 hr for 4 doses. Patients should also be treated with diphenhydramine 50 mg IV and cimetidine 300 mg IV 30 minutes before the rechallenge.

6. Medical personnel should be readily available at the time of drug administration. Emergency equipment, including Ambu bag, EKG machine, IV fluids, pressors, and other drugs for resuscitation, must be at bedside before initiation of treatment.

7. Monitor patient's vital signs every 15 minutes during the first hour of drug administration. HSR usually occurs within 2–3 minutes of start of infusion and almost always within the first 10 minutes.

8. Patients who have received >6 courses of weekly paclitaxel should be advised to avoid exposure of their skin as well as their fingernails and toenails to the sun as they are at increased risk for developing onycholysis. This side effect is not observed with the every-3-week schedule.

9. Pregnancy category D. Breast-feeding should be avoided.

Toxicity 1

Myelosuppression. Dose-limiting neutropenia with nadir at day 8–10 and recovery by day 15–21. Decreased incidence of neutropenia with 3-hour schedule when compared to 24-hour schedule.

Toxicity 2

HSR. Occurs in up to 20%–40% of patients. Characterized by generalized skin rash, flushing, erythema, hypotension, dyspnea, and/or bronchospasm. Usually occurs within the first 2–3 minutes of an infusion and almost always within the first 10 minutes. Incidence of HSR is the same with 3- and 24-hour schedules. Premedication regimen, as outlined in Special Considerations, has significantly decreased incidence.

Toxicity 3

Neurotoxicity mainly in the form of sensory neuropathy with numbness and paresthesias. Dose-dependent effect. Other risk factors include prior exposure to known neurotoxic agents (e.g., cisplatin) and pre-existing medical disorders such as diabetes mellitus and chronic alcoholism. Also more frequent with longer infusions and at doses >175 mg/m². Motor and autonomic neuropathy observed at high doses. Optic nerve disturbances with scintillating scotomata observed rarely.

Toxicity 4

Transient asymptomatic sinus bradycardia is most commonly observed cardiotoxicity. Occurs in 30% of patients. Other rhythm disturbances are seen, including Mobitz type I, Mobitz type II, and third-degree heart block, as well as ventricular arrhythmias.

Toxicity 5

Alopecia. Occurs in nearly all patients, with loss of total body hair.

Toxicity 6

Mucositis and/or diarrhea seen in 30%–40% of patients. Mucositis is more common with the 24-hour schedule. Mild to moderate nausea and vomiting, usually of brief duration.

Toxicity 7

Transient elevations in serum transaminases, bilirubin, and alkaline phosphatase.

Toxicity 8

Onycholysis. Mainly observed in those receiving >6 courses on the weekly schedule. Not seen with the every-3-week schedule.

Panitumumab

Trade Name

Vectibix

Classification

Monoclonal antibody, anti-EGFR antibody

Category

Biologic response modifier agent

Drug Manufacturer

Amgen

Mechanism of Action

- Fully human IgG2 monoclonal antibody directed against the EGFR.
- Precise mechanism(s) of action remains unknown.
- Binds with nearly 40-fold higher affinity to EGFR than normal ligands EGF and TGF-α, which results in inhibition of EGFR. Prevents both homodimerization and heterodimerization of the EGFR, which leads to inhibition of autophosphorylation and inhibition of EGFR signaling.
- Inhibition of the EGFR signaling pathway results in inhibition of critical mitogenic and anti-apoptotic signals involved in proliferation, growth, invasion/metastasis, and angiogenesis.
- Inhibition of the EGFR pathway enhances the response to chemotherapy and/or radiation therapy.

Mechanism of Resistance

- Mutations in the EGFR leading to decreased binding affinity to panitumumab.
- Decreased expression of EGFR.
- Presence of KRAS mutations, which mainly occur in codons 12 and 13.
- BRAF mutations.
- Activation/induction of alternative cellular signaling pathways, such as PI3K/Akt and IGF-1R.

Distribution

Distribution in the body is not well characterized.

Metabolism

Metabolism of panitumumab has not been extensively characterized. Pharmacokinetic studies showed clearance of antibody was saturated at a weekly dose of 2 mg/kg. Half-life is on the order of 6 to 7 days with minimal clearance by the liver or kidneys.

Indications

1. FDA-approved as monotherapy for the treatment of advanced colorectal cancer following fluoropyrimidine-, oxaliplatin-, and irinotecan-containing regimens. Use of panitumumab is not recommended in mutant KRAS CRC.

2. Approved in Europe as monotherapy for advanced, refractory disease in wild-type KRAS CRC.

Dosage Range

1. Recommended dose for the treatment of advanced colorectal cancer is 6 mg/kg IV on an every 2 week schedule.

2. An alternative schedule is 2.5 mg/kg IV every week.

Drug Interactions

No formal drug interactions have been characterized to date.

Special Considerations

1. The incidence of infusion reactions is lower when compared with cetuximab anti-EGFR therapy, as panitumumab is a fully human antibody.

2. The level of EGFR expression does not correlate with clinical activity, and as such, EGFR testing should not be required for clinical use.

3. KRAS testing should be performed in all patients to determine KRAS status. Only patients whose tumors express wild-type KRAS should receive panitumumab therapy.

4. Development of skin toxicity appears to be a surrogate marker for panitumumab clinical activity.

5. Use with caution in patients with underlying interstitial lung disease as these patients are at increased risk for developing worsening of their interstitial lung disease.

6. In patients who develop a skin rash, topical antibiotics such as Cleocin gel or either oral Cleocin and/or oral minocycline may help. Patients should be warned to avoid sunlight exposure.

7. Electrolyte status (magnesium and calcium) should be closely monitored during therapy and for up to 8 weeks after completion of therapy.

8. Pregnancy category C. Breast-feeding should be avoided.

Toxicity 1

Pruritus, dry skin with mainly a pustular, acneiform skin rash. Presents mainly on the face and upper trunk. Improves with continued treatment and resolves upon cessation of therapy.

Toxicity 2

Infusion-related symptoms with fever, chills, urticaria, flushing, and headache. Usually minor in severity and observed most commonly with administration of the first infusion.

Toxicity 3

Pulmonary toxicity in the form of ILD manifested by increased cough, dyspnea, and pulmonary infiltrates. Observed rarely in less than 1% of patients and more frequent in patients with underlying pulmonary disease.

Toxicity 4

Hypomagnesemia.

Toxicity 5

Diarrhea.

Toxicity 6

Asthenia and generalized malaise observed in up to 10% to 15%.

Toxicity 7

Paronychial inflammation with swelling of the lateral nail folds of the toes and fingers. Usually occurs with prolonged use of panitumumab.

Pegfilgrastim

Trade Names

Neulasta, PEG-rHuG-CSF

Classification

Colony-stimulating growth factor, cytokine

Category

Biologic response modifier agent

Drug Manufacturer

Amgen

Mechanism of Action

- Covalent conjugate of recombinant methionyl human G-CSF (filgrastim) and monomethoxypolyethylene glycol. The molecular weight of pegfilgrastim is approximately 39 kDa.
- Pleiotropic cytokine that binds to specific surface receptors of hematopoietic progenitor cells.
- Stimulates the proliferation, differentiation, and activation of granulocyte progenitor cells and the activity of mature granulocytes.
- Enhances neutrophil chemotaxis and phagocytosis.
- Does not possess antitumor activity.

Absorption

Pegfilgrastim is rapidly and completely absorbed into the circulation after an SC dose, with peak plasma concentration achieved 2–8 hours after administration.

Distribution

Distributes into blood and bone marrow. Binding to plasma proteins not known.

Metabolism

Metabolized in both the liver and the kidney. Pegfilgrastim has reduced renal clearance and prolonged persistence in vivo when compared with filgrastim. The terminal half-life ranges from 15 to 80 hours.

Indications

Adjunct to myelosuppressive chemotherapy—Prophylactic use in patients with non-myeloid malignancies receiving chemotherapy with either previous history of drug-related neutropenia and/or fever or in patients receiving drugs associated with a significant incidence of severe neutropenia and fever.

Dosage Range

Prevention of chemotherapy-induced neutropenia: single SC injection of 6 mg, administered once per chemotherapy cycle.

Drug Interactions

Steroids, lithium—Caution should be exercised when using these drugs concurrently with pegfilgrastim as they may potentiate the release of neutrophils during pegfilgrastim therapy.

Special Considerations

1. Contraindicated in patients with known hypersensitivity to *E. coli*-derived products, pegfilgrastim, filgrastim, and/or any component contained within the product.

2. Concurrent administration with chemotherapy is contraindicated as an increased incidence of serious adverse events has been observed. Pegfilgrastim should **NOT** be administered in the period between 14 days before and 24 hours after administration of chemotherapy as the stimulatory effects of G-CSF on the hematopoietic precursors render them more susceptible to chemotherapy.

3. Blood counts should be monitored closely following pegfilgrastim therapy.

4. Pegfilgrastim is incompatible with saline-containing solutions.

5. Use with caution in patients receiving steroids or lithium as these drugs may potentiate the release of neutrophils.

6. Use with caution in patients with sickle cell disease as severe sickle cell crises have been observed in patients receiving filgrastim therapy. Patients with sickle cell disease who receive pegfilgrastim should be well hydrated and closely monitored.

7. Pegfilgrastim is **NOT** indicated for mobilization of peripheral blood progenitor cells.

8. Rare cases of splenic rupture have been reported following filgrastim therapy. Patients who report left upper quadrant abdominal pain and/or shoulder pain should be immediately evaluated for an enlarged spleen and/or splenic rupture.

9. Closely monitor patients for the onset of fever, pulmonary infiltrates, or respiratory distress as ARDS has been reported in neutropenic patients with sepsis receiving filgrastim, the parent compound of pegfilgrastim.

10. Premedication with acetaminophen helps to relieve the bone pain that arises due to bone marrow expansion in response to treatment.

11. Pregnancy category C. Breast-feeding should be avoided.

Toxicity 1

Transient bone pain occurs in up to 25% of patients. Usually mild to moderate and well controlled with non-narcotic medications.

Toxicity 2

HSR in the form of skin rash, urticaria, and anaphylaxis is uncommon.

Toxicity 3

Leukocytosis observed in less than 1% of patients and usually not associated with any adverse effects.

Toxicity 4

Transient elevations in serum lactate dehydrogenase, alkaline phosphatase, and uric acid.

Pemetrexed

Trade Names

Alimta, LY231514

Classification

Antimetabolite

Category

Chemotherapy drug

Drug Manufacturer

Eli Lilly

Mechanism of Action

- Pyrrolopyrimidine antifolate analog with activity in the S-phase of the cell cycle.

- Transported into the cell primarily via the RFC and to a smaller extent by the folate-receptor protein (FRP).

- Metabolized intracellularly to higher polyglutamate forms by the enzyme folylpolyglutamate synthase (FPGS). The pentaglutamate form is the predominant intracellular species. Pemetrexed polyglutamates are approximately 60-fold more potent than the parent monoglutamate compound, and they exhibit prolonged cellular retention.

- Inhibition of the folate-dependent enzyme thymidylate synthase (TS) resulting in inhibition of de novo thymidylate and DNA synthesis. This represents the main site of action of the drug.

- Inhibition of TS leads to accumulation of dUMP and subsequent incorporation of dUTP into DNA, resulting in inhibition of DNA synthesis and function.

- Inhibition of dihydrofolate reductase, resulting in depletion of reduced folates and of critical one-carbon carriers for cellular metabolism.

- Inhibition of de novo purine biosynthesis through inhibition of glycinamide ribonucleotide formyltransferase (GART) and aminoimidazole carboxamide ribonucleotide formyltransferase (AICART).

Mechanism of Resistance

- Increased expression of the target enzyme TS.
- Alterations in the binding affinity of TS for pemetrexed.
- Decreased transport of drug into cells through decreased expression of the RFC and/or FRP.
- Decreased polyglutamation of drug, resulting in decreased formation of cytotoxic metabolites.

Absorption

Pemetrexed is given only by the IV route.

Distribution

Peak plasma levels are reached in less than 30 minutes. Widely distributed throughout the body. Tissue concentrations highest in liver, kidneys, small intestine, and colon.

Metabolism

Significant intracellular metabolism of drug to the polyglutamated species. Metabolism in the liver through as yet undefined mechanisms. Principally cleared by renal excretion with as much as 90% of the drug in the urine unchanged during the first 24 hours after administration. Short distribution half-life in plasma with a mean of 3 hours. However, relatively prolonged terminal half-life of about 20 hours and a prolonged intracellular half-life as a result of pemetrexed polyglutamates.

Indications

1. Mesothelioma—FDA-approved in combination with cisplatin for treatment of locally advanced or metastatic non-squamous non-small cell lung cancer.

2. Non–small cell lung cancer—FDA-approved in combination with cisplatin for the initial treatment of locally advanced or metastatic non-squamous non-small cell lung cancer.

3. Non–small cell lung cancer—FDA-approved as second-line monotherapy for locally advanced or metastatic non-squamous non-small cell lung cancer.

4. Non–small cell lung cancer—FDA-approved as maintenance treatment of locally advanced or metastatic non-squamous non-small cell lung cancer whose disease has not progressed after 4 cycles of platinum-based first-line chemotherapy.

5. Pemetrexed should not be used in patients with squamous cell non-small cell lung cancer.

Dosage Range

1. Recommended dose as a single agent is 500 mg/m^2 IV every 3 weeks.

2. When used in combination with cisplatin, recommended dose is 500 mg/m^2 IV every 3 weeks.

Drug Interaction 1

Thymidine—Thymidine rescues against the host toxic effects of pemetrexed.

Drug Interaction 2

5-FU—Pemetrexed may enhance the antitumor activity of 5-FU. Precise mechanism of interaction remains unknown.

Drug Interaction 3

Leucovorin—Administration of leucovorin may decrease the antitumor activity of pemetrexed.

Drug Interaction 4

NSAIDs and aspirin—Concomitant administration of NSAIDs and aspirin may inhibit the renal excretion of pemetrexed, resulting in enhanced drug toxicity.

Special Considerations

1. Use with caution in patients with abnormal renal function. Dose should be reduced in proportion to the creatinine clearance. Important to obtain baseline creatinine clearance and to monitor renal function before each cycle of therapy.

2. Dose reduction is not necessary in patients with mild to moderate liver impairment.

3. Monitor CBCs on a periodic basis.

4. Dietary folate status of patient may be an important factor in determining risk for clinical toxicity. Patients with insufficient folate intake may be at increased risk for host toxicity. Evaluation of serum homocysteine and folate levels at baseline and during therapy may be helpful. A baseline serum homocysteine level >10 is a good predictor for the development of grade 3/4 toxicities.

5. All patients should receive vitamin supplementation with 350 µg/day of folic acid PO and 1,000 µg of vitamin B12 SC every three cycles to reduce the risk and incidence of toxicity while on drug therapy. Folic acid supplementation should begin 7 days prior to initiation of pemetrexed treatment, and the first vitamin B12 injection should be administered at least 1 week prior to the start of pemetrexed. No evidence that vitamin supplementation reduces clinical efficacy.

6. Prophylactic use of steroids may ameliorate and/or completely eliminate the development of skin rash. Dexamethasone can be given at a dose of 4 mg PO bid for 3 days beginning the day before therapy.

7. NSAIDs and aspirin should be discontinued for at least 2 days before therapy with pemetrexed and should not be restarted for at least 2 days after a drug dose. These agents may inhibit the renal clearance of pemetrexed, resulting in enhanced toxicity.

8. Pregnancy category D.

Toxicity 1

Myelosuppression. Dose-limiting, dose-related toxicity with neutropenia and thrombocytopenia being most commonly observed.

Toxicity 2

Skin rash, usually in the form of the hand-foot syndrome.

Toxicity 3

Mucositis, diarrhea, and nausea and vomiting.

Toxicity 4

Transient elevation in serum transaminases and bilirubin. Occurs in 10%–15% of patients. Clinically asymptomatic in most cases.

Toxicity 5

Fatigue.

Pentostatin

Trade Names

2'-Deoxycoformycin, Nipent, dCF

Classification

Antimetabolite

Category

Chemotherapy drug

Drug Manufacturer

SuperGen

Mechanism of Action

- Fermentation product of *Streptomyces antibioticus*.
- Both cell cycle–specific and cell cycle–nonspecific effects.
- Inhibits the enzyme adenosine deaminase, which results in accumulation of deoxyadenosine and deoxyadenosine triphosphate (dATP). dATP is cytotoxic to lymphocytes.
- Feedback inhibition of ribonucleotide reductase by dATP resulting in inhibition of DNA synthesis and function.
- Inhibits S-adenosyl-L-homocysteine hydrolase resulting in inhibition of one-carbon dependent methylation reactions.

Mechanism of Resistance

- Decreased nucleoside transport resulting in decreased intracellular accumulation of drug.
- Increased expression of ribonucleotide reductase.

Absorption

Not orally bioavailable due to rapid degradation in acidic conditions. Given only by the IV route.

Distribution

Widely distributed in total body water. Does not cross the blood-brain barrier. About 5%–15% of drug is bound to plasma proteins. After 1 hour of administration, plasma drug levels far exceed the inhibitory concentration for adenosine deaminase by approximately six orders of magnitude.

Metabolism

Metabolism occurs to only a very small degree. Greater than 90% of drug is eliminated in unchanged form and/or metabolites in urine. Elimination half-life is about 5–6 hours. Significant correlation between plasma levels and creatinine clearance.

Indications

1. Hairy cell leukemia.
2. Chronic lymphocytic leukemia.
3. Cutaneous T-cell lymphoma.
4. Acute lymphoblastic leukemia.

Dosage Range

Usual dose is 4 mg/m^2 IV every other week.

Drug Interaction 1

Vidarabine—Pentostatin enhances the activity and toxicity of vidarabine by preventing its inactivation.

Drug Interaction 2

Fludarabine—Combination of pentostatin and fludarabine has been associated with fatal pulmonary toxicity and is absolutely contraindicated.

Special Considerations

1. Use with caution in patients with abnormal renal function. Dose reduction is recommended in this setting and should be done in proportion to the creatinine clearance. Important to obtain baseline creatinine clearance and to monitor renal function before each cycle of therapy.
2. Fluid status of patient is important, and hydration with at least 2 liters of D5NS is required to ensure sufficient urine output (2 liters) on the day of drug administration.
3. Use with caution in patients on sedative and hypnotic drugs as CNS toxicity may be enhanced.
4. Pregnancy category D.

Toxicity 1

Myelosuppression. Dose-limiting leukopenia observed more commonly than thrombocytopenia. Leukopenia nadir at days 10–14 with recovery by days 21–27.

Toxicity 2

Immunosuppression. Both B and T lymphocytes are suppressed. Increased risk of viral, bacterial, fungal, and parasitic infections.

Toxicity 3

Nausea and vomiting. Common but usually not severe.

Toxicity 4

Mild elevations in serum bilirubin and transaminases. Usually reversible.

Toxicity 5

Dose-related headache, lethargy, and fatigue.

Toxicity 6

Allergic/hypersensitivity reaction in the form of fever, chills, myalgias, and arthralgias.

Toxicity 7

Conjunctivitis, photophobia, and diplopia. Ototoxicity in the form of ear pain, labyrinthitis, and tinnitus is rare.

Procarbazine

$$CH_3NHNHCH_2 - \text{(ring)} - \overset{\overset{O}{\|}}{C}NHCH \overset{CH_3}{\underset{CH_3}{<}}$$

Trade Names

Matulane, N-Methylhydrazine

Classification

Nonclassic alkylating agent

Category

Chemotherapy drug

Drug Manufacturer

Roche

Mechanism of Action

- Hydrazine analog that acts as an alkylating agent. Weak monoamine oxidase (MAO) inhibitor and a relative of the MAO inhibitor 1-methyl-2-benzylhydrazine.
- Requires metabolic activation for cytotoxicity. Occurs spontaneously through a non-enzymatic process and/or by an enzymatic reaction mediated by the liver cytochrome P450 system.
- While the precise mechanism of cytotoxicity is unclear, this drug inhibits DNA, RNA, and protein synthesis.
- Cell cycle–nonspecific drug.

Mechanism of Resistance

1. Enhanced DNA repair secondary to increased expression of O6-alkylguanine-DNA transferase (AGAT).
2. Enhanced DNA repair secondary to AGAT-independent mechanisms.

Absorption

Rapid and complete absorption from the GI tract, reaching peak plasma levels within 1 hour.

Distribution

Rapidly and extensively metabolized by the liver cytochrome P450 microsomal system. Procarbazine metabolites cross the blood-brain barrier, and peak CSF levels of drug occur within 30–90 min after drug administration.

Metabolism

Metabolized to active and inactive metabolites by two main pathways, chemical breakdown in aqueous solution and liver microsomal P450 system. Possible formation of free radical intermediates. About 70% of procarbazine is excreted in urine within 24 hours. Less than 5%–10% of the drug is eliminated in an unchanged form. The elimination half-life is short, being less than 1 hour after oral administration.

Indications

1. Hodgkin's lymphoma.
2. Non-Hodgkin's lymphoma.
3. Brain tumors—adjuvant and/or advanced disease.
4. Cutaneous T-cell lymphoma.

Dosage Range

1. Hodgkin's lymphoma: 100 mg/m² PO daily for 14 days, as part of MOPP regimen.
2. Brain tumors: 60 mg/m² PO daily for 14 days, as part of PCV regimen.

Drug Interaction 1

Alcohol- or tyramine-containing foods—Concurrent use with procarbazine can result in nausea, vomiting, increased CNS depression, hypertensive crisis, visual disturbances, and headache.

Drug Interaction 2

Antihistamines, CNS depressants—Concurrent use of procarbazine with antihistamines can result in CNS and/or respiratory depression.

Drug Interaction 3

Levodopa, meperidine—Concurrent use of procarbazine with levodopa or meperidine results in hypertension.

Drug Interaction 4

Tricyclic antidepressants—Concurrent use of procarbazine with sympathomimetics and tricyclic antidepressants may result in CNS excitation, hypertension, tremors, palpitations, and in severe cases, hypertensive crisis and/or angina.

Drug Interaction 5

Antidiabetic agents—Concurrent use of procarbazine with antidiabetic agents such as sulfonylurea compounds and insulin may potentiate hypoglycemic effect.

Special Considerations

1. Monitor CBC while on therapy.

2. Prophylactic use of antiemetics 30 minutes before drug administration to decrease risk of nausea and vomiting. Incidence and severity of nausea usually decrease with continued therapy.

3. Important to review patient's list of concurrent medications as procarbazine has several potential drug–drug interactions.

4. Instruct patients against ingestion of alcohol while on procarbazine. May result in Antabuse-like effect.

5. Instruct patients about specific types of food to avoid during drug therapy (e.g., dark beer, wine, cheese, bananas, yogurt, and pickled and smoked foods).

6. Pregnancy category D. Breast-feeding not recommended.

Toxicity 1

Myelosuppression. Dose-limiting toxicity. Thrombocytopenia is most pronounced effect with nadir in 4 weeks and return to normal in 4–6 weeks. Leukopenia usually occurs after thrombocytopenia. Patients with G6PD deficiency may present with hemolytic anemia while on procarbazine therapy.

Toxicity 2

Nausea and vomiting. Usually develop in the first days of therapy and improve with continued therapy. Diarrhea may also be observed.

Toxicity 3

Flu-like syndrome in the form of fever, chills, sweating, myalgias, and arthralgias. Usually occurs with initial therapy.

Toxicity 4

CNS toxicity in the form of paresthesias, neuropathies, ataxia, lethargy, headache, confusion, and/or seizures.

Toxicity 5

Hypersensitivity reaction with pruritus, urticaria, maculopapular skin rash, flushing, eosinophilia, and pulmonary infiltrates. Skin rash responds to steroid therapy, and drug treatment may be continued. However, procarbazine-induced interstitial pneumonitis usually mandates discontinuation of therapy.

Toxicity 6

Amenorrhea and azoospermia.

Toxicity 7

Immunosuppressive activity with increased risk of infections.

Toxicity 8

Increased risk of secondary malignancies in the form of acute leukemia. The drug is teratogenic, mutagenic, and carcinogenic.

Rituximab

Trade Names

Rituxan

Classification

Monoclonal antibody

Category

Biologic response modifier agent

Drug Manufacturer

Biogen-IDEC and Genentech

Mechanism of Action

- Chimeric anti-CD20 antibody consisting of human IgG1-κ constant regions and variable regions from the murine monoclonal anti-CD20 antibody.

- Targets the CD20 antigen, a 35 kDa cell surface non-glycosylated phosphoprotein expressed during early pre–B cell development until the plasma cell stage. Binding of antibodies to CD20 induces a transmembrane signal that blocks cell activation and cell cycle progression.

- CD20 is expressed on more than 90% of all B-cell non-Hodgkin's lymphomas and leukemias.

- CD20 is not expressed on early pre–B cells, plasma cells, normal bone marrow stem cells, antigen-presenting dendritic reticulum cells, or other normal tissues.

- Chimeric antibody mediates complement-dependent cell lysis (CDCC) in the presence of human complement and antibody-dependent cellular cytotoxicity (ADCC) with human effector cells.

Absorption

Rituximab is given only by the IV route.

Distribution

Peak and trough levels of rituximab correlate inversely with the number of circulating CD20-positive B cells.

Metabolism

Plasma half-life of rituximab is dose-dependent. The median plasma half-life is 76 hours after the first infusion as compared to 206 hours after the fourth infusion. This change in half-life may reflect changes in either the tumor burden or the number of circulating CD20-positive cells. Antibody can be detected in serum up to 3–6 months after completion of therapy.

Elimination pathway has not been well characterized, although antibody-coated cells are reported to undergo elimination via Fc-receptor binding and phagocytosis by the reticuloendothelial system.

Indications

1. Relapsed and/or refractory low-grade or follicular, CD20+, B-cell non-Hodgkin's lymphoma.

2. Intermediate- and/or high-grade, CD20+, B-cell non-Hodgkin's lymphoma—Used as a single agent or in combination with anthracycline-based chemotherapy regimens such as EPOCH or CHOP.

3. FDA-approved for first-line treatment of patients with low-grade or follicular CD20-positive, B-cell non-Hodgkin's lymphoma in combination with CVP chemotherapy or after CVP chemotherapy.

Dosage Range

Recommended dose is 375 mg/m² IV on a weekly schedule for 4 or 8 weeks.

Drug Interactions

None characterized to date.

Special Considerations

1. Contraindicated in patients with known type I hypersensitivity or anaphylactic reactions to murine proteins or product components.

2. Patients should be premedicated with acetaminophen and diphenhydramine to reduce the incidence of infusion-related reactions.

3. Infusion should be started at an initial rate of 50 mg/hour. If no toxicity is observed during the first hour, the infusion rate can be escalated by increments of 50 mg/hour every 30 minutes to a maximum of 400 mg/hour. If the first treatment is well tolerated, the starting infusion rate for the second and subsequent infusions can be administered at 100 mg/hour with 100 mg/hour increments at 30-minute intervals up to 400 mg/hour. Rituximab should **NOT** be given by IV push.

4. Monitor for infusion-related events, which usually occur 30–120 minutes after the start of the first infusion. Infusion should be immediately stopped if signs or symptoms of an allergic reaction are observed. Immediate institution of diphenhydramine, acetaminophen, corticosteroids, IV fluids, and/or vasopressors may be necessary. In most instances, the infusion can be restarted at a reduced rate (50%) once symptoms have completely resolved. Resuscitation equipment should be readily available at bedside.

5. Infusion-related deaths within 24 hours have been reported. Usually occur with the first infusion. Other risk factors include female gender, patients with pre-existing pulmonary disease, and patients with CLL or mantle cell lymphoma.

6. Monitor for tumor lysis syndrome, especially in patients with high numbers of circulating cells (>25,000/mm^3) or high tumor burden. In this case, the first dose of rituximab can be split into two doses with 50% of the total dose to be given on days 1 and 2.

7. Use with caution in patients with pre-existing heart disease, including arrhythmias and angina, as there is an increased risk of cardiotoxicity. The development of cardiac arrhythmias requires cardiac monitoring with subsequent infusion of drug. Patients should be monitored during the infusion and in the immediate post-transfusion period.

8. Monitor for the development of skin reactions. Patients experiencing severe skin reactions should not receive further therapy, and skin biopsies may be required to guide future treatment.

9. Pregnancy category C. Breast-feeding should be avoided.

Toxicity 1

Infusion-related symptoms, including fever, chills, urticaria, flushing, fatigue, headache, bronchospasm, rhinitis, dyspnea, angioedema, nausea, and/or hypotension. Usually occur within 30 minutes to 2 hours after the start of the first infusion. Usually resolves upon slowing or interrupting the infusion and with supportive care. Incidence decreases with subsequent infusion.

Toxicity 2

Tumor lysis syndrome. Characterized by hyperkalemia, hyperuricemia, hyperphosphatemia, hypocalcemia, and renal insufficiency. Usually occurs within the first 12–24 hours of treatment. Risk is increased in patients with high numbers of circulating malignant cells (>25,000/mm^3) and/or high tumor burden.

Toxicity 3

Skin reactions, including pemphigus, Stevens-Johnson syndrome, lichenoid dermatitis, and toxic epidermal neurolysis. Usual onset ranges from 1 to 13 weeks following drug treatment.

Toxicity 4

Arrhythmias and chest pain, usually occurring during drug infusion. Increased risk in patients with pre-existing cardiac disease.

Toxicity 5

Myelosuppression is rarely observed.

Nausea and vomiting. Generally mild.

Sargramostim

Trade Names

Granulocyte-macrophage colony-stimulating factor, GM-CSF, Leukine

Classification

Colony-stimulating growth factor

Category

Biologic response modifier agent

Drug Manufacturer

Genzyme

Mechanism of Action

- No known antitumor activity.
- Stimulates proliferation and differentiation of hematopoietic progenitor cells. Induces partially committed progenitor cells to differentiate along the granulocyte-macrophage pathways.
- Activates mature granulocytes and macrophages.
- Promotes the growth and differentiation of megakaryocytic and erythroid progenitor cells.

Distribution

Distributed into various tissues of the body, including liver, spleen, and kidney. Peak plasma concentration occurs during or immediately after an IV infusion and 1–3 hours after SC administration. Appears to be highly protein-bound.

Metabolism

Metabolism has not been completely characterized. Initial half-life 12–17 minutes with a terminal half-life of 1.6–2.6 hours.

Indications

1. Use following induction chemotherapy in AML.
2. Mobilization of peripheral blood stem cells for either autologous or allogeneic stem cell transplant.
3. Use after bone marrow or stem cell transplant (autologous or allogeneic) to accelerate myeloid recovery.
4. Use in bone marrow transplantation failure or engraftment delay.
5. Use in chemotherapy-induced neutropenia for solid tumors.

Dosage Range

1. Following induction chemotherapy for AML: 250 µg/m²/day IV over 4 hours starting 4 days after completion of induction chemotherapy.

2. Mobilization of peripheral blood stem cells: 250 µg/m²/day IV over 24 hours or SC once daily.

3. Use after peripheral blood stem cell transplant: 250 µg/m²/day IV over 24 hours or SC once daily starting immediately after infusion of progenitor stem cells.

4. Use after bone marrow transplant: 250 µg/m²/day IV over 2 hours beginning 2–4 hours after bone marrow infusion.

5. Use after bone marrow transplant failure or engraftment delay: 250 µg/m²/day IV over 2 hours for 14 days.

6. Use in chemotherapy-induced neutropenia for solid tumors: 250 µg/m²/day SC beginning no earlier than 24 hours after chemotherapy.

Drug Interactions

Steroids, lithium—Concurrent use with steroids and/or lithium may potentiate the release of neutrophils in response to sargramostim.

Special Considerations

1. Contraindicated in patients with excess number of leukemic blasts in peripheral blood (>10%) and/or bone marrow.

2. Contraindicated in patients with known hypersensitivity to GM-CSF or yeast-derived products.

3. Concurrent administration with chemotherapy or radiation therapy is contraindicated as an increased incidence of serious adverse events has been observed. Sargramostim must be given at least 24 hours after the last dose of chemotherapy and 12 hours after radiation therapy.

4. Premedication with acetaminophen helps to relieve the bone pain that arises due to bone marrow expansion in response to treatment.

5. Associated with higher incidence of fever and fluid retention than observed with G-CSF.

6. Monitor CBC at least twice per week during treatment. Therapy should be terminated once total WBC >10,000/mm³ or ANC >1,000/mm³ for 3 days.

7. Therapy should be discontinued immediately if leukemic growth or disease progression occurs.

8. Use with caution in the presence of steroids and lithium as they may potentiate the release of neutrophils following sargramostim therapy.

9. Use with caution in patients with pre-existing heart disease, congestive heart failure, and pulmonary infiltrates as sargramostim may aggravate fluid retention.

10. Pregnancy category C.

Toxicity 1

Flu-like syndrome characterized by fever, chills, lethargy, malaise, and headache.

Toxicity 2

Transient bone pain. May be prevented by acetaminophen.

Toxicity 3

Fluid retention syndrome. Presents as pleural and/or pericardial effusions and peripheral edema. Results from migration of neutrophils into the lung with release of various cytokines.

Toxicity 4

Injection reaction manifested by transient flushing, myalgias, dyspnea, nausea and vomiting, tachycardia, and rarely hypotension. Occurs usually with the first dose and tends not to recur with subsequent doses.

Toxicity 5

Transient elevation in serum bilirubin and liver transaminases.

Sorafenib

Trade Name

Nexavar, BAY 43-9006

Classification

Signal transduction inhibitor

Category

Chemotherapy drug

Drug Manufacturer

Bayer and Onyx

Mechanism of Action

- Inhibits multiple receptor tyrosine kinases (RTKs), some of which are involved in tumor growth, tumor angiogenesis, and metastasis.
- Potent inhibitor of intracellular kinases, including c-Raf and wild-type and mutant B-Raf.
- Targets vascular endothelial growth factor receptors, VEGFR2 and VEGFR3, and platelet-derived growth factor receptor-β (PDGFR-β), and in so doing, inhibits angiogenesis.

Mechanism of Resistance

None well characterized to date.

Absorption

Rapidly absorbed after an oral dose with peak plasma levels achieved within 2 to 7 hours. Oral administration should be without food at least 1 hour before or 2 hours after eating, as food with a high fat content reduces oral bioavailability by up to 30%.

Distribution

Extensive binding (99%) to plasma proteins. Steady-state drug concentrations are reached in 7 days.

Metabolism

Metabolized in the liver primarily by CYP3A4 microsomal enzymes and by glucuronidation mediated by UGT1A9. Parent drug accounts for 70%–85% at steady-state, while the pyridine-N-oxide metabolite, which has similar biological activity to sorafenib, accounts for 10%–16%. Elimination is hepatic with excretion in feces (~80%), with renal elimination of the glucuronidated metabolites accounting for 16% of the administered dose. The terminal half-life of sorafenib is approximately 25 to 48 hours.

Indications

1. FDA-approved for the treatment of advanced renal cell cancer.
2. FDA approved for the treatment of unresectable hepatocellular cancer (HCC).

Dosage Range

Recommended dose is 400 mg PO bid. Dose may need to be reduced in Asian patients, as they experience increased toxicity to sorafenib.

Drug Interaction 1

Drugs such as ketoconazole, itraconazole, erythromycin, clarithromycin, atazanavir, indinavir, nefazodone, nelfinavir, ritonavir, saquinavir, telithromycin, and voriconazole decrease the rate of metabolism of sorafenib, resulting in increased drug levels and potentially increased toxicity.

Drug Interaction 2

Drugs such as rifampicin, phenytoin, phenobarbital, carbamazepine, and St. John's wort increase the rate of metabolism of sorafenib, resulting in its inactivation.

Special Considerations

1. Sorafenib should be taken without food at least 1 hour before or 2 hours after a meal.
2. No dose adjustment is necessary in patients with Child-Pugh A and B liver dysfunction. However, sorafenib has not been studied in patients with Child-Pugh C liver disease, and caution should be used in this setting.
3. No dose adjustments are necessary in patients with mild to moderate renal dysfunction. Sorafenib has not been studied in patients undergoing dialysis.
4. Use with caution when administering sorafenib with agents that are metabolized and/or eliminated by the UGT1A1 pathway, such as irinotecan, as sorafenib is an inhibitor of UGT1A1.
5. Patients receiving sorafenib along with oral warfarin anticoagulant therapy should have their coagulation parameters (PT and INR)

monitored frequently as elevations in INR and bleeding events have been observed.

6. Closely monitor blood pressure while on therapy, especially during the first 6 weeks of therapy, and treat as needed with standard oral anti-hypertensive medication.

7. Skin toxicities, including rash and hand-foot reaction, should be managed early in the course of therapy with topical treatments for symptomatic relief, temporary interruption, dose reduction, and/or discontinuation. Sun exposure should be avoided, and periodic dermatologic evaluation is recommended.

8. Sorafenib therapy should be interrupted in patients undergoing major surgical procedures.

9. Avoid grapefruit and grapefruit juice while on sorafenib therapy.

10. Pregnancy category D. Breast-feeding should be avoided.

Toxicity 1

Hypertension occurs in nearly 30% of patients. Usually occurs within 6 weeks of starting therapy and well-controlled with oral anti-hypertensive medication.

Toxicity 2

Skin rash occurs in up to 2/3 of patients. Hand-foot skin reaction occurs in up to 30%. Rare cases of actinic keratoses and cutaneous squamous cell cancer have been reported.

Toxicity 3

Bleeding complications with epistaxis most commonly observed.

Toxicity 4

Wound healing complications.

Toxicity 5

Constitutional side effects with fatigue and asthenia.

Toxicity 6

Diarrhea and nausea are the most common GI side effects.

Toxicity 7

Hypophosphatemia occurs in up to 45% of patients, but usually clinically asymptomatic.

Streptozocin

Trade Names

Streptozotocin, Zanosar

Classification

Alkylating agent

Category

Chemotherapy drug

Drug Manufacturer

Teva Pharmaceuticals

Mechanism of Action

- Cell cycle–nonspecific nitrosourea analog.
- Formation of intrastrand cross-links of DNA resulting in inhibition of DNA synthesis and function.
- Selectively targets pancreatic β cells, possibly due to the presence of a glucose moiety on the compound.
- In contrast with other nitrosourea analogs, no effect on RNA or protein synthesis.

Mechanism of Resistance

- Decreased cellular uptake of drug.
- Increased intracellular thiol content due to glutathione and/or glutathione-related enzymes.
- Enhanced activity of DNA repair enzymes.

Absorption

Not absorbed orally.

Distribution

Rapidly cleared from plasma with an elimination half-life of 35 minutes. Drug concentrates in the liver and kidney, reaching concentrations equivalent to those in plasma. Drug metabolites cross the blood-brain barrier and enter the CSF. Selectively concentrates in pancreatic β cells presumably due to the glucose moiety on the molecule.

Metabolism

Metabolized primarily by the liver to active metabolites. The elimination half-life of the drug is short, being less than 1 hour. About 60%–70% of drug is excreted in urine, 20% in unchanged form. Less than 1% of drug is eliminated in stool.

Indications

1. Pancreatic islet cell cancer.
2. Carcinoid tumors.

Dosage Range

1. Weekly schedule: 1,000–1,500 mg/m^2 IV weekly for 6 weeks followed by 4 weeks of observation.
2. Daily schedule: 500 mg/m^2 IV for 5 days every 6 weeks.

Drug Interaction 1

Steroids—Concurrent use of steroids and streptozocin may result in severe hyperglycemia.

Drug Interaction 2

Phenytoin—Phenytoin antagonizes the antitumor effect of streptozocin.

Drug Interaction 3

Nephrotoxic drugs—Avoid concurrent use of streptozocin with nephrotoxic agents as renal toxicity may be enhanced.

Special Considerations

1. Use with caution in patients with abnormal renal function. Dose reduction is recommended in this setting as nephrotoxicity is dose-limiting and can be severe and/or fatal. Baseline creatinine clearance is required, as is monitoring of renal function before each cycle of therapy. Hydration with 1–2 liters of fluid is recommended to prevent nephrotoxicity.
2. Monitor CBC while on therapy.
3. Avoid the use of other nephrotoxic agents in combination with streptozocin.
4. Carefully administer drug to minimize and/or avoid burning, pain, and extravasation.
5. Pregnancy category D. Breast-feeding should be avoided.

Toxicity 1

Renal toxicity is dose-limiting. Seen in 40%–60% of patients and manifested initially by proteinuria and azotemia. Can also present as glucosuria, hypophosphatemia, and nephrogenic diabetes insipidus. Permanent renal damage can occur in rare instances.

Toxicity 2

Nausea and vomiting occur in 90% of patients. More frequently observed with the daily dosage schedule and can be severe.

Toxicity 3

Myelosuppression. Usually mild with nadir occurring at 3–4 weeks.

Toxicity 4

Pain and/or burning at the injection site.

Toxicity 5

Altered glucose metabolism resulting in either hypoglycemia or hyperglycemia.

Toxicity 6

Mild and transient increases in SGOT, alkaline phosphatase, and bilirubin. Usual onset is within 2–3 weeks of starting therapy.

Sunitinib

Trade Name

Sutent, SU11248

Classification

Signal transduction inhibitor

Category

Chemotherapy drug

Drug Manufacturer

Pfizer

Mechanism of Action

- Inhibits multiple RTKs, some of which are involved in tumor growth, tumor angiogenesis, and metastasis.
- Potent inhibitor of platelet-derived growth factor receptors (PDGFR-α and PDGFR-β), vascular endothelial growth factor receptors (VEGFR1, VEGFR2, and VEGFR3), stem cell factor receptor (KIT), Fms-like tyrosine kinase-3 (FLT3), colony-stimulating factor receptor type 1 (CSF-1R), and the glial cell-line derived neurotrophic factor receptor (RET).

Mechanism of Resistance

- Increased expression of PDGFR-α, PDGFR-β, VEGFR1, VEGFR2, VEGFR3, KIT, CSF-1R, and RET.
- Alterations in binding affinity of the drug to the RTK resulting from mutations in the RTKs.
- Increased degradation and/or metabolism of the drug through as yet ill-defined mechanisms.

Absorption

Oral bioavailability is nearly 100%. Sunitinib may be taken with or without food, as food does not affect oral bioavailability.

Distribution

Extensive binding (90%–95%) of sunitinib and its primary metabolite to plasma proteins. Peak plasma levels are achieved 6 to 12 hours after ingestion. Steady-state drug concentrations of sunitinib and its primary active metabolite are reached in 10 to 14 days.

Metabolism

Metabolized in the liver primarily by CYP3A4 microsomal enzymes to produce its primary active metabolite, which is further metabolized by CYP3A4. The primary active metabolite comprises 23% to 37% of the total exposure. Elimination is hepatic with excretion in feces (~60%), with renal elimination accounting for 16% of the administered dose. The terminal half-lives of sunitinib and its primary active metabolite are approximately 40 to 60 hours and 80 to 110 hours, respectively. With repeated daily administration, sunitinib accumulates 3- to 4-fold, while the primary metabolite accumulates 7- to 10-fold.

Indications

1. FDA-approved for the treatment of GIST after disease progression on or intolerance to imatinib.
2. FDA-approved for the treatment of advanced renal cell cancer.

Dosage Range

Recommended dose is 50 mg/day PO for 4 weeks followed by 2 weeks off.

Drug Interaction 1

Drugs such as ketoconazole, itraconazole, erythromycin, clarithromycin, atazanavir, indinavir, nefazodone, nelfinavir, ritonavir, saquinavir, telithromycin, and voriconazole decrease the rate of metabolism of sunitinib, resulting in increased drug levels and potentially increased toxicity.

Drug Interaction 2

Drugs such as rifampicin, Dilantin, phenobarbital, carbamazepine, and St. John's wort increase the rate of metabolism of sunitinib, resulting in its inactivation.

Special Considerations

1. Baseline and periodic evaluations of LVEF should be performed while on sunitinib therapy.
2. Use with caution in patients with underlying cardiac disease, especially those who presented with cardiac events within 12 months prior to initiation of sunitinib, such as myocardial infarction

(including severe/unstable angina), coronary/peripheral artery bypass graft, and CHF.

3. In the presence of clinical manifestations of CHF, discontinuation of sunitinib is recommended. The dose of sunitinib should be interrupted and/or reduced in patients without clinical evidence of CHF but with an ejection fraction <50% and >20% below baseline.

4. Closely monitor blood pressure while on therapy and treat as needed with standard oral anti-hypertensive medication. In cases of severe hypertension, temporary suspension of sunitinib is recommended until hypertension is controlled.

5. Monitor for adrenal insufficiency in patients who experience increased stress such as surgery, trauma, or severe infection.

6. Closely monitor thyroid function tests and TSH at 2 to 3-month intervals, as sunitinib treatment results in hypothyroidism. The incidence of hypothyroidism is increased with prolonged duration of therapy.

7. Avoid grapefruit and grapefruit juice while on sunitinib therapy.

8. Pregnancy category D. Breast-feeding should be avoided.

Toxicity 1

Hypertension occurs in up to nearly 30% of patients. Usually occurs within 3–4 weeks of starting therapy and well-controlled with oral anti-hypertensive medication.

Toxicity 2

Yellowish discoloration of the skin occurs in approximately 30% of patients. Skin rash, dryness, thickness, and/or cracking of skin. Depigmentation of hair and/or skin may also occur.

Toxicity 3

Bleeding complications with epistaxis most commonly observed.

Toxicity 4

Constitutional side effects with fatigue and asthenia, which may be significant in some patients.

Toxicity 5

Diarrhea, stomatitis, altered taste, and abdominal pain are the most common GI side effects. Pancreatitis has been reported rarely with elevations in serum lipase and amylase.

Toxicity 6

Myelosuppression with neutropenia and thrombocytopenia.

Toxicity 7

Increased risk of left ventricular dysfunction, which in some cases results in CHF.

Toxicity 8

Adrenal insufficiency and hypothyroidism.

Tamoxifen

$$O\diagup NMe_2$$

Trade Names

Nolvadex

Classification

Antiestrogen

Category

Hormonal agent

Drug Manufacturer

AstraZeneca

Mechanism of Action

- Nonsteroidal antiestrogen with weak estrogen agonist effects.
- Competes with estrogen for binding to ERs. Binding of tamoxifen to ER leads to ER dimerization. The tamoxifen-bound ER dimer is transported to the nucleus, where it binds to DNA sequences referred to as ER elements. This interaction results in inhibition of critical transcriptional processes and signal transduction pathways that are required for cellular growth and proliferation.
- Cell cycle–specific agent that blocks cells in the mid-G1 phase of the cell cycle. Effect may be mediated by cyclin D.
- Stimulates the secretion of transforming growth factor-β (TGF-β), which then acts to inhibit the expression and/or activity of TGF-α and IGF-1, two genes that are involved in cell growth and proliferation.

Mechanism of Resistance

- Decreased expression of ER.
- Mutations in the ER leading to decreased binding affinity to tamoxifen.
- Overexpression of growth factor receptors, such as TGF-α or IGF-1, that counteract the inhibitory effects of tamoxifen.

Absorption

Rapidly and completely absorbed in the GI tract. Peak plasma levels are achieved within 4–6 hours after oral administration.

Distribution

Distributes to most body tissues, especially in those expressing estrogen receptors. Present in very low concentrations in CSF. Nearly all of drug is bound to plasma proteins.

Metabolism

Extensively metabolized by liver cytochrome P450 enzymes after oral administration. The main metabolite, N-desmethyl tamoxifen, has biologic activity similar to that of the parent drug. Both tamoxifen and its metabolites are excreted primarily (75%) in feces with minimal clearance in urine. The terminal half-lives of tamoxifen and its metabolites are relatively long, approaching 7–14 days.

Indications

1. Adjuvant therapy in axillary node-negative breast cancer following surgical resection.

2. Adjuvant therapy in axillary node-positive breast cancer in postmenopausal women following surgical resection.

3. Adjuvant therapy in women with ductal carcinoma in situ (DCIS) after surgical resection and radiation therapy.

4. Metastatic breast cancer in women and men.

5. Approved as a chemopreventive agent for women at high risk for breast cancer. "High-risk" women are defined as women >35 years and with a 5-year predicted risk of breast cancer ≥1.67%, according to the Gail model.

6. Endometrial cancer.

Dosage Range

Recommended dose for treatment of breast cancer patients is 20 mg PO every day.

Drug Interaction 1

Warfarin—Tamoxifen can inhibit metabolism of warfarin by the liver P450 system leading to increased anticoagulant effect. Coagulation parameters, including PT and INR, must be closely monitored, and dose adjustments may be required.

Drug Interaction 2

Drugs activated by liver P450 system—Tamoxifen and its metabolites are potent inhibitors of hepatic P450 enzymes and may inhibit the metabolic activation of drugs utilizing this pathway, including cyclophosphamide.

Drug Interaction 3

Drugs metabolized by liver P450 system—Tamoxifen and its metabolites are potent inhibitors of hepatic P450 enzymes and may inhibit the metabolism of various drugs, including erythromycin, calcium channel blockers, and cyclosporine.

Special Considerations

1. Instruct patients to notify physician about menstrual irregularities, abnormal vaginal bleeding, and pelvic pain and/or discomfort while on therapy.

2. Patients should have routine follow-up with a gynecologist as tamoxifen therapy is associated with an increased risk of endometrial hyperplasia, polyps, and endometrial cancer.

3. Use with caution in patients with abnormal liver function as there may be an increased risk of drug accumulation resulting in toxicity.

4. Use with caution in patients with either personal history or family history of thromboembolic disease or hypercoagulable states as tamoxifen is associated with an increased risk of thromboembolic events. Tamoxifen therapy is associated with antithrombin III deficiency.

5. Initiation of treatment with tamoxifen may induce a transient tumor flare. Tamoxifen should not be given in patients with impending ureteral obstruction, spinal cord compression, or in those with extensive painful bone metastases.

6. Premenopausal patients should be warned about the possibility of developing menopausal symptoms with tamoxifen therapy.

7. Monitor CBC during therapy with tamoxifen as myelosuppression can occur, albeit rarely.

8. Pregnancy category D.

Toxicity 1

Menopausal symptoms, including hot flashes, nausea, vomiting, vaginal bleeding, and menstrual irregularities. Vaginal discharge and vaginal dryness also observed.

Toxicity 2

Fluid retention and peripheral edema observed in about 30% of patients.

Toxicity 3

Tumor flare usually occurs within the first 2 weeks of starting therapy. May observe increased bone pain, urinary retention, back pain with spinal cord compression, and/or hypercalcemia.

Toxicity 4

Headache, lethargy, dizziness occur rarely. Visual disturbances, including cataracts, retinopathy, and decreased visual acuity, have been described.

Toxicity 5

Skin rash, pruritus, hair thinning, and/or partial hair loss.

Toxicity 6

Myelosuppression is rare, with transient thrombocytopenia and leukopenia. Usually resolves after the first week of treatment.

Toxicity 7

Thromboembolic complications, including deep vein thrombosis, pulmonary embolism, and superficial phlebitis. Incidence of thromboembolic events may be increased when tamoxifen is given concomitantly with chemotherapy.

Toxicity 8

Elevations in serum triglycerides.

Toxicity 9

Increased incidence of endometrial hyperplasia, polyps, and endometrial cancer.

Temozolomide

Trade Names

Temodar

Classification

Nonclassic alkylating agent

Category

Chemotherapy drug

Drug Manufacturer

Schering

Mechanism of Action

- Imidazotetrazine analog that is structurally and functionally similar to dacarbazine.
- Cell cycle–nonspecific agent.
- Metabolic activation to the reactive compound MTIC is required for antitumor activity.
- Although the precise mechanism of cytotoxicity is unclear, this drug methylates guanine residues in DNA and inhibits DNA, RNA, and protein synthesis. Does not cross-link DNA strands.

Mechanism of Resistance

Increased activity of DNA repair enzymes such as O6-alkylguanine DNA alkyltransferase.

Absorption

Widely distributed in body tissues. Rapidly and completely absorbed with an oral bioavailability approaching 100%. Maximum plasma concentrations are reached within 1 hour after administration. Food reduces the rate and extent of drug absorption.

Distribution

Because temozolomide is lipophilic, it crosses the blood-brain barrier. Levels in brain and CSF are 30%–40% of those achieved in plasma.

Metabolism

Metabolized primarily by non-enzymatic hydrolysis at physiologic pH. Undergoes conversion to the metabolite MTIC, which is further hydrolyzed to AIC, a known intermediate in purine de novo synthesis, and methylhydrazine, the presumed active alkylating species. The elimination half-life of the drug is 2 hours. About 40%–50% of the parent drug is excreted in urine within 6 hours of administration, and tubular secretion is the predominant mechanism of renal excretion. No specific guidelines for drug dosing in the setting of hepatic and/or renal dysfunction. However, dose modification should be considered in patients with moderately severe hepatic and/or renal dysfunction.

Indications

1. FDA-approved for refractory anaplastic astrocytomas at first relapse following treatment with a nitrosourea and procarbazine-containing regimen.

2. FDA-approved for newly diagnosed glioblastoma multiformae (GBM) in combination with radiotherapy and then as maintenance treatment.

3. Metastatic melanoma.

Dosage Range

- Usual dose is 150 mg/m² PO daily for 5 days every 28 days.

- Dose is adjusted to nadir neutrophil and platelet counts. If nadir of ANC is acceptable, the dose may be increased to 200 mg/m² PO daily for 5 days. If ANC falls below acceptable levels during any cycle, the next dose should be reduced by 50 mg/m² PO daily.

- Temozolomide is given at 75 mg/m² PO daily for 42 days along with radiotherapy (60 Gy in 30 fractions) for newly diagnosed GBM. During the maintenance phase, which is started 4 weeks after completion of the combined modality therapy, temozolomide is given on cycle 1 at 150 mg/m² PO daily for five days followed by 23 days without treatment. For cycles 2–6, the dose of temozolomide may be escalated to 200 mg/m² if tolerated.

Drug Interactions

None known.

Special Considerations

1. Temozolomide is a moderately emetogenic agent. Aggressive use of antiemetics prior to drug administration is required to decrease the risk of nausea and vomiting.

2. Patients should be warned to avoid sun exposure for several days after drug treatment.

3. Use with caution in elderly patients (age >65) as they are at increased risk for myelosuppression.

4. Patients should be monitored closely for the development of PCP, and those receiving temozolomide and radiotherapy require PCP prophylaxis.

5. Pregnancy category D. Breast-feeding should be discontinued.

Toxicity 1

Myelosuppression. Dose-limiting toxicity. Leukopenia and thrombocytopenia are commonly observed.

Toxicity 2

Nausea and vomiting. Mild to moderate, usually occurring within 1–3 hours and lasting for up to 12 hours. Aggressive antiemetic therapy strongly recommended.

Toxicity 3

Headache and fatigue.

Toxicity 4

Mild elevation in hepatic transaminases.

Toxicity 5

Photosensitivity.

Toxicity 6

Teratogenic, mutagenic, and carcinogenic.

Temsirolimus

Trade Names

Torisel, CCI-779

Classification

Signal transduction inhibitor

Category

Chemotherapy drug

Drug Manufacturer

Wyeth

Mechanism of Action

- Potent inhibitor of the mammalian target of rapamycin (mTOR) kinase, which is a key component of cellular signaling pathways involved in the growth and proliferation of tumor cells.
- Inhibition of mTOR signaling results in cell cycle arrest, induction of apoptosis, and inhibition of angiogenesis.

Mechanism of Resistance

None well characterized to date.

Absorption

Not available for oral use and is administered only by the IV route.

Distribution

Widely distributed in tissues. Steady-state drug concentrations are reached in 7 to 8 days.

Metabolism

Metabolism in the liver primarily by the CYP3A4 microsomal enzyme. The main metabolite is sirolimus, which is a potent inhibitor of mTOR signaling, with the other metabolites accounting for <10% of all metabolites measured. Elimination is mainly hepatic with excretion in the feces, and renal elimination of parent drug and its metabolites accounts for only 5% of an administered dose. The terminal half-life of the parent drug is 17 hours, while that of sirolimus is 55 hours.

Indications

FDA-approved for the treatment of advanced renal cell cancer.

Dosage Range

Recommended dose is 25 mg IV administered on a weekly schedule.

Drug Interaction 1

Dilantin and other drugs that stimulate the liver microsomal CYP3A4 enzyme, including carbamazepine, rifampin, phenobarbital, and St. John's wort—These drugs may increase the rate of metabolism of temsirolimus, resulting in its inactivation.

Drug Interaction 2

Drugs that inhibit the liver microsomal CYP3A4 enzyme, including ketoconazole, itraconazole, erythromycin, and clarithromycin—These drugs may decrease the rate of metabolism of temsirolimus, resulting in increased drug levels and potentially increased toxicity.

Special Considerations

1. Use with caution in patients with hepatic impairment, and dose reduction and/or interruption should be considered.

2. Patients should be premedicated with an H1 antihistamine (diphenhydramine 25 to 50 mg IV) 30 minutes before the start of therapy to reduce the incidence of hypersensitivity reactions.

3. Closely monitor serum glucose levels in all patients, especially those with diabetes mellitus.

4. Closely monitor patients for new or progressive pulmonary symptoms, including cough, dyspnea, and fever. Temsirolimus therapy should be interrupted pending further diagnostic evaluation.

5. Patients are at increased risk for developing opportunistic infections while on temsirolimus.

6. Closely monitor serum triglyceride and cholesterol levels while on therapy.

7. Patients should be advised to report the development of fever, abdominal pain, and/or bloody stools, as temsirolimus may cause bowel perforation on rare occasions.

8. Closely monitor renal function during therapy, as temsirolimus can cause progressive and severe renal failure, especially in patients with pre-existing renal impairment.

9. Use with caution after surgical procedures, as temsirolimus can impair the process of wound healing.

10. Avoid grapefruit and grapefruit juice while on temsirolimus.

11. Avoid the use of live vaccines and/or close contact with those who have received live vaccines while on temsirolimus.

12. Pregnancy category D.

Toxicity 1
Asthenia and fatigue.

Toxicity 2
Pruritus, dry skin with mainly a pustular, acneiform skin rash.

Toxicity 3
Nausea/vomiting, mucositis, and anorexia. On rare occasions, bowel perforations can occur and present as fever, abdominal pain, and bloody stools.

Toxicity 4
Hyperlipidemia with increased serum triglycerides and/or cholesterol in up to 90% of patients.

Toxicity 5
Hyperglycemia in up to 80% to 90% of patients.

Toxicity 6
Allergic, hypersensitivity reactions occur in 10% of patients.

Toxicity 7
Pulmonary toxicity in the form of ILD manifested by increased cough, dyspnea, fever, and pulmonary infiltrates. Observed in less than 1% of patients and more frequent in patients with underlying pulmonary disease.

Toxicity 8
Renal toxicity with elevation in serum creatinine.

Toxicity 9
Peripheral edema.

Thalidomide

Trade Names

Thalomid

Classification

Immunomodulatory agent, anti-angiogenic agent

Category

Unclassified therapeutic agent, biologic response modifier agent

Drug Manufacturer

Celgene

Mechanism of Action

- Mechanism of action is not fully characterized.
- Inhibition of TNF-α synthesis and down-modulation of selected cell surface adhesion molecules.
- May exert an anti-angiogenic effect through inhibition of bFBG and VEGF as well as through as yet undefined mechanisms.

Mechanism of Resistance

None known.

Absorption

Oral bioavailability of thalidomide is not known due to poor aqueous solubility. Slowly absorbed from the GI tract with peak plasma levels reached 3–6 hours after oral administration.

Distribution

The apparent volume of distribution varies by dose level: 67 L and 166 L at doses of 200 and 1,200 mg/day. Remains unclear whether thalidomide is present in the ejaculate of males. The extent of binding to plasma proteins is not known.

Metabolism

Non-enzymatic hydrolysis appears to be the principal mechanism of thalidomide breakdown. However, the exact metabolic pathway(s) has not been fully characterized. The precise route of drug excretion is not well defined.

Indications

1. FDA-approved in combination with dexamethasone for the treatment of newly diagnosed multiple myeloma.

2. FDA-approved for the treatment of the cutaneous manifestations of erythema nodosum leprosum (ENL).

3. Thalidomide has activity in MDS and in a broad range of solid tumors.

Dosage Range

No standard dose recommendations for use in cancer patients have been established. When used in combination with chemotherapy, doses are typically titrated up to 400 mg PO daily given as a single bedtime dose. As a single agent, doses have been in the range of 100 mg to 1,200 mg daily.

Drug Interaction 1

Barbiturates, chlorpromazine, and reserpine—Sedative effect of thalidomide is enhanced with concurrent use of these medications.

Drug Interaction 2

Alcohol—Sedative effect of thalidomide is enhanced with concurrent use of alcohol.

Special Considerations

1. Pregnancy category X. Severe fetal malformations can occur if even one capsule is taken by a pregnant woman. All women should have a baseline β-human chorionic gonadotropin before starting therapy with thalidomide. All women of childbearing potential should practice two forms of birth control throughout treatment with thalidomide: one highly effective (intrauterine device, hormonal contraception, partner's vasectomy) and one additional barrier method (latex condom, diaphragm, cervical cap). It is strongly recommended that these precautionary measures begin 4 weeks before initiation of therapy, that they continue while on therapy, and continue for at least 4 weeks after therapy is discontinued.

2. Breast-feeding while on therapy should be avoided given the potential for serious adverse reactions from thalidomide in nursing infants. It remains unknown whether thalidomide is excreted in human milk.

3. Men taking thalidomide must use latex condoms for every sexual encounter with a woman of childbearing potential since thalidomide may be present in semen.

4. Patients with AIDS should have their HIV mRNA levels monitored after the first and third months after treatment initiation with

thalidomide, then every 3 months thereafter, as HIV mRNA levels may be increased while on thalidomide.

5. Instruct patients to avoid operating heavy machinery or driving a car while on thalidomide as the drug can cause drowsiness.

6. Patients who develop a skin rash during therapy with thalidomide should have prompt medical evaluation. Serious skin reactions, including Stevens-Johnson syndrome, which may be fatal, have been reported.

7. There is an increased risk of thromboembolic complications, including DVT and PE, and prophylaxis with low molecular weight heparin, Coumadin, or aspirin can help to prevent and/or reduce the incidence.

Toxicity 1

Teratogenic effect is most serious toxicity. Severe birth defects or death to an unborn fetus. Manifested as absent or defective limbs, hypoplasia or absence of bones, facial palsy, absent or small ears, absent or shrunken eyes, congenital heart defects, and GI and renal abnormalities.

Toxicity 2

General neurologic-related events that occur frequently include fatigue, orthostatic hypotension, and dizziness. Specific peripheral neuropathy in the form of numbness, tingling, and pain in the feet or hands does not appear to be dose- or duration-related. Prior exposure to neurotoxic agents increases the risk of occurrence.

Toxicity 3

Constipation is most common GI toxicity.

Toxicity 4

No known direct myelosuppressive effects. Effects on blood cell counts may occur indirectly through its effect on TNF-α or other cytokines that influence blood cell regulation, recruitment, and activation. Certain treatment populations (ENL and HIV) have reported a higher incidence of abnormalities in blood counts.

Toxicity 5

Maculopapular skin rash, urticaria, and dry skin. Serious dermatologic reactions, including Stevens-Johnson syndrome, have been reported. Patients who develop a skin rash during therapy with thalidomide should discontinue therapy. Therapy can be restarted with caution if the rash was not exfoliative, purpuric, or bullous or otherwise suggestive of a serious skin condition.

Toxicity 6

Daytime sedation or fatigue following an evening dose often associated with larger initial doses. Doses can be reduced until the patient accommodates to the effect.

Toxicity 7

Increased risk of thromboembolic complications, including DVT and PE.

Thioguanine

$$\text{structure: purine ring with } S \text{ (thione), } NH_2 \text{, and } N \text{ atoms}$$

Trade Names

6-Thioguanine, 6-TG

Classification

Antimetabolite

Category

Chemotherapy drug

Drug Manufacturer

GlaxoSmithKline

Mechanism of Action

- Cell cycle–specific purine analog with activity in the S-phase.
- Parent drug is inactive. Requires intracellular phosphorylation by the enzyme HGPRT to the cytotoxic monophosphate form, which is then eventually metabolized to the triphosphate metabolite form.
- Inhibits de novo purine synthesis by inhibiting PRPP amidotransferase.
- Incorporation of thiopurine triphosphate nucleotides into DNA resulting in inhibition of DNA synthesis and function.
- Incorporation of thiopurine triphosphate nucleotides into RNA resulting in alterations in RNA processing and/or translation.

Mechanism of Resistance

- Decreased expression of the activating enzyme HGPRT.
- Increased expression of the catabolic enzyme alkaline phosphatase or the conjugating enzyme TPMT.
- Decreased cellular transport of drug.
- Decreased expression of mismatch repair enzymes (e.g., hMLH1, hMSH2).
- Cross-resistance between thioguanine and mercaptopurine.

Absorption

Oral absorption of drug is incomplete and variable. Only 30% of an oral dose is absorbed. Peak plasma levels are reached in 2–4 hours after ingestion.

Distribution

Distributes widely into the RNA and DNA of peripheral blood and bone marrow cells. Crosses the placenta but does not appear to cross the blood-brain barrier.

Metabolism

Metabolized in the liver by the processes of deamination and methylation. Main pathway of inactivation is catalyzed by guanine deaminase (guanase). In contrast with mercaptopurine, metabolism of thioguanine does not involve xanthine oxidase. Metabolites are eliminated in both feces and urine. Plasma half-life is on the order of 80–90 minutes.

Indications

1. Acute myelogenous leukemia.
2. Acute lymphoblastic leukemia.
3. Chronic myelogenous leukemia.

Dosage Range

1. Induction: 100 mg/m^2 PO every 12 hours on days 1–5, usually in combination with cytarabine.
2. Maintenance: 100 mg/m^2 PO every 12 hours on days 1–5, every 4 weeks, usually in combination with other agents.
3. Single-agent: 1–3 mg/kg PO daily.

Drug Interactions

None known.

Special Considerations

1. Dose of drug does not need to be reduced in patients with abnormal liver and/or renal function.
2. In contrast with 6-mercaptopurine, dose of drug does not need to be reduced in the presence of concomitant allopurinol therapy.
3. Administer on an empty stomach to facilitate absorption.
4. Use with caution in the presence of other hepatotoxic drugs as the risk of thioguanine-associated hepatotoxicity is increased.
5. Pregnancy category D.

Toxicity 1

Myelosuppression. Dose-limiting toxicity. Leukopenia tends to precede thrombocytopenia with nadir at 10–14 days and recovery by day 21.

Toxicity 2

Nausea and vomiting. Dose-related, usually mild.

Toxicity 3

Mucositis and diarrhea. May be severe, requiring dose reduction.

Toxicity 4

Hepatotoxicity in the form of elevated serum bilirubin and transaminases. Veno-occlusive disease has been reported rarely.

Toxicity 5

Immunosuppression. Increased risk of bacterial, fungal, and parasitic infections.

Toxicity 6

Transient renal toxicity.

Toxicity 7

Mutagenic, teratogenic, and carcinogenic.

T Thiotepa

Trade Names

Triethylenethiophosphoramide, Thioplex

Classification

Alkylating agent

Category

Chemotherapy drug

Drug Manufacturer

Immunex

Mechanism of Action

- Ethylenimine analog chemically related to nitrogen mustard.
- Functions as an alkylating agent by alkylating the N-7 position of guanine.
- Cell cycle–nonspecific agent.
- Inhibits DNA, RNA, and protein synthesis.

Mechanism of Resistance

- Decreased uptake of drug into cell.
- Increased activity of DNA repair enzymes.
- Increased expression of sulfhydryl proteins, including glutathione and glutathione-related proteins.

Absorption

Incomplete and erratic absorption via the oral route. Thiotepa is primarily administered by the IV route. Also given by intravesical route where the absorption from the bladder is variable, ranging from 10%–100% of an administered dose.

Distribution

Widely distributed throughout the body. About 40% of drug is bound to plasma proteins.

Metabolism

Extensively metabolized by the liver microsomal P450 system to both active and inactive metabolites. About 60% of a dose is eliminated in urine within 24–72 hours with only a small amount excreted as parent drug. Elimination half-life is on the order of 2–3 hours.

Indications

1. Breast cancer.
2. Ovarian cancer.
3. Superficial transitional cell cancer of the bladder.
4. Hodgkin's and non-Hodgkin's lymphoma.
5. High-dose transplant setting for breast and ovarian cancer.

Dosage Range

1. Usual dose is 10–20 mg/m^2 IV given every 3–4 weeks.
2. High-dose transplant setting: Doses range from 180 to 1,100 mg/m^2 IV.
3. Intravesical instillation: Dose for bladder instillation is 60 mg administered in 60 mL sterile water weekly for up to 4 weeks.

Drug Interactions

Myelosuppressive agents—Bone marrow toxicity of thiotepa is enhanced when combined with other myelosuppressive anticancer agents.

Special Considerations

1. Monitor CBC while on therapy as thiotepa is highly toxic to the bone marrow.
2. Use with caution in regimens including other myelosuppressive agents as the risk of bone marrow toxicity is significantly increased.
3. Resuscitation equipment and medications should be available during administration of drug as there is a risk of hypersensitivity reaction.
4. Monitor CBC after intravesical administration of drug into the bladder as severe bone marrow depression can arise from systemically absorbed drug.
5. Caution patients about the risk of skin changes such as rash, urticaria, bronzing, flaking, and desquamation that can occur following high-dose therapy. Topical skin care should be initiated promptly.
6. Pregnancy category D.

Toxicity 1

Myelosuppression. Dose-limiting toxicity. Leukopenia nadir 7–10 days with recovery by day 21. Platelet count nadir occurs at day 21 with usual recovery by day 28–35.

Toxicity 2

Nausea and vomiting. Dose-dependent. Usual onset is 6–12 hours after treatment.

Toxicity 3

Mucositis. May be dose-limiting with high-dose therapy.

Toxicity 4

Allergic reaction in the form of skin rash, hives, and rarely bronchospasm.

Toxicity 5

Chemical and/or hemorrhagic cystitis. Occurs rarely following intravesical treatment.

Toxicity 6

Skin changes with rash and bronzing of skin, erythema, flaking, and desquamation developing after high-dose therapy.

Toxicity 7

Thiotepa is teratogenic, mutagenic, and carcinogenic. Increased risk of secondary malignancies, usually in the form of acute myelogenous leukemia. Breast cancer and non–small cell lung cancer have also been reported.

Topotecan

Trade Names

Hycamtin

Classification

Topoisomerase I inhibitor

Category

Chemotherapy drug

Drug Manufacturer

GlaxoSmithKline

Mechanism of Action

- Semisynthetic derivative of camptothecin, an alkaloid extract from the *Camptotheca acuminata* tree.

- Inhibits topoisomerase I function. Binds to and stabilizes the topoisomerase I-DNA complex and prevents the religation of DNA after it has been cleaved by topoisomerase I. The collision between this stable cleavable complex and the advancing replication fork results in double-strand DNA breaks and cellular death.

- Antitumor activity of drug requires the presence of topoisomerase I and ongoing DNA synthesis.

Mechanism of Resistance

- Decreased expression of topoisomerase I.

- Mutations in topoisomerase I enzyme with decreased binding affinity to drug.

- Increased expression of the multidrug-resistant phenotype with overexpression of P170 glycoprotein. Results in enhanced efflux of drug and decreased intracellular accumulation of drug.

- Decreased accumulation of drug into cells through non–multidrug-resistant-related mechanisms.

Absorption

Administered only by the IV route.

Distribution

Widely distributed in body tissues. Binding to plasma proteins is on the order of 10%–35%. Levels of drug in the CSF are only 30% of those in plasma. Peak drug levels are achieved within 1 hour after drug administration.

Metabolism

Rapid conversion of topotecan in plasma and in aqueous solution from the lactone ring form to the carboxylate acid form. At acidic pH, topotecan is mainly in the lactone ring, while at physiologic and basic pH, the carboxylate form predominates. Only about 20% to 30% of a given dose is present as the active lactone metabolite at 1 hour after drug administration. The major route of elimination of topotecan is renal excretion accounting for 40%–68% of drug clearance. Metabolism in the liver appears to be minimal and is mediated by the liver microsomal P450 system. The elimination half-life is approximately 3 hours.

Indications

1. Ovarian cancer—FDA-approved in patients with advanced ovarian cancer who failed platinum-based chemotherapy.

2. Small cell lung cancer—FDA-approved in patients with sensitive disease who failed first-line chemotherapy.

3. Acute myelogenous leukemia.

Dosage Range

Usual dose is 1.5 mg/m^2 IV for 5 consecutive days given every 21 days.

Drug Interactions

None known.

Special Considerations

1. Use with caution in patients with abnormal renal function. Dose reduction is necessary in this setting. Baseline creatinine clearance is critical, as is periodic monitoring of renal function.

2. Monitor CBC on a weekly basis.

3. Carefully monitor administration of drug as it is a mild vesicant. The infusion site should be carefully monitored for extravasation, in which case flushing with sterile water, elevation of the extremity, and local application of ice are recommended. In severe cases, a plastic surgeon should be consulted.

4. If granulocyte nadir count is low, begin G-CSF or GM-CSF 24 hours after the completion of topotecan therapy.

5. Pregnancy category D. Breast-feeding should be avoided.

Toxicity 1

Myelosuppression. Dose-limiting with neutropenia being most commonly observed. Typical nadir occurs at days 7–10 with full recovery by days 21–28.

Toxicity 2

Nausea and vomiting. Mild to moderate and dose-related. Occur in 60%–80% of patients. Diarrhea with abdominal pain also observed.

Toxicity 3

Headache, fever, malaise, arthralgias, and myalgias.

Toxicity 4

Microscopic hematuria. Seen in 10% of patients.

Toxicity 5

Alopecia.

Toxicity 6

Transient elevation in serum transaminases, alkaline phosphatase, and bilirubin.

Toremifene

Trade Names
Fareston

Classification
Antiestrogen

Category
Hormonal agent

Drug Manufacturer
Orion and GTx

Mechanism of Action
- Synthetic analog of tamoxifen.
- Nonsteroidal antiestrogen that directly binds to estrogen receptors on breast cancer cells. Affinity for estrogen receptor is 4- to 5-fold higher than tamoxifen. Blocks downstream intracellular signal transduction pathways, leading to inhibition of cell growth and induction of apoptosis.

Mechanism of Resistance
None known.

Absorption
Well-absorbed after oral administration. Food does not interfere with oral absorption.

Distribution
Widely distributed to body tissues. Extensive (>99%) binding to plasma proteins, mainly albumin. Steady-state plasma concentrations are reached in 4–6 weeks.

Metabolism

Extensive metabolism in the liver by the cytochrome P450 system. Major metabolites, N-demethyltoremifene and 4-hydroxytoremifene, have long terminal half-lives of 4–6 days secondary to enterohepatic recirculation. Parent drug and metabolites are excreted mainly in bile and feces. Minimal excretion in urine.

Indications

Metastatic breast cancer in postmenopausal women with ER+ tumors or in cases where ER status is not known. Not recommended in ER- tumors.

Dosage Range

Recommended dose is 60 mg PO daily until disease progression.

Drug Interaction 1

Thiazide diuretics—Decreases renal clearance of calcium and increases the risk of hypercalcemia associated with toremifene.

Drug Interaction 2

Warfarin—Toremifene inhibits liver P450 metabolism of warfarin resulting in an increased anticoagulant effect. Coagulation parameters, PT and INR, should be closely monitored, and dose adjustments made accordingly.

Drug Interaction 3

Phenobarbital, carbamazepine, phenytoin—Liver P450 metabolism of toremifene may be enhanced by phenobarbital, carbamazepine, and phenytoin resulting in reduced blood levels and reduced clinical efficacy.

Drug Interaction 4

Ketoconazole and erythromycin—Liver P450 metabolism of toremifene may be inhibited by ketoconazole and erythromycin, resulting in elevated blood levels and enhanced clinical efficacy.

Drug Interaction 5

Tamoxifen—Cross-resistance between toremifene, tamoxifen, and other anti-estrogen agents.

Special Considerations

1. Patients with a prior history of thromboembolic events must be carefully monitored while on therapy as toremifene is thrombogenic.

2. Use with caution in the setting of brain and/or vertebral body metastases as tumor flare with bone and/or muscular pain, erythema, and transient increase in tumor volume can occur upon initiation of therapy.

3. Monitor CBC, LFTs, and serum calcium on a regular basis.

4. Contraindicated in patients with a prior history of endometrial hyperplasia. Increased risk of endometrial cancer associated with therapy. Onset of vaginal bleeding during therapy requires immediate gynecologic evaluation.

5. Baseline and biannual eye exams are recommended as toremifene can lead to cataract formation.

6. Pregnancy category D. Not known whether toremifene is excreted in breast milk.

Toxicity 1

Hot flashes, sweating, menstrual irregularity, milk production in breast, and vaginal discharge and bleeding are commonly observed.

Toxicity 2

Transient tumor flare manifested by bone and/or tumor pain.

Toxicity 3

Ocular toxicity with cataract formation and xerophthalmia.

Toxicity 4

Nausea, vomiting, and anorexia.

Toxicity 5

Myelosuppression is usually mild.

Toxicity 6

Rare skin toxicity in the form of rash, alopecia, and peripheral edema.

Tositumomab

Trade Names

Bexxar

Classification

Monoclonal antibody

Category

Biologic response modifier agent

Drug Manufacturer

Corixa and GlaxoSmithKline

Mechanism of Action

- Radioimmunotherapeutic monoclonal antibody-based regimen composed of the tositumomab monoclonal antibody and the radiolabeled monoclonal antibody I-131 tositumomab, a radio-iodinated derivative of tositumomab that has been covalently linked to I-131.

- The antibody moiety is tositumomab, which targets the CD20 antigen, a 35 kDa cell surface non-glycosylated phosphoprotein expressed during early pre–B cell development until the plasma cell stage. Binding of the antibody to CD20 induces a transmembrane signal that blocks cell activation and cell cycle progression.

- CD20 is expressed on more than 90% of all B-cell non-Hodgkin's lymphomas and leukemias. CD20 is not expressed on early pre–B cells, plasma cells, normal bone marrow stem cells, antigen-presenting dendritic reticulum cells, or other normal tissues.

- Ionizing radiation from the I-131 radioisotope results in cell death.

Absorption

Tositumomab is given only by the IV route.

Distribution

Higher clearance, shorter terminal half-life, and larger volumes of distribution observed in patients with higher tumor burden, splenomegaly, and/or bone marrow involvement.

Metabolism

Elimination of I-131 occurs by decay and excretion in the urine. The total body clearance is 67% of an administered dose, and nearly 100% of the clearance is accounted for in the urine.

Indications

Relapsed and/or refractory CD20-positive, follicular non-Hodgkin's lymphoma with and without transformation-disease is refractory to rituximab therapy and has relapsed following chemotherapy.

Dosage Range

The treatment schema is as follows: Day 0: Begin Lugol's solution or oral potassium iodide solution; Day 1, Dosimetric dose: 450 mg unlabeled tositumomab, followed by 5 mCi of I-131 tositumomab (35 mg). Measurement of whole body counts and calculation of therapeutic dose; Day 7 up to Day 14, Therapeutic dose: 450 mg unlabeled tositumomab, followed by calculated therapeutic dose of I-131 tositumomab to deliver 75 cGy; Days 8–21: Continue Lugol's solution or oral potassium iodide solution.

Drug Interactions

None characterized to date.

Special Considerations

1. Contraindicated in patients with known type I hypersensitivity or known hypersensitivity to any component of the BEXXAR therapeutic regimen.

2. TSH levels should be monitored before treatment and on an annual basis thereafter.

3. Before receiving the dosimetric dose of I-131, patients must receive at least three doses of SSKI, three doses of Lugol's solution, or one dose of 130 mg potassium iodide (at least 24 hours prior to the dosimetric dose).

4. This therapy should be used only by physicians and health care professionals who are qualified and experienced in the safe use and handling of radioisotopes.

5. Patients should be premedicated with acetaminophen and diphenhydramine before each administration of tositumomab in the dosimetric and therapeutic steps to reduce the incidence of infusion-related reactions.

6. The same IV tubing set and filter must be used throughout the dosimetric and therapeutic step as a change in filter can result in loss of effective drug delivery.

7. Monitor for infusion-related events resulting from tositumomab infusion, which usually occur during or within 48 hours of infusion. Infusion rate should be reduced by 50% for mild to moderate allergic reaction and immediately stopped for a severe reaction. Immediate institution of diphenhydramine, acetaminophen, corticosteroids, IV fluids, and/or vasopressors may be necessary. In the setting of a severe reaction, the infusion can be restarted at a reduced rate (50%)

once symptoms have completely resolved. Resuscitation equipment should be readily available at bedside.

8. Tositumomab therapy should not be given to patients with >25% involvement of the bone marrow by lymphoma and/or impaired bone marrow reserve or to patients with platelet count <100,000/mm^3 or neutrophil count <15,000/mm^3.

9. Complete blood counts and platelet counts should be monitored weekly following tositumomab therapy for up to 10–12 weeks after therapy.

10. The tositumomab regimen should be given only as a single-course treatment.

11. The tositumomab regimen may have direct toxic effects on the male and female reproductive organs, and effective contraception should be used during therapy and for up to 12 months following the completion of therapy.

12. Pregnancy category X. Contraindicated in women who are pregnant.

13. Breast-feeding should be discontinued immediately prior to starting therapy.

Toxicity 1

Infusion-related symptoms, including fever, chills, urticaria, flushing, fatigue, headache, bronchospasm, rhinitis, dyspnea, angioedema, nausea, and/or hypotension. Usually resolve upon slowing and/or interrupting the infusion and with supportive care.

Toxicity 2

Myelosuppression is most common side effect with neutropenia, thrombocytopenia, and anemia. The time to nadir is typically 4–7 weeks, and the duration of cytopenias is 30 days. In 5%–7% of patients, severe cytopenias persist beyond 12 weeks after therapy.

Toxicity 3

Mild asthenia and fatigue occur in up to 40% of patients.

Toxicity 4

Infections develop in up to 45% of patients. Majority of infection events are viral and relatively minor, but up to 10% of patients experience infections that require hospitalization.

Toxicity 5

Mild nausea and vomiting.

Toxicity 6

Hypothyroidism.

Toxicity 7

Secondary malignancies occur in about 2%–3% of patients. Acute myelogenous leukemia and myelodysplastic syndrome have been reported with a cumulative incidence of 1.4% at 2 years and 4.8% at 4 years following therapy.

Toxicity 8

Development of HAMAs. Rare event in less than 1%–2% of patients.

Trastuzumab

Trade Names

Herceptin, Anti-HER-2-antibody

Classification

Monoclonal antibody

Category

Biologic response modifier agent

Drug Manufacturer

Genentech

Mechanism of Action

- Recombinant humanized monoclonal antibody directed against the extracellular domain of the HER-2/neu growth factor receptor. This receptor is overexpressed in several human cancers, including 25%–30% of breast cancers and up to 20% of gastric cancers.
- Precise mechanism(s) of action remains unknown.
- Downregulates expression of HER-2/neu receptor.
- Inhibits HER-2/neu intracellular signaling pathways.
- Induction of apoptosis through as yet undetermined mechanisms.
- Immunologic mechanisms may also be involved in antitumor activity, and they include recruitment of antibody-dependent cellular cytotoxicity (ADCC) and/or complement-mediated cell lysis.

Mechanism of Resistance

- Mutations in the HER-2/neu growth factor receptor leading to decreased binding affinity to trastuzumab.
- Decreased expression of HER-2/neu receptors.
- Activation/induction of alternative cellular signaling pathways, such as IGF-1R.

Distribution

Distribution in body is not well characterized.

Metabolism

Metabolism of trastuzumab has not been extensively characterized. Half-life is on the order of 5–6 days with the every-2-week schedule and a mean life of 16 days with the every-3-week schedule.

Indications

1. Metastatic breast cancer—First-line therapy in combination with paclitaxel. Patient's tumor must express HER-2/neu protein to be treated with this monoclonal antibody.

2. Metastatic breast cancer—Second- and third-line therapy as a single agent in patients whose tumors overexpress the HER-2/neu protein.

3. FDA-approved for the adjuvant therapy of node-positive, HER2-overexpressing breast cancer as part of a treatment regimen containing doxorubicin, cyclophosphamide, and either paclitaxel or docetaxel.

Dosage Range

1. Recommended loading dose of 4 mg/kg IV administered over 90 minutes, followed by maintenance dose of 2 mg/kg IV on a weekly basis.

2. Alternative schedule is to give a loading dose of 8 mg/kg IV administered over 90 minutes, followed by maintenance dose of 6 mg/kg IV every 3 weeks.

Drug Interactions

Anthracyclines, taxanes—Increased risk of cardiotoxicity when trastuzumab is used in combination with anthracyclines and/or taxanes.

Special Considerations

1. Caution should be exercised in treating patients with pre-existing cardiac dysfunction. Careful baseline assessment of cardiac function (LVEF) before treatment and frequent monitoring (every 3 months) of cardiac function while on therapy. Trastuzumab should be held for ≥16% absolute decrease in LVEF from a normal baseline value. Trastuzumab therapy should be stopped immediately in patients who develop clinically significant congestive heart failure. When trastuzumab is used in the adjuvant setting, cardiac function should be assessed every 6 months for at least 2 years following the completion of therapy.

2. Carefully monitor for infusion reactions, which typically occur during or within 24 hours of drug administration. Administer initial loading dose over 90 minutes and then observe patient for 1 hour following completion of the loading dose. May need to treat with benadryl and acetaminophen. Rarely, in severe cases, may need to treat with IV fluids and/or pressors.

3. Maintenance doses are administered over 30 minutes if loading dose was well tolerated without fever and chills. However, if fever and chills were experienced with loading dose, need to administer over 90 minutes.

4. Pregnancy category B.

Toxicity 1

Infusion-related symptoms with fever, chills, urticaria, flushing, fatigue, headache, bronchospasm, dyspnea, angioedema, and hypotension. Occur in 40%–50% of patients. Usually mild to moderate in severity and observed most commonly with administration of the first infusion.

Toxicity 2

Nausea and vomiting, diarrhea. Generally mild.

Toxicity 3

Cardiotoxicity in the form of dyspnea, peripheral edema, and reduced left ventricular function. Significantly increased risk when used in combination with an anthracycline-based regimen. In most instances, cardiac dysfunction is readily reversible.

Toxicity 4

Myelosuppression. Increased risk and severity when trastuzumab is administered with chemotherapy.

Toxicity 5

Generalized pain, asthenia, and headache.

Toxicity 6

Pulmonary toxicity in the form of increased cough, dyspnea, rhinitis, sinusitis, pulmonary infiltrates, and/or pleural effusions.

Tretinoin

$$CH_3 \quad CH_3 \qquad CH_3 \qquad CH_3$$

Trade Names

All-*trans*-retinoic acid, ATRA, Vesanoid

Classification

Retinoid

Category

Differentiating agent

Drug Manufacturer

Roche

Mechanism of Action

- Precise mechanism of action has not been fully elucidated.
- Induces differentiation of acute promyelocytic cells to normal myelocyte cells, thereby decreasing cellular proliferation.
- Upon entry into cells, tretinoin binds to the cytoplasmic protein, cellular retinoic acid binding protein (CRABP). The retinoid CRABP complex is transported to the nucleus where it binds to retinoid-dependent receptors known as RAR and/or RXR. This process affects the transcription and subsequent expression of various target cellular genes involved in growth, proliferation, and differentiation.
- Effects on the immune system may also contribute to antitumor activity.
- Induces apoptosis through as yet undetermined mechanisms.

Mechanism of Resistance

- Alteration in drug metabolism by the liver P450 system. Tretinoin induces the activity of cytochrome P450 enzymes, which are responsible for its oxidative metabolism. Plasma concentrations decrease to about one-third of their day one values after 1 week of continuous therapy.
- Increased expression of CRABP, which acts to sequester tretinoin within the cell, preventing its subsequent delivery to the nucleus.

Absorption

Well absorbed by the GI tract, reaching peak plasma concentration between 1 and 2 hours after oral administration.

Distribution

Binds extensively (>95%) to plasma proteins, mainly to albumin. The apparent volume of distribution has not been determined.

Metabolism

Undergoes oxidative metabolism by the liver cytochrome P450 system. Several metabolites have been identified, including 13-cis retinoic acid, 4-oxo *trans* retinoic acid, 4-oxo cis retinoic acid, and 4-oxo *trans* retinoic acid glucuronide. Excreted in urine (63%) and in feces (31%). The terminal elimination half-life is approximately 40 to 120 minutes.

Indications

Acute promyelocytic leukemia (APL)—induction of remission in patients with APL characterized by the t(15;17) translocation and/or the presence of the PML/RAR-α gene following progression and/or relapse with anthracycline-based chemotherapy or for whom anthracycline-based chemotherapy is contraindicated.

Dosage Range

Recommended dose is 45 mg/m^2/day PO divided in two daily doses for a minimum of 45 days and a maximum of 90 days.

Drug Interaction 1

Drugs metabolized by liver P450 system—Tretinoin is metabolized by hepatic cytochrome P450 enzymes. Caution should be exercised when using drugs that induce this enzyme system, such as rifampin and phenobarbital, and drugs that inhibit this system, including ketoconazole, cimetidine, erythromycin, verapamil, diltiazem, and cyclosporine.

Drug Interaction 2

Vitamin A supplements—Use of vitamin A supplements may increase toxicity of tretinoin.

Special Considerations

1. Contraindicated in patients with a known hypersensitivity to retinoids.

2. Monitor for new-onset fever, respiratory symptoms, and leukocytosis as 25% of patients develop the retinoic acid syndrome. Tretinoin should be stopped immediately, and high-dose dexamethasone, 10 mg IV q 12 hours should be given for 3 days or until resolution of symptoms. In most cases, therapy can be resumed once the syndrome has completely resolved. Usually occurs during the first month of treatment.

3. Use with caution in patients with pre-existing hypertriglyceridemia and in those with diabetes mellitus, obesity, and/or predisposition to excessive alcohol intake. Serum triglyceride and cholesterol levels should be closely monitored.

4. Monitor CBC, coagulation profile, and LFTs on a frequent basis during therapy.

5. Oral absorption of tretinoin may be increased when taken with food.

6. Pregnancy category D.

Toxicity 1

Vitamin A toxicity. Nearly universal. Most common side effects are headache, usually occurring in the first week of therapy with improvement thereafter, fever, dryness of the skin and mucous membranes, skin rash, peripheral edema, mucositis, pruritus, and conjunctivitis.

Toxicity 2

Retinoic acid syndrome. Can be dose-limiting and occurs in 25% of patients. Varies in severity but has resulted in death. Characterized by fever, leukocytosis, dyspnea, weight gain, diffuse pulmonary infiltrates on chest x-ray, and pleural and/or pericardial effusions. More commonly observed with WBC >10,000/mm^3. Usually observed during the first month of therapy but may follow the initial drug dose.

Toxicity 3

Flushing, hypotension, hypertension, phlebitis, and congestive heart failure. Cardiac ischemia, myocardial infarction, stroke, myocarditis, pericarditis, and pulmonary hypertension are rarer events, each being reported in less than 3% of patients.

Toxicity 4

Increased serum cholesterol and triglyceride levels occur in up to 60% of patients. Usually reversible upon completion of treatment.

Toxicity 5

CNS toxicity in the form of dizziness, anxiety, paresthesias, depression, confusion, and agitation. Hallucinations, agnosia, aphasia, slow speech, asterixis, cerebellar disorders, convulsion, coma, dysarthria, encephalopathy, facial paralysis, hemiplegia, and hyporeflexia are less often seen.

Toxicity 6

GI toxicity. Relatively common and manifested by abdominal pain, constipation, diarrhea, and GI bleeding. Elevations in serum transaminases and alkaline phosphatase occur in 50%–60% of patients and usually resolve after completion of therapy.

Toxicity 7

Alterations in hearing sensation with hearing loss. About 25% of patients describe earache or a fullness in the ears.

Toxicity 8

Renal dysfunction and dysuria occur rarely.

Toxicity 9

Pseudotumor cerebri. Benign intracranial hypertension with papilledema, headache, nausea and vomiting, and visual disturbances.

Toxicity 10

Teratogenic.

Vinblastine

Trade Names

Velban

Classification

Vinca alkaloid, anti-microtubule agent

Category

Chemotherapy drug

Drug Manufacturer

Eli Lilly

Mechanism of Action

- Plant alkaloid extracted from the periwinkle plant *Catharanthus roseus*.
- Cell cycle–specific with activity in the mitosis (M) phase.
- Inhibits tubulin polymerization, disrupting formation of microtubule assembly during mitosis. This results in an arrest in cell division, ultimately leading to cell death.
- May also inhibit DNA, RNA, and protein synthesis.

Mechanism of Resistance

- Overexpression of the P170 glycoprotein encoded by the multidrug-resistant gene, resulting in enhanced efflux of drug and decreased intracellular drug accumulation. Cross-resistance may be observed with other natural products, such as taxanes, epipodophyllotoxins, anthracyclines, and actinomycin-D.
- Mutations in $\alpha \propto$ and β-tubulin proteins with decreased binding affinity to vinblastine.

Absorption

Poorly and erratically absorbed by the oral route.

Distribution

Widely and rapidly distributed into most body tissues. Binds extensively to platelets, RBCs, and WBCs within 30 minutes of administration. Poor penetration into the CSF.

Metabolism

Metabolized in the liver by the cytochrome P450 microsomal system. Small quantities of at least one metabolite, desacetyl vinblastine, may be as active as the parent drug. Majority of vinblastine is excreted in metabolite form via the enterohepatic biliary system. Only about 10% of the parent drug is excreted in feces. Approximately 14% of the drug is eliminated by the kidneys. Plasma terminal half-life of about 25 hours.

Indications

1. Hodgkin's and non-Hodgkin's lymphoma.
2. Testicular cancer.
3. Breast cancer.
4. Kaposi's sarcoma.
5. Renal cell carcinoma.

Dosage Range

1. Hodgkin's lymphoma: 6 mg/m^2 IV on days 1 and 15, as part of the ABVD regimen.
2. Testicular cancer: 0.15 mg/kg IV on days 1 and 2, as part of the PVB regimen.

Drug Interaction 1

Drugs metabolized by liver P450 system—Vinblastine should be used cautiously in patients receiving medications that inhibit drug metabolism via the hepatic cytochrome P450 system, including calcium channel blockers, cimetidine, cyclosporine, erythromycin, metoclopramide, and ketoconazole.

Drug Interaction 2

Phenytoin—Vinblastine reduces blood levels of phenytoin through either reduced absorption of phenytoin or an increase in the rate of its metabolism and elimination.

Drug Interaction 3

Bleomycin—Risk of Raynaud's syndrome may be increased with the combination of vinblastine and bleomycin.

Special Considerations

1. Use with caution in patients with abnormal liver function as toxicity of vinblastine may be significantly enhanced. Dose reduction is recommended in this setting.

2. Vinblastine should be infused as a rapid push in a free-flowing IV line to avoid extravasation. If extravasation occurs, the infusion should be discontinued immediately. Flushing with sterile water, elevation of the involved extremity, and local application of ice are recommended. In severe cases, a plastic surgeon should be consulted.

3. Patients should be warned about the risk of constipation upon starting therapy, and a bowel regimen including a high-fiber diet and a stool softener should be initiated.

4. Observe for hypersensitivity reactions, especially when the drug is administered in association with mitomycin-C.

5. Contamination of the eye may lead to severe irritation and even corneal ulceration. If accidental contamination occurs, the eyes should be immediately and thoroughly washed.

6. Pregnancy category D. Not known if excreted in milk.

Toxicity 1

Myelosuppression. Dose-limiting toxicity with neutropenia being most commonly observed with nadir at days 4–6. Thrombocytopenia and anemia are less common.

Toxicity 2

Mucositis and stomatitis. More frequently observed with vinblastine than with vincristine. Nausea, vomiting, anorexia, and diarrhea may also occur.

Toxicity 3

Alopecia is common. Usually mild and reversible.

Toxicity 4

Hypertension. Most common cardiovascular side effect and occurs as a consequence of autonomic dysfunction.

Toxicity 5

Neurotoxicity. Occurs much less frequently than with vincristine. Presents with the same manifestations as seen with vincristine: peripheral neuropathy (paresthesias, paralysis, loss of deep tendon reflexes, and constipation) and autonomic nervous system dysfunction (orthostatic hypotension, paralytic ileus, and urinary retention). Less commonly, cranial nerve paralysis, ataxia, cortical blindness, seizures, and coma may occur.

Toxicity 6

Vesicant. Extravasation may cause local skin damage.

Toxicity 7

SIADH.

Toxicity 8

Headache and depression.

Toxicity 9

Vascular events, such as stroke, myocardial infarction, and Raynaud's syndrome.

Toxicity 10

Acute pulmonary edema, bronchospasm, acute respiratory distress, interstitial pulmonary infiltrates, and dyspnea have been reported on rare occasion.

Vincristine

Trade Names

Oncovin, VCR

Classification

Vinca alkaloid, anti-microtubule agent

Category

Chemotherapy drug

Drug Manufacturer

Eli Lilly

Mechanism of Action

- Plant alkaloid derived from the periwinkle plant *Catharanthus roseus*.
- Cell cycle–specific with activity in the mitosis (M) phase.
- Inhibits tubulin polymerization, disrupting formation of microtubule assembly during mitosis. This results in an arrest in cell division, ultimately leading to cell death.
- May also inhibit DNA, RNA, and protein synthesis.

Mechanism of Resistance

- Overexpression of the P170 glycoprotein encoded by the multidrug-resistant gene, resulting in enhanced efflux of drug and decreased intracellular drug accumulation. Cross-resistance may be observed with other natural products, such as taxanes, epipodophyllotoxins, anthracyclines, and actinomycin-D.
- Mutations in α- and β-tubulin proteins with decreased affinity to vincristine.

Absorption

Not available for oral use and administered only by the IV route.

Distribution

Widely and rapidly distributed into body tissues within 30 minutes of administration. Poor penetration across the blood-brain barrier and into the CSF.

Metabolism

Metabolized in the liver by the cytochrome P450 microsomal system. The majority of vincristine (80%) is excreted in bile and feces. Only 15%–20% of the drug is recovered in urine. Terminal half-life is long, on the order of 85 hours.

Indications

1. Acute lymphoblastic leukemia.
2. Hodgkin's and non-Hodgkin's lymphoma.
3. Multiple myeloma.
4. Rhabdomyosarcoma.
5. Neuroblastoma.
6. Ewing's sarcoma.
7. Wilms' tumor.
8. Chronic leukemias.
9. Thyroid cancer.
10. Brain tumors.
11. Trophoblastic neoplasms.

Dosage Range

1. Doses usually vary between 0.5 and 1.4 mg/m^2. The total individual dose should be limited to 2 mg to prevent the development of neurotoxicity.
2. Continuous infusion: 0.4 mg/day IV continuous infusion for 4 days, as part of the VAD regimen for multiple myeloma.

Drug Interaction 1

Drugs metabolized by liver P450 system—Vincristine should be used with caution in patients receiving medications that inhibit drug metabolism via the hepatic cytochrome P450 system.

Drug Interaction 2

Phenytoin—Vincristine reduces the blood levels of phenytoin and its subsequent efficacy through either reduced absorption of phenytoin or an increase in the rate of its metabolism and/or elimination.

Drug Interaction 3

Digoxin—Vincristine reduces the blood levels of digoxin resulting in decreased efficacy.

Drug Interaction 4

Cisplatin and paclitaxel—Concurrent administration of vincristine with other neurotoxic agents such as cisplatin and paclitaxel may increase the risk and severity of neurotoxicity.

Drug Interaction 5

L-Asparaginase—When used in combination with L-asparaginase, vincristine should be administered 12–24 hours before as L-asparaginase inhibits vincristine clearance.

Drug Interaction 6

Methotrexate—Vincristine increases the cellular uptake of methotrexate resulting in enhanced antitumor activity and host toxicity.

Drug Interaction 7

Filgrastim—Concurrent use of vincristine with filgrastim may result in severe atypical neuropathy.

Special Considerations

1. Use with caution in patients with abnormal liver function as increased toxicity may be observed. Dose reduction is necessary in this setting.

2. Vincristine should be infused as a rapid push over 1 minute in a side port of a free-flowing IV line to avoid extravasation. If extravasation occurs, the infusion should be discontinued immediately. Application of ice to the area of leakage along with elevation of involved extremity may minimize discomfort and the possibility of cellulitis. In severe cases, a plastic surgeon should be consulted.

3. Contamination of the eye may lead to severe irritation and even corneal ulceration. If accidental contamination occurs, the eyes should be washed immediately and thoroughly.

4. Patients should be warned about the risk of constipation upon starting therapy, and a bowel regimen including stool softeners and high-fiber diet should be initiated. Patients should be advised to seek medical attention if persistent nausea, vomiting, and abdominal pain develop after beginning therapy.

5. Careful baseline neurologic evaluation should be performed before starting therapy and at the start of each cycle. The onset of severe signs and/or symptoms of neurotoxicity warrants immediate discontinuation of the drug. Avoid the simultaneous use of drugs associated with neurologic toxicity. Risk factors for neurotoxicity

include elderly patients and those with pre-existing neuropathies and/or neuromuscular disorders.

6. Overdose of vincristine may be treated with leucovorin 100 mg IV every 3 hours for the first 24 hours and then every 6 hours for 48 hours. Other supportive measures should be considered, including prevention of SIADH; use of anticonvulsants, enemas, or cathartics to prevent ileus; monitoring of the cardiovascular system; and monitoring of CBC.

7. Pregnancy category D. Not known if excreted in milk.

Toxicity 1

Neurotoxicity. Most commonly observed dose-limiting toxicity. Clinical manifestations are variable, and include peripheral neuropathy (paresthesias, paralysis, and loss of deep tendon reflexes), autonomic nervous system dysfunction (orthostasis, sphincter problems, and paralytic ileus), cranial nerve palsies, ataxia, cortical blindness, seizures, and coma. Bone, back, limb, jaw, and parotid gland pain may also occur.

Toxicity 2

Constipation, abdominal pain, and paralytic ileus are common. A prophylactic bowel regimen for constipation is recommended. Nausea, vomiting, and diarrhea can also occur, but are rare.

Toxicity 3

Alopecia, skin rash, and fever.

Toxicity 4

Vesicant. Extravasation may cause local tissue injury, inflammation, and necrosis.

Toxicity 5

Myelosuppression. Generally mild and much less significant than with vinblastine.

Toxicity 6

SIADH.

Toxicity 7

Hypersensitivity reactions.

Toxicity 8

Azoospermia and amenorrhea may be permanent.

Vinorelbine

Trade Names

Navelbine

Classification

Vinca alkaloid, anti-microtubule agent

Category

Chemotherapy drug

Drug Manufacturer

GlaxoSmithKline

Mechanism of Action

- Semisynthetic alkaloid derived from vinblastine.
- Cell cycle–specific with activity in mitosis (M) phase.
- Inhibits tubulin polymerization, disrupting formation of microtubule assembly during mitosis. This results in an arrest in cell division, ultimately leading to cell death.
- Relatively high specificity for mitotic microtubules with lower affinity for axonal microtubules.
- May also inhibit DNA, RNA, and protein synthesis.

Mechanism of Resistance

- Overexpression of the P170 glycoprotein encoded by the multidrug-resistant gene, resulting in enhanced efflux of drug and decreased intracellular drug accumulation. Cross-resistance may be observed with other natural products, such as taxanes, epipodophyllotoxins, anthracyclines, and actinomycin-D.
- Mutations in α- and β-tubulin proteins with decreased binding affinity to vinorelbine.

Absorption

Administered only by the IV route.

Distribution

Widely and rapidly distributed into most body tissues with a large apparent volume of distribution (>30 L/kg). Extensive binding to plasma proteins (about 80%).

Metabolism

Metabolized in the liver by the cytochrome P450 microsomal system. Small quantities of at least one metabolite, desacetyl vinorelbine, have antitumor activity similar to that of parent drug. Majority of vinorelbine excreted in feces via the enterohepatic biliary system (50%). About 15%–20% of the drug is eliminated by the kidneys. Prolonged terminal half-life of 27–43 hours secondary to relatively slow efflux of drug from peripheral tissues.

Indications

1. Non–small cell lung cancer.
2. Breast cancer.
3. Ovarian cancer.

Dosage Range

Usual dose is 30 mg/m² IV on a weekly schedule either as a single agent or in combination with cisplatin. Dose adjustment on day of treatment according to ANC.

Drug Interaction 1

Drugs metabolized by the liver P450 system—Vinorelbine should be used cautiously in patients receiving medications that inhibit drug metabolism via the hepatic cytochrome P450 system.

Drug Interaction 2

Phenytoin—Vinorelbine reduces blood levels of phenytoin through either reduced absorption of phenytoin or an increase in the rate of its metabolism and elimination.

Drug Interaction 3

Cisplatin—Risk of myelosuppression increases when vinorelbine is used in combination with cisplatin.

Drug Interaction 4

Mitomycin-C—Increased risk of acute allergic reactions when vinorelbine is used in combination with mitomycin-C.

Special Considerations

1. Use with caution in patients with abnormal liver function as toxicity of vinorelbine may be significantly enhanced. Dose reduction is recommended in this setting.

2. Use with caution in patients previously treated with chemotherapy and/or radiation therapy as their bone marrow reserve may be compromised.

3. Vinorelbine should be infused as a rapid push in a free-flowing IV line to avoid extravasation. If extravasation occurs, the infusion should be discontinued immediately. Flushing with sterile water, elevation of the extremity, and local application of ice are recommended. In severe cases, a plastic surgeon should be consulted.

4. Contamination of the eye may lead to severe irritation and even corneal ulceration. If accidental contamination occurs, the eyes should be immediately and thoroughly washed.

5. Pregnancy category D. Breast-feeding should be avoided.

Toxicity 1

Myelosuppression. Dose-limiting toxicity. Readily reversible once treatment is stopped. Neutropenia is most commonly observed. Nadirs occur by day 7, with recovery by day 14. Thrombocytopenia and anemia are less common.

Toxicity 2

Nausea and vomiting. Usually moderate and occur within first 24 hours after treatment.

Toxicity 3

GI toxicities in the form of constipation (35%), diarrhea (17%), stomatitis (<20%), and anorexia (<20%).

Toxicity 4

Transient elevation in LFTs, including SGOT and bilirubin. Usually clinically asymptomatic.

Toxicity 5

Vesicant. Extravasation may cause local tissue injury and inflammation.

Toxicity 6

Neurotoxicity. Usually mild in severity and occurs much less frequently than with other vinca alkaloids. Vinorelbine has lower affinity for axonal microtubules than observed with vincristine or vinblastine. Increased risk in patients with pre-existing neuromuscular disease.

Toxicity 7

Alopecia. Observed in 10%–15% of patients.

Toxicity 8

SIADH.

Toxicity 9

Hypersensitivity and/or allergic reactions presenting as dyspnea and bronchospasm. Incidence is increased when used in combination with mitomycin-C.

Toxicity 10

Generalized fatigue. Occurs in 35% of patients and incidence increases with cumulative doses.

Vorinostat

Trade Names

Zolinza

Classification

Histone deacetylase (HDAC) inhibitor

Category

Chemotherapy drug

Drug Manufacturer

Merck

Mechanism of Action

- Potent inhibitor of histone deacetylases HDAC1, HDAC2, and HDAC3 (Class I) and HDAC6 (Class II).
- Inhibition of HDAC activity leads to accumulation of acetyl groups on the histone lysine residues, resulting in open chromatin structure and transcriptional activation. Induction of cell cycle arrest and/or apoptosis may then occur.
- The precise mechanisms by which vorinostat exerts its antitumor activity has not been fully characterized.

Mechanism of Resistance

None well characterized to date.

Absorption

Oral absorption is not significantly affected when administered with food.

Distribution

Significant binding (75%) to plasma proteins and extensive tissue distribution. Peak plasma levels are achieved 4 hours after ingestion.

Metabolism

Metabolism involves glucuronidation and hydrolysis followed by β-oxidation. In vitro studies suggest minimal biotransformation by the cytochrome P450 system. Elimination is mainly via metabolism, and renal elimination of parent drug accounts for <1% of an administered dose. The terminal half-life of the parent drug is 2 hours.

Indications

FDA-approved for the treatment of patients with CTCL who have progressive, persistent, or recurrent disease on or after two systemic therapies.

Dosage Range

Recommended dose is 400 mg PO daily.

Drug Interaction 1

Warfarin—Patients receiving coumarin-derived anticoagulants should be closely monitored for alterations in their clotting parameters (PT and INR) and/or bleeding, as prolongation of PT and INR has been observed with concomitant use of vorinostat. The dose of warfarin may require careful adjustment in the presence of vorinostat therapy.

Drug Interaction 2

HDAC inhibitors—Severe thrombocytopenia and GI bleeding have been reported when vorinostat and other HDAC inhibitors, such as valproic acid, are used together. CBC and platelet counts should be monitored every 2 weeks for the first 2 months of therapy.

Special Considerations

1. Use with caution in patients with hepatic impairment, although no specific dose recommendations have been provided.

2. Patients should be instructed to drink at least 2 L/day of fluids to maintain hydration.

3. Closely monitor CBC and platelet count every 2 weeks during the first 2 months of therapy and at monthly intervals thereafter.

4. Monitor EKG with QT measurement at baseline and periodically during therapy, as QTc prolongation has been observed. Use with caution in patients at risk of developing QT prolongation, including hypokalemia, hypomagnesemia, congenital long QT syndrome, patients taking antiarrhythmic medications or any other products that may cause QT prolongation, and cumulative high-dose anthracycline therapy.

5. Closely monitor serum glucose levels, especially in diabetic patients, as hyperglycemia may develop while on therapy. Alterations in diet and/or therapy for increased glucose may be necessary.

6. Pregnancy category D.

Toxicity 1

Nausea/vomiting and diarrhea are the most common GI toxicities.

Toxicity 2

Myelosuppression with thrombocytopenia and anemia more common than neutropenia.

Toxicity 3

Fatigue and anorexia.

Toxicity 4

Cardiac toxicity with QTc prolongation.

Toxicity 5

Hyperglycemia.

Toxicity 6

Increased risk of thromboembolic complications, including DVT and PE.

3

Guidelines for Chemotherapy and Dosing Modifications

M. Sitki Copur, Dawn Tiedemann, and Edward Chu

Successful administration of chemotherapy relies on several critical factors: patient's age; performance status; co-morbid illnesses; prior therapy; and baseline hematologic, hepatic, and renal status. The dose of a given chemotherapeutic agent must be adjusted accordingly to reflect these parameters, as well as any specific drug-induced toxicities that may have been experienced with prior treatment. This chapter outlines performance scales that have been established to determine a patient's functional status; reviews methods to determine creatinine clearance, body surface area, and drug dose; and provides recommendations for dosing in the setting of hepatic and renal dysfunction. General guidelines for dialyzing chemotherapeutic agents in the setting of drug overdose or renal failure are provided. A more detailed review for each individual drug is provided in Chapter 2, and the reader is advised to refer to the published literature for further details regarding specific guidelines for drug precautions and dose modifications.

Table 1. Performance Scales

Karnofsky

(%)	Performance
100	Normal, no evidence of disease
90	Able to carry on normal activity, minor signs or symptoms of disease
80	Normal activity with effort, some signs or symptoms of disease
70	Unable to perform normal activity, cares for self
60	Requires occasional assistance
50	Requires considerable assistance and frequent medical care
40	Disabled, requires special care and assistance
30	Severely disabled, hospitalization may be required
20	Hospitalization necessary for support, very sick
10	Moribund, rapid progression of disease
0	Dead

ECOG

(%)	Performance
0	Asymptomatic, normal activity
1	Fully ambulatory, symptomatic, able to perform activities of daily living
2	Symptomatic, up and about, in bed less than 50% of time
3	Symptomatic, capable of only limited self-care, in bed more than 50% of time
4	Completely disabled, cannot perform any self-care, bedridden 100% of time
5	Dead

Table 2. Determination of Creatinine Clearance

- The creatinine clearance is determined by the Cockcroft-Gault formula (Cockcroft, DW, Gault, MH. *Nephron* 1976; 16:31–34), which takes into account age, weight, and serum creatinine.

$$\text{Males: Creatinine Clearance (mL/min)} = \frac{\text{weight (kg)} \times (140 - \text{age})}{72 \times \text{serum creatinine (mg/dL)}}$$

Females: Creatinine Clearance (mL/min) $= \dfrac{\text{weight (kg)} \times (140 - \text{age}) \times 0.85}{72 \times \text{serum creatinine (mg/dL)}}$

- The creatinine clearance can also be determined from a timed urine collection.

Creatinine Clearance $= \dfrac{\text{urine creatinine}}{\text{serum creatinine}} \times \dfrac{\text{urine volume}}{\text{time}}$

Table 3. Determination of Target Area Under the Curve (AUC)

AUC refers to the area under the drug concentration × time curve, and it provides a measure of total drug exposure. It is expressed in concentration × units (mg/mL × min).

A formula for quantifying exposure to carboplatin based on dose and renal function was developed by Calvert et al. (Calvert, H, et al. *J Clin Oncol* 1989; 7:1748–1756) and is as follows:

Carboplatin Dose (mg) = target AUC (mg/mL × min) × [GFR (mL/min) + 25].

It is important to note that the total dose is in mg and NOT mg/m². Target AUC is usually between 5 and 7 mg/mL/min for previously untreated patients. In previously treated patients, lower AUCs (between 4 and 6 mg/mL/min) are recommended. AUCs >7 are generally not associated with improved response rates.

Table 4. Determination of Drug Dose

- Drug doses are usually calculated according to body surface area (BSA, mg/m²).

- BSA is determined by using a nomogram scale or by using a BSA calculator.

- Once the BSA is determined, multiply the BSA by the amount of drug specified in the regimen to give the total dose of drug to be administered.

- For obese patients, ideal body weight (IBW), as opposed to the actual body weight, may be used to calculate BSA. It is important to refer to an IBW table to determine the IBW based on the individual's actual height. Once the IBW is determined, add one-third of the IBW to the IBW, which is then used to determine the BSA.

- IBW can be calculated from the following formulas: IBW for men (kg): 50.0 kg + 2.3 kg per inch over = feet; IBW for women (kg): 45.5 kg + 2.3 kg per inch over = feet.

Taken from: Olin, B (Ed.): "Drug Facts and Comparisons," St. Louis, Missouri, 1996.

Table 5. Calculation of Body Surface Area in Adult Amputees

Body Part	% Surface Area of Amputated Part
Hand and five fingers	3.0
Lower part of arm	4.0
Upper part of arm	6.0
Foot	3.0
Lower part of leg	6.0
Thigh	12.0

BSA (m^2) = BSA - [(BSA) × (%BSA$_{part}$)], where BSA = body surface area, BSA$_{part}$ = body surface area of amputated part.

Taken from: Colangelo, PM, et al. *Am J Hosp Pharm* 1984; 41:2650–2655.

Table 6. General Guidelines for Chemotherapy Dosage Based on Hepatic Function

Drug	Recommended Dose Reduction for Hepatic Dysfunction
Alemtuzumab	N/A
Altretamine	No dose reduction is necessary.
Amifostine	No dose reduction is necessary.
Aminoglutethimide	No dose reduction is necessary.
Amsacrine	Reduce dose by 25% if bilirubin >2.0 mg/dL.
Anastrozole	No formal recommendation for dose reduction. Dose reduction may be necessary in patients with hepatic dysfunction.
Arsenic trioxide	No dose reduction is necessary.
Asparaginase	No dose reduction is necessary.
Azacitidine	No dose reduction is necessary.
Bendamustine	Omit if SGOT or SGPT 2.5–10 × ULN and total bilirubin >1.5 × ULN.
Bevacizumab	N/A

Drug	Recommended Dose Reduction for Hepatic Dysfunction
Bicalutamide	No formal recommendation for dose reduction. Dose reduction may be necessary if bilirubin >3.0 mg/dL.
Bleomycin	No dose reduction is necessary.
Buserelin	No dose reduction is necessary.
Busulfan	No dose reduction is necessary.
Capecitabine	No formal recommendation for dose reduction. Patients need to be closely monitored in the setting of moderate-to-severe hepatic dysfunction.
Carboplatin	No dose reduction is necessary.
Carmustine	No dose reduction is necessary.
Cetuximab	No dose reduction is necessary.
Chlorambucil	No dose reduction is necessary.
Cisplatin	No dose reduction is necessary.
Cladribine	No dose reduction is necessary.
Cyclophosphamide	Reduce by 25% if bilirubin 3.0–5.0 mg/dL or SGOT >180 mg/dL. Omit if bilirubin >5.0 mg/dL.
Cytarabine	No formal recommendation for dose reduction. Dose reduction may be necessary in patients with hepatic dysfunction.
Dacarbazine	No dose reduction is necessary.
Dactinomycin	Reduce dose by 50% if bilirubin >3.0 mg/dL.
Daunorubicin	Reduce dose by 25% if bilirubin 1.5–3.0 mg/dL. Reduce dose by 50% if bilirubin >3.0 mg/dL. Omit if bilirubin >5.0 mg/dL.
Decitabine	N/A
Docetaxel	Omit if bilirubin >1.5 mg/dL, SGOT >60 mg/dL, or alkaline phosphatase >2.5 × ULN.
Doxorubicin	Reduce dose by 50% if bilirubin 1.5–3.0 mg/dL. Reduce dose by 75% if bilirubin 3.1–5.0 mg/dL. Omit if bilirubin >5.0 mg/dL.
Doxorubicin liposome	Reduce dose by 50% if bilirubin 1.5–3.0 mg/dL. Reduce dose by 75% if bilirubin 3.1–5.0 mg/dL. Omit if bilirubin >5.0 mg/dL.

Drug	Recommended Dose Reduction for Hepatic Dysfunction
Erlotinib	No formal recommendations for dose reduction. Dose reduction or interruption should be considered in patients with severe hepatic dysfunction and/or in those with a bilirubin >3 x ULN.
Estramustine	No dose reduction is necessary.
Etoposide	Reduce dose by 50% if bilirubin 1.5–3.0 mg/dL or SGOT 60–180 mg/dL. Omit if bilirubin >3 mg/dL or SGOT >180 mg/dL.
Etoposide phosphate	Reduce dose by 50% if bilirubin 1.5–3.0 mg/dL or SGOT 60–180 mg/dL. Omit if bilirubin >3 mg/dL or SGOT >180 mg/dL.
Everolimus	Reduce dose to 5 mg/day in setting of moderate hepatic dysfunction (Child-Pugh class B) Omit in setting of severe hepatic dysfunction (Child-Pugh class C).
Floxuridine	No dose reduction is necessary.
Fludarabine	No dose reduction is necessary.
5-Fluorouracil	Omit if bilirubin >5.0 mg/dL.
Flutamide	No formal recommendation for dose reduction. Dose reduction may be necessary if bilirubin >3.0 mg/dL.
Gefitinib	No formal recommendations for dose reduction. Dose reduction or interruption should be considered in patients with severe hepatic dysfunction.
Gemcitabine	No dose reduction is necessary.
Goserelin	No dose reduction is necessary.
Hydroxyurea	No dose reduction is necessary.
Idarubicin	Reduce dose by 25% if bilirubin 1.5–3.0 mg/dL or SGOT 60–180 mg/dL. Reduce dose by 50% if bilirubin 3.0–5.0 or SGOT >180 mg/dL. Omit if bilirubin >5.0 mg/dL.
Ifosfamide	No dose reduction is necessary.
Imatinib	Omit if bilirubin >3 mg/dL or SGOT >5 x ULN.

Drug	Recommended Dose Reduction for Hepatic Dysfunction
	Once bilirubin <1.5 or SGOT <2.5 × ULN, reduce dose from 400 mg to 300 mg or from 600 mg to 400 mg.
Interferon-α	No dose reduction is necessary.
Interleukin-2	Omit if signs of hepatic failure (ascites, encephalopathy, jaundice) are observed. Do NOT restart sooner than 7 weeks after recovery from severe hepatic dysfunction.
Irinotecan	No formal recommendation for dose reduction in the presence of hepatic dysfunction. Dose reduction may be necessary. Omit if bilirubin >2.0 mg/dL.
Ixabepilone	Omit when used in combination with capecitabine if SGOT or SGPT >2.5 × ULN or bilirubin >1 × ULN. When used as monotherapy, dose reduce to 32 mg/m² if SGOT or SGPT ≤10 × ULN and bilirubin ≤1.5 × ULN and dose reduce to 20–30 mg/m² if SGOT or SGPT ≤10 × ULN and bilirubin >1.5 × ULN to ≤3 × ULN.
Isotretinoin	No formal recommendation for dose reduction in the presence of mild or moderate hepatic dysfunction. Dose reduction may be necessary.
Lapatinib	No formal recommendation for dose reduction in the presence of mild or moderate hepatic dysfunction. Reduce dose to 750 mg/day in setting of severe hepatic dysfunction (Child-Pugh class C).
Lenalidomide	No formal recommendations for dose reduction.
Leuprolide	No dose reduction is necessary.
Lomustine	No dose reduction is necessary.
Mechlorethamine	No dose reduction is necessary.
Megestrol acetate	No dose reduction is necessary.
Melphalan	No dose reduction is necessary.
6-Mercaptopurine	No dose reduction is necessary.
Methotrexate	Reduce dose by 25% if bilirubin 3.1–5.0 mg/dL or SGOT >180 mg/dL. Omit if bilirubin >5.0 mg/dL.
Mitomycin-C	No dose reduction is necessary.

Drug	Recommended Dose Reduction for Hepatic Dysfunction
Mitotane	No formal recommendation for dose reduction in the presence of hepatic dysfunction. Dose reduction may be necessary.
Mitoxantrone	Reduce dose by 25% if bilirubin >3.0 mg/dL.
Nilutamide	No formal recommendation for dose reduction. Dose reduction may be necessary if bilirubin >3.0 mg/dL.
Oxaliplatin	No dose reduction is necessary.
Paclitaxel	No formal recommendation for dose reduction if bilirubin 1.5–3.0 mg/dL or SGOT 60–180 mg/dL. Omit if bilirubin >5.0 mg/dL or SGOT >180 mg/dL.
Panitumumab	No dose reduction is necessary.
Pegasparaginase	No dose reduction is necessary.
Pemetrexed	No dose reduction is necessary.
Pentostatin	No dose reduction is necessary.
Procarbazine	No formal recommendation for dose reduction in the presence of hepatic dysfunction. Dose reduction may be necessary.
Rituximab	No dose reduction is necessary.
Sorafenib	No formal recommendation for dose reduction in the presence of hepatic dysfunction. Dose reduction may be necessary.
Streptozocin	No dose reduction is necessary.
Sunitinib	No dose reduction is necessary in patients with Child-Pugh Class A or B hepatic dysfunction. Dose reduction may be necessary in patients with Child-Pugh Class C hepatic dysfunction, although there are no formal recommendations.
Tamoxifen	No dose reduction is necessary.
Temozolomide	No dose reduction is necessary.
Thalidomide	N/A
Thioguanine	Omit if bilirubin >5.0 mg/dL.
Thiotepa	No formal recommendation for dose reduction in the presence of hepatic dysfunction. Dose reduction may be necessary.
Topotecan	No dose reduction is necessary.
Trastuzumab	No dose reduction is necessary.

Drug	Recommended Dose Reduction for Hepatic Dysfunction
Tretinoin	Reduce dose to a maximum of 25 mg/m^2 if bilirubin 3.1–5.0 mg/dL or SGOT >180 mg/dL.
	Omit if bilirubin >5.0 mg/dL.
Vinblastine	No dose reduction if bilirubin <1.5 mg/dL and SGOT <60 mg/dL.
	Reduce by 50% if bilirubin 1.5–3.0 mg/dL and SGOT 60–180 mg/dL.
	Omit if bilirubin >3.0 mg/dL or SGOT >180 mg/dL.
Vincristine	No dose reduction if bilirubin <1.5 mg/dL and SGOT <60 mg/dL.
	Reduce by 50% if bilirubin 1.5–3.0 mg/dL and SGOT 60–180 mg/dL.
	Omit if bilirubin >3.0 mg/dL or SGOT >180 mg/dL.
Vinorelbine	No dose reduction if bilirubin <2.0 mg/dL.
	Reduce dose by 50% if bilirubin 2.0–3.0 mg/dL.
	Reduce dose by 75% if bilirubin 3.1–5.0 mg/dL.
	Omit if bilirubin >5.0 mg/dL.
Vorinostat	N/A

N/A—not available

ULN—upper limit of normal

Table 7. General Guidelines for Chemotherapy Dosage Based on Renal Function

Drug	Recommended Dose Reduction for Renal Dysfunction
Alemtuzumab	N/A
Altretamine	N/A
Aminoglutethimide	N/A
Anastrozole	No dose reduction is necessary.

Drug	Recommended Dose Reduction for Renal Dysfunction
Arsenic trioxide	No formal recommendation for dose reduction in the presence of renal dysfunction. Dose reduction may be necessary.
L-Asparaginase	Omit if CrCl <60 mL/min.
Bendamustine	Omit if CrCl <40 mL/min.
Bevacizumab	N/A
Bicalutamide	No dose reduction is necessary.
Bleomycin	No dose reduction if CrCl >60 mL/min. Reduce dose by 25% if CrCl 10–60 mL/min. Reduce dose by 50% if CrCl <10 mL/min.
Buserelin	N/A
Busulfan	No dose reduction is necessary.
Capecitabine	Reduce dose by 25% if CrCl 30–50 mL/min. Omit if CrCl <30 mL/min.
Carboplatin	No dose reduction if CrCl >60 mL/min. AUC dose is modified according to CrCl.
Carmustine	Omit if CrCl <60 mL/min.
Chlorambucil	No dose reduction is necessary.
Cisplatin	No dose reduction if CrCl >60 mL/min. Reduce dose by 50% if CrCl 30–60 mL/min. Omit if CrCl <30 mL/min.
Cetuximab	No dose reduction is necessary.
Cladribine	No formal recommendation for dose reduction in the presence of renal dysfunction. Dose reduction may be necessary.
Cyclophosphamide	No dose reduction if CrCl >50 mL/min. Reduce dose by 25% if CrCl 10–50 mL/min. Reduce dose by 50% if CrCl <10 mL/min.
Cytarabine	No formal recommendation for dose reduction in the presence of renal dysfunction. Dose reduction may be necessary.
Dacarbazine	No formal recommendation for dose reduction in the presence of renal dysfunction. Dose reduction may be necessary.
Dactinomycin	N/A
Dasatinib	No dose reduction is necessary.

Drug	Recommended Dose Reduction for Renal Dysfunction
Daunorubicin	Reduce dose by 50% if serum creatinine >3.0 mg/dL.
Decitabine	N/A
Docetaxel	No dose reduction is necessary.
Doxorubicin	No dose reduction is necessary.
Doxorubicin liposome	No dose reduction is necessary.
Erlotinib	No dose reduction is necessary.
Estramustine	N/A
Etoposide	No dose reduction if CrCl >50 mL/min.
	Reduce dose by 25% if CrCl 10–50 mL/min.
	Reduce dose by 50% if CrCl <10 mL/min.
Etoposide phosphate	No dose reduction if CrCl >50 mL/min.
	Reduce dose by 25% if CrCl 10–50 mL/min.
	Reduce dose by 50% if CrCl <10 mL/min.
Everolimus	No dose reduction is necessary.
Floxuridine	No dose reduction is necessary.
Fludarabine	No formal recommendation for dose reduction in the presence of renal dysfunction. Dose reduction may be necessary.
5-Fluorouracil	No dose reduction is necessary.
Flutamide	N/A
Gefitinib	No dose reduction is necessary.
Gemcitabine	No dose reduction is necessary.
Goserelin	No dose reduction is necessary.
Hydroxyurea	Reduce dose by 80% if CrCl <10 mL/min.
Idarubicin	No dose reduction is necessary.
Ifosfamide	N/A
Imatinib	No dose reduction is necessary.
Interferon-α	No dose reduction is necessary.
Interleukin-2	Omit or discontinue if serum creatinine >4.5 mg/dL or serum creatinine >4.0 mg/dL in the presence of fluid overload.
Irinotecan	No dose reduction is necessary.
Isotretinoin	N/A
Ixabepilone	No formal recommendation for dose reduction.
Lapatinib	No dose reduction is necessary.

Drug	Recommended Dose Reduction for Renal Dysfunction
Lenalidomide	No formal recommendation for dose reduction. In the setting of moderate to severe renal dysfunction, dose reduction may be necessary.
Leuprolide	N/A
Lomustine	Omit if CrCl <60 mL/min.
Mechlorethamine	N/A
Megestrol acetate	N/A
Melphalan	No formal recommendation for dose reduction. However, use with caution in the presence of renal dysfunction.
6-Mercaptopurine	No formal recommendation for dose reduction in the presence of renal dysfunction. Adjust for renal dysfunction by either increasing the interval or decreasing the dose.
Methotrexate	No dose reduction is necessary if CrCl >60 mL/min. Reduce by 50% if CrCl 30–60 mL/min. Omit if CrCl <30 mL/min.
Mitomycin-C	No dose reduction is necessary if CrCl >60 mL/min. Reduce dose by 25% if CrCl 10–60 mL/min. Reduce dose by 50% if CrCl <10 mL/min.
Mitotane	N/A
Mitoxantrone	No dose reduction is necessary.
Nilotinib	No dose reduction is necessary.
Nilutamide	No dose reduction is necessary.
Oxaliplatin	No formal recommendation for dose reduction. Omit if CrCl <20 mL/min.
Paclitaxel	No dose reduction is necessary.
Panitumumab	No dose reduction is necessary.
Pegasparaginase	N/A
Pemetrexed	Dose reduction is necessary when CrCl <60 mL/min and in proportion to the reduction in CrCl.
Pentostatin	No formal recommendation for dose reduction in the presence of renal dysfunction. Dose reduction may be necessary if CrCl 30–60 mL/min.
Procarbazine	Omit if CrCl <30 mL/min.

Drug	Recommended Dose Reduction for Renal Dysfunction
Rituximab	N/A
Sorafenib	No dose reduction is necessary.
Streptozocin	Omit if CrCl <60 mL/min.
Sunitinib	N/A
Tamoxifen	No dose reduction is necessary.
Temozolomide	N/A
Temsirolimus	No dose reduction is necessary.
Thalidomide	No formal recommendation for dose reduction in the presence of renal dysfunction. Dose reduction may be necessary.
Thioguanine	N/A
Thiotepa	No formal recommendation for dose reduction in the presence of renal dysfunction. Dose reduction may be necessary.
Topotecan	No dose reduction is necessary if CrCl >60 mL/min. Reduce dose by 50% if CrCl 10–60 mL/min. Omit if CrCl <10 mL/min.
Trastuzumab	N/A
Tretinoin	Give a maximum of 25 mg/m² in the presence of renal dysfunction. No dose reduction is necessary.
Vinblastine	No dose reduction is necessary.
Vincristine	No dose reduction is necessary.
Vinorelbine	No dose reduction is necessary.
Vorinostat	No dose reduction is necessary.

CrCl—creatinine clearance

N/A—not available

Table 8. Guidelines for Dialysis of Chemotherapy Drugs

	Hemodialysis			Peritoneal Dialysis		
Drug	YES	NO	UNKNOWN	YES	NO	UNKNOWN
Alemtuzumab			X			X
Altretamine			X			X
Aminoglutethimide	X					X
Amsacrine			X			X
Anastrozole			X			X
Arsenic trioxide			X			X
Azacitidine			X			X
Bevacizumab			X			X
Bicalutamide			X			X
Bleomycin		X				X
Bortezomib			X			X
Buserelin			X			X
Busulfan			X			X
Capecitabine			X			X
Carboplatin	X				X	
Carmustine		X				X
Cetuximab			X			X
Chlorambucil			X			X
Cisplatin	X					X
Cladribine			X			X
Cyclophosphamide	X					X
Cytarabine			X		X	
Dacarbazine			X			X
Dactinomycin			X			X
Daunorubicin			X			X
Docetaxel			X			X
Doxorubicin		X				X
Doxorubicin liposome			X			X
Estramustine			X			X
Etoposide	X					X
Etoposide phosphate		X				X

Drug	Hemodialysis			Peritoneal Dialysis		
	YES	NO	UNKNOWN	YES	NO	UNKNOWN
Floxuridine		X				X
Fludarabine		X				X
5-Fluorouracil		X				X
Flutamide		X				X
Gemcitabine		X				X
Goserelin		X				X
Hydroxyurea		X				X
Idarubicin		X				X
Ifosfamide		X				X
Imatinib		X				X
Irinotecan		X				X
Isotretinoin		X				X
Lapatinib			X			X
Lenalidomide			X			X
Leuprolide		X				X
Lomustine	X					X
Mechlorethamine			X			X
Megestrol acetate			X			X
Melphalan			X			X
6-Mercaptopurine			X			X
Methotrexate		X			X	
Mitomycin-C			X			X
Mitotane			X			X
Mitoxantrone			X			X
Nilutamide			X			X
Oxaliplatin			X			X
Paclitaxel			X			X
Pemetrexed		X				X
Pentostatin			X			X
Procarbazine			X			X
Rituximab			X			X
Sorafenib			X			X
Streptozocin			X			X
Sunitinib			X			X
Tamoxifen			X			X

Drug	Hemodialysis			Peritoneal Dialysis		
	YES	NO	UNKNOWN	YES	NO	UNKNOWN
Temozolomide			X			X
Temsirolimus			X			X
Thalidomide			X			X
Thioguanine			X			X
Thiotepa			X			X
Topotecan			X			X
Trastuzumab			X			X
Vinblastine			X			X
Vincristine			X			X
Vinorelbine			X			X

Table 9. Classification of Teratogenic Potential and Use in Pregnancy for Chemotherapy Agents

Pregnancy Category A. Controlled studies show no risk in pregnancy.

Controlled studies in pregnant women have not shown an increased risk of fetal abnormalities when the drug is administered during pregnancy. The possibility of fetal harm appears remote when the drug is used during pregnancy.

Pregnancy Category B. No evidence of risk in pregnancy.

(a) Controlled studies in animals have shown that the drug poses a risk to the fetus. However, studies in pregnant women have failed to show such a risk.

(b) Controlled studies in animals do not show evidence of impaired fertility or harm to the fetus. However, similar studies have not been performed in humans. Because animal studies are not entirely predictive of human response, the drug should be used during pregnancy only if clearly needed.

Pregnancy Category C. Risk in pregnancy cannot be ruled out.

Controlled studies either have not been conducted in animals or show that the drug is teratogenic or has an embryocidal effect and/or other adverse effect in animals. However, there are no adequate and well-controlled studies in pregnant women. The drug should be used during pregnancy only if the potential benefit justifies the potential risk to the fetus.

Pregnancy Category D. Clear evidence of risk in pregnancy.

The drug can cause fetal harm when administered to a pregnant woman. If the drug is used during pregnancy, or if a patient becomes pregnant while taking this drug, the patient should be informed of the potential hazard to the fetus. However, the potential benefits of treatment may outweigh any potential risk.

Pregnancy Category X. Absolutely contraindicated in pregnancy.

The drug has been shown to cause fetal harm when administered to a pregnant woman. The drug is absolutely contraindicated in women who are or may become pregnant. If this drug is used during pregnancy, or if a patient becomes pregnant while taking this drug, the patient should be informed of the potential hazard to the fetus. The potential risk, in this case, outweighs any potential benefit from treatment.

4

Common Chemotherapy Regimens in Clinical Practice

M. Sitki Copur, Edward Chu, Laurie J. Harrold,
Hari Deshpande, and Arthur L. Levy

This chapter provides some of the common combination regimens as well as selected single-agent regimens for solid tumors and hematologic malignancies. They are organized alphabetically by the specific cancer type. In each case, the regimens selected are based on the published literature and are used in clinical practice in the medical oncology community. It should be emphasized that not all of the drugs and dosages in the regimens have been officially approved by the Food and Drug Administration (FDA) for the treatment of a particular tumor. As such, the reader should be aware that some of these treatment regimens may not be approved for reimbursement. This chapter should serve as a quick reference for physicians and health care providers actively engaged in the practice of cancer treatment and provides several options for treating an individual tumor type. It is not intended to be an all-inclusive review of current treatments nor is it intended to endorse and/or prioritize any particular combination or single-agent regimen.

It is important to emphasize that the reader should carefully review the original reference for each of the regimens cited to confirm the specific doses and schedules and to check the complete prescribing information contained within the package insert for each agent.

While considerable efforts have been made to ensure the accuracy of the regimens presented, printing and/or typographical errors may have been made in the preparation of this book. As a result, no liability can be assumed for their use. Moreover, the reader should be reminded that several variations in combination and single-agent regimens exist based on institutional and/or individual experience. Additionally, modifications in dose and schedule may be required according to individual performance status, co-morbid illnesses, baseline blood counts, baseline hepatic and/or renal function, and development of toxicity.

ANAL CANCER

5-Fluorouracil + Mitomycin-C + Radiation Therapy (RTOG/ECOG regimen)

5-Fluorouracil:	1,000 mg/m^2/day IV continuous infusion on days 1–4 and 29–32
Mitomycin-C:	10 mg/m^2 IV (maximum of 20 mg) on days 1 and 29
Radiation therapy:	180 cGy/day, 5 days/week for a total of 5 weeks (total dose, 4,500 cGy)

Chemotherapy is given concurrently with radiation therapy (1).

5-Fluorouracil + Mitomycin-C + Radiation Therapy (EORTC regimen)

5-Fluorouracil:	200 mg/m^2/day IV continuous infusion on days 1–26
Mitomycin-C:	10 mg/m^2 IV on day 1
Radiation therapy:	180 cGy/day, 5 days/week for a total of 4 weeks (total dose, 3,600 cGy)

Chemotherapy is given concurrently with radiation therapy (2). There is a 2-week break following the completion of this first treatment, after which the second treatment is initiated with concurrent chemotherapy and radiation therapy.

5-Fluorouracil:	200 mg/m^2/day IV continuous infusion on days 1–17
Mitomycin-C:	10 mg/m^2 IV on day 1
Radiation therapy:	Total dose, 2,340 cGy over 17 days

5-Fluorouracil + Cisplatin + Radiation Therapy

5-Fluorouracil:	250 mg/m^2/day IV continuous infusion on days 1–5 of each week of radiation therapy
Cisplatin:	4 mg/m^2/day IV continuous infusion on days 1–5 of each week of radiation therapy
Radiation therapy:	Total dose, 5,500 cGy over 6 weeks

Chemotherapy is given concurrently with radiation therapy (3).

XELOX + Radiation Therapy

Capecitabine:	825 mg/m^2 PO bid on Monday-Friday for 6 weeks
Oxaliplatin:	50 mg/m^2 IV on days 1, 8, 22, 29

Radiation therapy: 180 cGy/day, 5 days/week for a total of 6 weeks
Chemotherapy is given concurrently with radiation therapy (4) .

Metastatic Disease and/or Salvage Chemotherapy

5-Fluorouracil + Cisplatin
5-Fluorouracil: 1,000 mg/m^2/day IV continuous infusion on
                               days 1–5
Cisplatin: 100 mg/m^2 IV on day 2
Repeat cycle every 21–28 days (5) .

BILIARY TRACT CANCER

Combination Regimens

Gemcitabine + Cisplatin
Gemcitabine: 1,250 mg/m^2 IV on days 1 and 8
Cisplatin: 75 mg/m^2 on day 1
Repeat cycle every 21 days (6) .
or
Gemcitabine: 1,000 mg/m^2 IV on days 1 and 8
Cisplatin: 25 mg/m^2 on day 1 and 8
Repeat cycle every 21 days for 8 cycles (7) .

Gemcitabine + Capecitabine
Gemcitabine: 1,000 mg/m^2 IV on days 1 and 8
Capecitabine: 650 mg/m^2 PO bid on days 1–14
Repeat cycle every 21 days (8) .

Gemcitabine + Oxaliplatin
Gemcitabine: 1,000 mg/m^2 IV on day 1
Oxaliplatin: 100 mg/m^2 on day 2
Repeat cycle every 14 days (9) .

5-Fluorouracil + Cisplatin
5-Fluorouracil: 400 mg/m^2 IV on day 1, followed by 600 mg/
                               m^2 IV infusion over 22 hours on days 1 and 2
Cisplatin: 50 mg/m^2 IV on day 2
Repeat cycle every 21 days (10) .

Capecitabine + Cisplatin
Capecitabine: $1,250$ mg/m^2 PO bid on days 1–14
Cisplatin: 60 mg/m^2 IV on day 2
Repeat cycle every 21 days (11) .

Single-Agent Regimens

Capecitabine
Capecitabine: $1,000$ mg/m^2 PO bid on days 1–14
Repeat cycle every 21 days (12) . Dose may be reduced to 825–900 mg/m^2
PO bid on days 1–14.

Docetaxel
Docetaxel: 100 mg/m^2 IV on day 1
Repeat cycle every 21 days (13) .

Gemcitabine
Gemcitabine: $1,000$ mg/m^2 IV on days 1 and 8
Repeat cycle every 21 days (14) .

BLADDER CANCER

Combination Regimens

ITP
Ifosfamide: $1,500$ mg/m^2 IV on days 1–3
Paclitaxel: 200 mg/m^2 IV over 3 hours on day 1
Cisplatin: 70 mg/m^2 IV on day 1
Repeat cycle every 21 days (15) . G-CSF support is recommended. Regimen
can also be administered every 28 days.

Gemcitabine + Cisplatin
Gemcitabine: $1,000$ mg/m^2 IV on days 1, 8, and 15
Cisplatin: 75 mg/m^2 IV on day 1
Repeat cycle every 28 days (16) .

Gemcitabine + Carboplatin
Gemcitabine: $1,000$ mg/m^2 IV on days 1 and 8
Carboplatin: AUC of 4, IV on day 1
Repeat cycle every 21 days up to 6 cycles (17) .

Gemcitabine + Paclitaxel

Gemcitabine:	1,000 mg/m^2 IV on days 1, 8, and 15
Paclitaxel:	200 mg/m^2 IV on day 1

Repeat cycle every 21 days (18).
or

Gemcitabine:	2,500 mg/m^2 IV on day 1
Paclitaxel:	150 mg/m^2 IV on day 1

Repeat cycle every 14 days (19).

Gemcitabine + Docetaxel

Gemcitabine:	1,000 mg/m^2 IV on days 1, 8, and 15
Docetaxel:	60 mg/m^2 IV on day 1

Repeat cycle every 28 days (20).

MVAC

Methotrexate:	30 mg/m^2 IV on days 1, 15, and 22
Vinblastine:	3 mg/m^2 IV on days 2, 15, and 22
Doxorubicin:	30 mg/m^2 IV on day 2
Cisplatin:	70 mg/m^2 IV on day 2

Repeat cycle every 28 days (21).

CMV

Cisplatin:	100 mg/m^2 IV on day 2 (give 12 hours after methotrexate)
Methotrexate:	30 mg/m^2 IV on days 1 and 8
Vinblastine:	4 mg/m^2 IV on days 1 and 8

Repeat cycle every 21 days (22).

Docetaxel + Cisplatin

Docetaxel:	75 mg/m^2 IV on day 1
Cisplatin:	75 mg/m^2 IV on day 1

Repeat cycle every 21 days up to 6 cycles (23).

Paclitaxel + Carboplatin

Paclitaxel:	225 mg/m^2 IV over 3 hours on day 1
Carboplatin:	AUC of 6, IV on day 1, given 15 minutes after paclitaxel

Repeat cycle every 21 days (24).

CAP

Cyclophosphamide:	400 mg/m^2 IV on day 1
Doxorubicin:	40 mg/m^2 IV on day 1

Cisplatin: 75 mg/m² IV on day 2
Repeat cycle every 21 days (25) .

Single-Agent Regimens

Gemcitabine
Gemcitabine: 1,200 mg/m² IV on days 1, 8, and 15
Repeat cycle every 28 days (26) .

Paclitaxel
Paclitaxel: 250 mg/m² IV over 24 hours on day 1
Repeat cycle every 21 days (27) .
or
Paclitaxel: 80 mg/m² IV weekly for 3 weeks
Repeat cycle every 4 weeks (28) .

Pemetrexed
Pemetrexed: 500 mg/m² IV on day 1
Repeat cycle every 21 days (29) . Folic acid at 350–1,000 µg PO daily beginning 1–2 weeks prior to therapy and vitamin B12 at 1,000 µg IM to start 1–2
weeks prior to first dose of therapy and repeated every 3 cycles.

BRAIN CANCER

Adjuvant Therapy

Combination Regimens

Temozolomide + Radiation Therapy
Radiation therapy: 200 cGy/day for 5 days per week for total of 6
                             weeks
Temozolomide: 75 mg/m² PO daily for 6 weeks with radiation
                             therapy, followed by 150 mg/m² PO on days 1–5
Repeat cycle every 28 days up to 6 cycles (30) . If well tolerated can increase
dose to 200 mg/m².

PCV
Procarbazine: 60 mg/m² PO on days 8–21
Lomustine: 130 mg/m² PO on day 1
Vincristine: 1.4 mg/m² IV on days 8 and 29
Repeat cycle every 8 weeks for 6 cycles (31) .

Single-Agent Regimens

BCNU
BCNU: 220 mg/m² IV on day 1
Repeat cycle every 6–8 weeks for 1 year (32) .
or
BCNU: 75–100 mg/m² IV on days 1 and 2
Repeat cycle every 6–8 weeks (32) .

Advanced Disease

Combination Regimens

PCV
Procarbazine: 75 mg/m² PO on days 8–21
Lomustine: 130 mg/m² PO on day 1
Vincristine: 1.4 mg/m² IV on days 8 and 29
Repeat cycle every 8 weeks (33) .

Irinotecan + Bevacizumab
Irinotecan: 125 mg/m² IV on day 1
Bevacizumab: 10 mg/kg IV on day 1
Repeat cycle every 2 weeks for 6 cycles (34) .

Temozolomide + Bevacizumab
Temozolomide: 150 mg/m² PO on days 1-5
Bevacizumab: 10 mg/kg IV on day 1 and 14
Repeat cycle every 28 days (35) .

Single-Agent Regimens

BCNU
BCNU: 200 mg/m² IV on day 1
Repeat cycle every 6–8 weeks (36) .

Procarbazine
Procarbazine: 150 mg/m² PO daily divided into 3 doses
Repeat daily (36) .

Temozolomide
Temozolomide: 150 mg/m² PO on days 1–5
Repeat cycle every 28 days (37) . If well tolerated, can increase dose to 200 mg/m².

Irinotecan

Irinotecan: 350 mg/m² IV over 90 min on day 1
Repeat cycle every 3 weeks (38) .
or
Irinotecan: 125 mg/m² IV weekly for 4 weeks
Repeat cycle every 6 weeks (39) .

BREAST CANCER

Neoadjuvant Therapy

Combination Regimens

ACT

Doxorubicin: 60 mg/m² IV on day 1
Cyclophosphamide: 600 mg/m² IV on day 1
Docetaxel: 100 mg/m² IV on day 1
Repeat cycle every 21 days for a total of 4 cycles, followed by surgery (40) .

Adjuvant Therapy

Combination Regimens: HER2-negative disease

AC

Doxorubicin: 60 mg/m² IV on day 1
Cyclophosphamide: 600 mg/m² IV on day 1
Repeat cycle every 21 days for a total of 4 cycles (41) .

AC→T

Doxorubicin: 60 mg/m² IV on day 1
Cyclophosphamide: 600 mg/m² IV on day 1
Repeat cycle every 21 days for a total of 4 cycles, followed by
Paclitaxel: 175 mg/m² IV on day 1
Repeat cycle every 21 days for a total of 4 cycles (42) .

AC→T (weekly)

Doxorubicin: 60 mg/m² IV on day 1
Cyclophosphamide: 600 mg/m² IV on day 1
Repeat cycle every 21 days for a total of 4 cycles, followed by
Paclitaxel: 80 mg/m² IV on day 1
Repeat on a weekly schedule for 12 weeks (43) .

AC→Docetaxel

Doxorubicin: 60 mg/m^2 IV on day 1
Cyclophosphamide: 600 mg/m^2 IV on day 1
Repeat cycle every 21 days for a total of 4 cycles, followed by
Docetaxel: 100 mg/m^2 IV on day 1
Repeat cycle every 21 days for a total of 4 cycles (44).

AC→Docetaxel (weekly)

Doxorubicin: 60 mg/m^2 IV on day 1
Cyclophosphamide: 600 mg/m^2 IV on day 1
Repeat cycle every 21 days for a total of 4 cycles, followed by
Docetaxel: 35 mg/m^2 IV on day 1
Repeat weekly for a total of 12 weeks (45).

TC

Docetaxel: 75 mg/m^2 IV on day 1
Cyclophosphamide: 600 mg/m^2 IV on day 1
Repeat cycle every 21 days for a total of 4 cycles (46).

TAC

Docetaxel: 75 mg/m^2 IV on day 1
Doxorubicin: 50 mg/m^2 IV on day 1
Cyclophosphamide: 500 mg/m^2 IV on day 1
Repeat cycle every 21 days for a total of 6 cycles (47).

CAF

Cyclophosphamide: 600 mg/m^2 IV on day 1
Doxorubicin: 60 mg/m^2 IV on day 1
5-Fluorouracil: 600 mg/m^2 IV on day 1
Repeat cycle every 28 days for a total of 4 cycles (48).

Epirubicin + CMF

Epirubicin: 100 mg/m^2 IV on day 1
Repeat cycle every 21 days for 4 cycles, followed by
Cyclophosphamide: 600 mg/m^2 IV on day 1
Methotrexate: 40 mg/m^2 IV on day 1
5-Fluorouracil: 600 mg/m^2 IV on day 1
Repeat cycle every 21 days for a total of 4 cycles (49).

FEC

5-Fluorouracil: 500 mg/m^2 IV on day 1

Epirubicin: 100 mg/m² IV on day 1
Cyclophosphamide: 500 mg/m² IV on day 1
Repeat cycle every 21 days for a total of 6 cycles (50) .

FEC→Docetaxel

5-Fluorouracil: 500 mg/m² IV on day 1
Epirubicin: 100 mg/m² IV on day 1
Cyclophosphamide: 500 mg/m² IV on day 1
Repeat cycle every 21 days for a total of 6 cycles (51) , followed by
Docetaxel: 100 mg/m² IV on day 1
Repeat cycle every 21 days for 3 cycles.

Dose-Dense Combination Regimens: HER2-negative disease

AC→T

Doxorubicin: 60 mg/m² IV on day 1
Cyclophosphamide: 600 mg/m² IV on day 1
Repeat cycle every 14 days for a total of 4 cycles, followed by
Paclitaxel: 175 mg/m² IV on day 1
Repeat cycle every 14 days for a total of 4 cycles (52) .
Administer pegfilgrastim 6 mg SC on day 2 of each treatment cycle.

A→T→C

Doxorubicin: 60 mg/m² IV on day 1
Repeat cycle every 2 weeks for 4 cycles, followed by
Paclitaxel: 175 mg/m² IV on day 1
Repeat cycle every 2 weeks for 4 cycles, followed by
Cyclophosphamide: 600 mg/m² IV on day 1
Repeat cycle every 2 weeks for 4 cycles.
Administer filgrastim 5 µg/kg SC on days 3–10 of each treament cycle (53) .

AC→Docetaxel

Doxorubicin: 60 mg/m² IV on day 1
Cyclophosphamide: 600 mg/m² IV on day 1
Repeat cycle every 14 days for a total of 4 cycles, followed by
Docetaxel: 75 mg/m² IV on day 1
Repeat cycle every 14 days for a total of 4 cycles (54) .
Administer pegfilgrastim 6 mg SC on day 2 of each treatment cycle.

Docetaxel→AC

Docetaxel: 75 mg/m² IV on day 1
Repeat cycle every 14 days for a total of 4 cycles, followed by

Doxorubicin: 60 mg/m² IV on day 1
Cyclophosphamide: 600 mg/m² IV on day 1
Repeat cycle every 14 days for a total of 4 cycles (54) .
Administer pegfilgrastim 6 mg SC on day 2 of each treatment cycle.

Combination Regimens: HER2-positive disease

AC→T + Trastuzumab

Doxorubicin: 60 mg/m² IV on day 1
Cyclophosphamide: 600 mg/m² IV on day 1
Repeat cycle every 21 days for a total of 4 cycles, followed by
Paclitaxel: 80 mg/m² IV over 1 hour on day 1
Trastuzumab: 4 mg/kg IV loading dose, then 2 mg/kg IV
                              weekly
Repeat weekly for 12 weeks, followed by
Trastuzumab: 2 mg/kg IV weekly
Repeat weekly for 40 weeks (55) .

AC→T + Trastuzumab (dose dense)

Doxorubicin: 60 mg/m² IV on day 1
Cyclophosphamide: 600 mg/m² IV on day 1
Repeat cycle every 14 days for a total of 4 cycles, followed by
Paclitaxel: 175 mg/m² IV on day 1
Repeat cycle every 14 days for a total of 4 cycles.
Trastuzumab: 4 mg/kg IV loading dose along with paclitaxel
                              and then 2 mg/kg IV weekly
Trastuzumab is administered for a total of 1 year (56) .

TCH

Docetaxel: 75 mg/m² IV on day 1
Carboplatin: AUC of 6, IV on day 1
Trastuzumab: 4 mg/kg IV loading dose and then 2 mg/kg IV
                              weekly
Repeat chemotherapy every 21 days for a total of 6 cycles. At the completion of chemotherapy, trastuzumab is administered at 6 mg/kg IV every 3 weeks for a total of 1 year (57) .

DH→FEC

Docetaxel: 100 mg/m² IV on day 1
Trastuzumab   4 mg/kg IV loading dose on day 1 and then 2
                              mg/kg IV weekly
Repeat cycle every 21 days for 3 cycles, followed by
5-Fluorouracil: 600 mg/m² IV on day 1

Epirubicin: 60 mg/m² IV on day 1
Cyclophosphamide: 600 mg/m² IV on day 1
Repeat cycle every 21 days for 3 cycles (58) .

Hormonal Regimens

Tamoxifen
Tamoxifen: 20 mg PO daily
Repeat daily for 5 years in patients with ER+ tumors or ER status unknown
(59) .

Anastrozole
Anastrozole: 1 mg PO daily
Repeat daily for 5 years in patients with ER+ tumors or ER status unknown
(60) .

Letrozole
Letrozole: 2.5 mg PO daily
Repeat daily for 5 years in patients with ER+ or PR+ tumors (61) .

Tamoxifen + Letrozole (62)
Tamoxifen: 20 mg PO daily for 5 years, followed by
Letrozole: 2.5 mg PO daily for 5 years

Tamoxifen + Exemestane (63)
Tamoxifen: 20 mg PO daily for 2–3 years, followed by
Exemestane: 25 mg PO daily for the remainder of 5 years

Tamoxifen + Goserelin + Zoledronic acid
Tamoxifen: 20 mg PO daily
Goserelin: 3.6 mg SC every 28 days
Zoledronic acid: 4 mg IV every 6 months
Continue treatment for a total of 3 years (64) .

Anastrozole + Goserelin + Zoledronic acid
Anastrozole: 1 mg PO daily
Goserelin: 3.6 mg SC every 28 days
Zoledronic acid: 4 mg IV every 6 months
Continue treatment for a total of 3 years (64) .

Metastatic Disease

Combination Regimens: HER2-negative disease

AC
Doxorubicin:	60 mg/m² IV on day 1
Cyclophosphamide:	600 mg/m² IV on day 1

Repeat cycle every 21 days (41) .

AT
Doxorubicin:	50 mg/m² IV on day 1
Paclitaxel:	150 mg/m² IV over 24 hours on day 1

Repeat cycle every 21 days (65) .

or

Doxorubicin:	60 mg/m² IV on day 1

Repeat cycle every 21 days up to a maximum of 8 cycles, followed by

Paclitaxel:	175 mg/m² IV on day 1

Repeat cycle every 21 days until disease progression (65) .

or

Paclitaxel:	175 mg/m² IV on day 1

Repeat cycle every 21 days until disease progression, followed by

Doxorubicin:	60 mg/m² IV on day 1

Repeat cycle every 21 days up to a maximum of 8 cycles (65) .

CAF
Cyclophosphamide:	600 mg/m² IV on day 1
Doxorubicin:	60 mg/m² IV on day 1
5-Fluorouracil:	600 mg/m² IV on day 1

Repeat cycle every 21 days (48) .

CEF
Cyclophosphamide:	75 mg/m² PO on days 1–14
Epirubicin:	60 mg/m² IV on days 1 and 8
5-Fluorouracil:	500 mg/m² IV on days 1 and 8

Repeat cycle every 28 days (66) .

CMF
Cyclophosphamide:	600 mg/m² IV on day 1
Methotrexate:	40 mg/m² IV on day 1
5-Fluorouracil:	600 mg/m² IV on day 1

Repeat cycle every 21 days (49) .

Capecitabine + Docetaxel (XT)

Capecitabine: 1,250 mg/m² PO bid on days 1–14
Docetaxel: 75 mg/m² IV on day 1
Repeat cycle every 21 days (67) . May decrease dose of capecitabine to 825–1,000 mg/m² PO bid on days 1–14 to reduce the risk of toxicity without compromising clinical efficacy.

Capecitabine + Paclitaxel (XP)

Capecitabine: 825 mg/m² PO bid on days 1–14
Paclitaxel: 175 mg/m² IV on day 1
Repeat cycle every 21 days (68) .

Capecitabine + Navelbine (XN)

Capecitabine: 1,000 mg/m² PO bid on days 1–14
Navelbine: 25 mg/m² IV on days 1 and 8
Repeat cycle every 21 days (68) .

Capecitabine + Ixabepilone (XI)

Capecitabine: 1,000 mg/m² PO bid on days 1–14
Ixabepilone: 40 mg/m² IV on day 1
Repeat cycle every 21 days (69) .

Docetaxel + Doxorubicin

Docetaxel: 75 mg/m² IV on day 1
Doxorubicin: 50 mg/m² IV on day 1
Repeat cycle every 21 days (70) .

Pegylated Liposomal Doxorubicin + Docetaxel

Pegylated Liposomal   30 mg/m² on day 1
Doxorubicin :
Docetaxel: 60 mg/m² on day 1
Repeat cycle every 21 days (71) .

FEC-100

5-Fluorouracil: 500 mg/m² IV on day 1
Epirubicin: 100 mg/m² IV on day 1
Cyclophosphamide: 500 mg/m² IV on day 1
Repeat cycle every 21 days (72) .

FEC-75

5-Fluorouracil: 500 mg/m² IV on day 1

Epirubicin: 75 mg/m² IV on day 1
Cyclophosphamide: 500 mg/m² IV on day 1
Repeat cycle every 21 days (73) .

FEC-50
5-Fluorouracil: 500 mg/m² IV on day 1
Epirubicin: 50 mg/m² IV on day 1
Cyclophosphamide: 500 mg/m² IV on day 1
Repeat cycle every 21 days (73) .

Gemcitabine + Paclitaxel
Gemcitabine: 1,250 mg/m² IV on days 1 and 8
Paclitaxel: 175 mg/m² IV on day 1
Repeat cycle every 21 days (74) .

Carboplatin + Paclitaxel
Carboplatin: AUC of 6, IV on day 1
Paclitaxel: 200 mg/m² IV over 3 hours on day 1
Repeat cycle every 21 days (75) .

Carboplatin + Docetaxel
Carboplatin: AUC of 6, IV on day 1
Docetaxel: 75 mg/m² IV on day 1
Repeat cycle every 21 days (76) .

Paclitaxel + Bevacizumab
Paclitaxel: 90 mg/m² IV on days 1, 8, and 15
Bevacizumab: 10 mg/kg on days 1 and 15
Repeat cycle every 28 days (77) .

Combination Regimens: HER2-positive disease

Trastuzumab-Paclitaxel
Trastuzumab: 4 mg/kg IV loading dose and then 2 mg/kg
                              weekly
Paclitaxel: 175 mg/m² IV over 3 hours on day 1
Repeat cycle every 21 days (78) .
or
Trastuzumab: 4 mg/kg IV loading dose and then 2 mg/kg
                              weekly
Paclitaxel: 80 mg/m² IV weekly
Repeat cycle every 4 weeks (79) .

Trastuzumab-Docetaxel

Trastuzumab: 4 mg/kg IV loading dose and then 2 mg/kg IV on days 8 and 15

Docetaxel: 35 mg/m² IV on days 1, 8, and 15

The first cycle is administered weekly for 3 weeks, with 1 week rest. For subsequent cycles,

Trastuzumab: 2 mg/kg IV weekly

Docetaxel: 35 mg/m² IV weekly

Repeat cycle every 4 weeks (80) .

TCH

Carboplatin: AUC of 6, IV on day 1

Docetaxel: 75 mg/m² IV on day 1

Trastuzumab: 4 mg/kg IV loading dose on day 1 and then 2 mg/kg IV on days 8 and 15, 2 mg/kg IV weekly thereafter

Repeat cycle every 21 days (81) .

Trastuzumab-Navelbine

Trastuzumab: 4 mg/kg IV loading dose and then 2 mg/kg IV weekly

Navelbine: 25 mg/m² IV weekly

Repeat on a weekly basis until disease progression (82) .

Trastuzumab-Gemcitabine

Trastuzumab: 4 mg/kg IV loading dose and then 2 mg/kg IV weekly

Gemcitabine: 1,200 mg/m² IV weekly for 2 weeks

Repeat cycle every 21 days (83) .

Trastuzumab-Capecitabine

Trastuzumab: 4 mg/kg IV loading dose and then 2 mg/kg IV weekly

Capecitabine: 1,250 mg/m² PO bid on days 1–14

Repeat cycle every 21 days (84) .

or

Trastuzumab: 8 mg/kg IV loading dose and then 6 mg/kg IV on day 1 of all subsequent cycles

Capecitabine: 1,250 mg/m² PO bid on days 1–14

Repeat cycle every 21 days (85) .

Trastuzumab-Lapatinib

| Trastuzumab: | 4 mg/kg IV loading dose and then 2 mg/kg IV weekly |
| Lapatinib: | 1,000 mg PO daily |

Continue until disease progression (86) .

Capecitabine + Lapatinib

| Capecitabine: | 1,000 mg/m^2 PO bid on days 1–14 |
| Lapatinib: | 1,250 mg PO daily |

Repeat cycle every 21 days (87) .

Single-Agent Regimens

Tamoxifen

| Tamoxifen: | 20 mg PO daily (88). |

Toremifene citrate

| Toremifene: | 60 mg PO daily (89). |

Exemestane

| Exemestane: | 25 mg PO daily (90). |

Anastrozole

| Anastrozole: | 1 mg PO daily (91). |

Letrozole

| Letrozole: | 2.5 mg PO daily (92). |

Fulvestrant

| Fulvestrant: | 250 mg IM on day 1 |

Repeat injection every month (93) .

or

| Fulvestrant: | 500 mg IM loading dose on day 1, then 250 mg IM on days 14 and 28 |

Continue on a monthly basis until disease progression (94) .

Megestrol

| Megestrol: | 40 mg PO qid (95). |

Trastuzumab

| Trastuzumab: | 4 mg/kg IV loading dose and then 2 mg/kg IV weekly |

Repeat cycle weekly for a total of 10 weeks. In the absence of disease progression, continue weekly maintenance dose of 2 mg/kg (96).
or

Trastuzumab: 8 mg/kg IV loading dose, then 6 mg/kg IV every 3 weeks

Continue 6 mg/kg every 3 weeks until disease progression (97).

Capecitabine

Capecitabine: 1,250 mg/m^2 PO bid for 2 weeks followed by 1-week rest period

Repeat cycle every 21 days (98). May decrease dose to 850–1,000 mg/m^2 PO bid on days 1–14 to reduce the risk of toxicity without compromising clinical efficacy.

Docetaxel

Docetaxel: 100 mg/m^2 IV on day 1

Repeat cycle every 21 days (99).
or

Docetaxel: 35–40 mg/m^2 IV weekly for 6 weeks

Repeat cycle every 8 weeks (100).

Paclitaxel

Paclitaxel: 175 mg/m^2 IV over 3 hours on day 1

Repeat cycle every 21 days (101).
or

Paclitaxel: 80–100 mg/m^2 IV weekly for 3 weeks

Repeat cycle every 4 weeks (102).

Ixabepilone

Ixabepilone: 40 mg/m^2 IV on day 1

Repeat cycle every 21 days (103).

Vinorelbine

Vinorelbine: 30 mg/m^2 IV on day 1

Repeat cycle every 7 days (104).

Doxorubicin

Doxorubicin: 20 mg/m^2 IV on day 1

Repeat cycle every 7 days (105).

Gemcitabine

Gemcitabine: 725 mg/m^2 IV weekly for 3 weeks
Repeat cycle every 28 days (106).

Pegylated Liposomal Doxorubicin
Pegylated Liposomal
Doxorubicin: 40 mg/m^2 IV on day 1
Repeat cycle every 28 days (107).

Abraxane
Abraxane: 260 mg/m^2 IV on day 1
Repeat cycle every 21 days (108).
or
Abraxane: 125 mg/m^2 IV on days 1, 8, and 15
Repeat cycle every 28 days (109).

CANCER OF UNKNOWN PRIMARY

PCE
Paclitaxel: 200 mg/m^2 IV over 1 hour on day 1
Carboplatin: AUC of 6, IV on day 1
Etoposide: 50 mg alternating with 100 mg PO on days 1–10
Repeat cycle every 21 days (110).

EP
Etoposide: 100 mg/m^2 IV on days 1–5
Cisplatin: 100 mg/m^2 IV on day 1
Repeat cycle every 21 days (111).

PEB
Cisplatin: 20 mg/m^2 IV on days 1–5
Etoposide: 100 mg/m^2 IV on days 1–5
Bleomycin: 30 units IV on days 1, 8, and 15
Repeat cycle every 21 days (112).

GCP
Gemcitabine: 1,000 mg/m^2 IV on days 1 and 8
Carboplatin: AUC of 5, IV on day 1
Paclitaxel: 200 mg/m^2 IV on day 1

Repeat cycle every 21 days for 4 cycles (113). This is to be followed by paclitaxel at 70 mg/m² IV every week for 6 weeks with a 2-week rest. Repeat for a total of 3 cycles.

Bevacizumab + Erlotinib
Bevacizumab: 10 mg/kg IV on day 1
Erlotinib: 150 mg PO daily
Continue until disease progression (114).

CARCINOID TUMORS

Combination Regimens

5-Fluorouracil + Streptozocin
5-Fluorouracil: 400 mg/m²/day IV on days 1–5
Streptozocin: 500 mg/m²/day IV on days 1–5
Repeat cycle every 6 weeks (115).

Doxorubicin + Streptozocin
Doxorubicin: 50 mg/m² IV on days 1 and 22
Streptozocin: 500 mg/m²/day IV on days 1–5
Repeat cycle every 6 weeks (115).

Cisplatin + Etoposide
Cisplatin: 45 mg/m²/day IV continuous infusion on days 2 and 3
Etoposide: 130 mg/m²/day IV continuous infusion on days 1–3
Repeat cycle every 21 days (116).

Single-Agent Regimens

Octreotide
Octreotide: 150–250 μg SC tid
Continue until disease progression (117).

Sunitinib
Sunitinib: 50 mg PO daily for 4 weeks
Repeat cycle every 6 weeks (118).

CERVICAL CANCER

Combination Regimens

Cisplatin + Radiation Therapy

Radiation therapy: 1.8 to 2 Gy per fraction (total dose, 45 Gy)

Cisplatin: 40 mg/m² IV weekly (maximal dose, 70 mg per week)

Cisplatin is given 4 hours before radiation therapy on weeks 1–6 (119) .

Paclitaxel + Cisplatin

Paclitaxel: 135 mg/m² IV over 24 hours on day 1

Cisplatin: 75 mg/m² IV on day 2

Repeat cycle every 21 days (120) .

Cisplatin + Topotecan

Cisplatin: 50 mg/m² IV on day 1

Topotecan: 0.75 mg/m²/day IV on days 1–3

Repeat cycle every 21 days (121) .

BIP

Bleomycin: 30 U IV over 24 hours on day 1

Ifosfamide: 5,000 mg/m² IV over 24 hours on day 2

Mesna: 6,000 mg/m² IV over 36 hours on day 2

Cisplatin: 50 mg/m² IV on day 2

Repeat cycle every 21 days (122) .

BIC

Bleomycin: 30 U IV on day 1

Ifosfamide: 2,000 mg/m² IV on days 1–3

Mesna: 400 mg/m² IV, 15 minutes before ifosfamide dose, then 400 mg/m² IV at 4 and 8 hours following ifosfamide

Carboplatin: 200 mg/m² IV on day 1

Repeat cycle every 21 days (123) .

Cisplatin + 5-Fluorouracil

Cisplatin: 75 mg/m² IV on day 1

5-Fluorouracil: 1,000 mg/m²/day IV continuous infusion on days 2–5

Repeat cycle every 21 days (124).

Cisplatin + Vinorelbine
Cisplatin: 80 mg/m² IV on day 1
Vinorelbine: 25 mg/m² IV on days 1 and 8
Repeat cycle every 21 days (125).

Cisplatin + Irinotecan
Cisplatin: 60 mg/m² IV on day 1
Irinotecan: 60 mg/m² IV on days 1, 8, and 15
Repeat cycle every 28 days (126).

Cisplatin + Gemcitabine
Cisplatin: 50 mg/m² IV on day 1
Gemcitabine: 1,000 mg/m² IV on days 1 and 8
Repeat cycle every 21 days for up to 6 cycles (127).

Carboplatin + Docetaxel
Carboplatin: AUC of 6, IV on day 1
Docetaxel: 60 mg/m² IV on day 1
Repeat cycle every 21 days (128).

Single-Agent Regimens

Docetaxel
Docetaxel: 100 mg/m² IV on day 1
Repeat cycle every 21 days (129).

Paclitaxel
Paclitaxel: 175 mg/m² IV over 3 hours on day 1
Repeat cycle every 21 days (130).

Irinotecan
Irinotecan: 125 mg/m² IV weekly for 4 weeks
Repeat cycle every 6 weeks (131).

Topotecan
Topotecan: 1.5 mg/m²/day on days 1–5
Repeat cycle every 21 days (132).

COLORECTAL CANCER

Neoadjuvant Combined Modality Therapy for Rectal Cancer

5-Fluorouracil + Radiation Therapy (German AIO regimen)

5-Fluorouracil: 1,000 mg/m²/day IV continuous infusion on days 1–5

Repeat infusional 5-FU on weeks 1 and 5.

Radiation therapy: 180 cGy/day for 5 days per week (total dose, 5,040 cGy)

Followed by surgical resection and then adjuvant chemotherapy with 5-FU at 500 mg/m² IV for 5 days every 28 days for a total of 4 cycles (133) .

Infusion 5-FU + Radiation Therapy

5-Fluorouracil: 225 mg/m²/day IV continuous infusion throughout entire course of radiation therapy

Radiation therapy: 180 cGy/day for 5 days per week (total dose, 5,040 cGy)

Followed by surgical resection and then adjuvant chemotherapy with capecitabine, 5-FU/LV, or FOLFOX4 for a total of 4 months (134) .

Capecitabine + Radiation Therapy

Capecitabine: 825 mg/m² PO bid throughout the entire course of radiation therapy or 900–1,000 mg/m² PO bid on days 1–5 of each week of radiation therapy

Radiation therapy: 180 cGy/day for 5 days per week (total dose, 5,040 cGy)

Followed by surgical resection and then adjuvant chemotherapy with capecitabine, 5-FU, or 5-FU/LV for a total of 4 cycles (135) .

5-FU/LV + Oxaliplatin + Radiation Therapy

5-Fluorouracil: 200 mg/m²/day IV continuous infusion throughout entire course of radiation therapy

Oxaliplatin: 60 mg/m² IV on days 1, 8, 15, 22, 29, and 36

Radiation therapy: 180 cGy/day for 5 days each week (total dose, 5,040 cGy)

Followed by surgical resection 4–6 weeks after completion of chemoradiotherapy and then adjuvant chemotherapy (136) .

XELOX + Radiation Therapy
Capecitabine: 825 mg/m² PO bid on days 1–14 and 22–35
Oxaliplatin: 50 mg/m² IV on days 1, 8, 22, and 29
Radiation therapy: 180 cGy/day for 5 days per week (total dose, 5,040 cGy)
Followed by surgical resection and then adjuvant chemotherapy with
Capecitabine: 1,000 mg/m² PO bid on days 1–14
Oxaliplatin: 130 mg/m² IV on day 1
Repeat cycle every 3 weeks for 4 cycles (137).

Adjuvant Therapy

5-Fluorouracil + Leucovorin (Mayo Clinic schedule)
5-Fluorouracil: 425 mg/m² IV on days 1–5
Leucovorin: 20 mg/m² IV on days 1–5, administered before 5-fluorouracil
Repeat cycle every 4–5 weeks for a total of 6 cycles (138).

5-Fluorouracil + Leucovorin (weekly schedule, high dose)
5-Fluorouracil: 500 mg/m² IV weekly for 6 weeks
Leucovorin: 500 mg/m² IV over 2 hours weekly for 6 weeks, administered before 5-fluorouracil
Repeat cycle every 8 weeks for a total of 4 cycles (32 weeks total) (139).

5-Fluorouracil + Leucovorin (weekly schedule, low dose)
5-Fluorouracil: 500 mg/m² IV weekly for 6 weeks
Leucovorin: 20 mg/m² IV weekly for 6 weeks, administered before 5-fluorouracil
Repeat cycle every 8 weeks for a total of 4 or 6 cycles (32 or 48 weeks total) (140).

Oxaliplatin + 5-Fluorouracil + Leucovorin (FOLFOX4)
Oxaliplatin: 85 mg/m² IV on day 1
5-Fluorouracil: 400 mg/m² IV bolus, followed by 600 mg/m² IV continuous infusion for 22 hours on days 1 and 2
Leucovorin: 200 mg/m² IV on days 1 and 2 as a 2-hour infusion before 5-fluorouracil
Repeat cycle every 2 weeks for a total of 12 cycles (6 months total) (141).

Oxaliplatin + 5-Fluorouracil + Leucovorin (mFOLFOX7)
Oxaliplatin: 100 mg/m² IV on day 1

| 5-Fluorouracil: | 3,000 mg/m² IV continuous infusion on days 1 and 2 for 46 hours |
| Leucovorin: | 200 mg/m² IV on day 1 as a 2-hour infusion before 5-fluorouracil |

Repeat cycle every 2 weeks for a total of 12 cycles (6 months total) (142) .

FLOX

5-Fluorouracil:	500 mg/m² IV weekly for 6 weeks, administered 1 hour after LV infusion begun
Leucovorin:	500 mg/m² IV over 2 hours weekly for 6 weeks, administered before 5-fluorouracil
Oxaliplatin:	85 mg/m² IV administered before 5-fluorouracil and LV and on days 1, 15, and 29

Repeat cycle every 8 weeks for a total of 3 cycles (6 months total) (143) .

Oxaliplatin + Capecitabine (XELOX)

| Oxaliplatin: | 130 mg/m² IV on day 1 |
| Capecitabine: | 1,000 mg/m² PO bid on days 1–14 |

Repeat cycle every 3 weeks for a total of 8 cycles (6 months total) (144) .
Dose may be decreased to 850 mg/m² PO bid days 1–14 to reduce risk of toxicity without compromising efficacy.

LV5FU2 (deGramont regimen)

5-Fluorouracil:	400 mg/m² IV bolus, followed by 600 mg/m² IV continuous infusion for 22 hours on days 1 and 2
Leucovorin:	200 mg/m² IV on days 1 and 2 as a 2-hour infusion before 5-fluorouracil
or	
L-Leucovorin	100 mg/m² IV on days 1 and 2 as a 2-hour infusion before 5-fluorouracil

Repeat cycle every 2 weeks for a total of 12 cycles (141) .

Capecitabine

| Capecitabine: | 1,250 mg/m² PO bid on days 1–14 |

Repeat cycle every 21 days for a total of 8 cycles (145) . Dose may be decreased to 850–1,000 mg/m² PO bid on days 1–14 to reduce the risk of toxicity without compromising clinical efficacy.

Metastatic Disease

Combination Regimens

Irinotecan + 5-Fluorouracil + Leucovorin (IFL Saltz regimen)

Irinotecan: 125 mg/m² IV over 90 minutes weekly for 4 weeks

5-Fluorouracil: 500 mg/m² IV weekly for 4 weeks

Leucovorin: 20 mg/m² IV weekly for 4 weeks

Repeat cycle every 6 weeks (146).

Irinotecan + 5-Fluorouracil + Leucovorin (IFL Saltz regimen) + Bevacizumab (BV)

Irinotecan: 125 mg/m² IV over 90 minutes weekly for 4 weeks

5-Fluorouracil: 500 mg/m² IV weekly for 4 weeks

Leucovorin: 20 mg/m² IV weekly for 4 weeks

Bevacizumab: 5 mg/kg IV every 2 weeks

Repeat cycle every 6 weeks (147).

Irinotecan + 5-Fluorouracil + Leucovorin (Modified IFL Saltz regimen)

Irinotecan: 125 mg/m² IV over 90 minutes weekly for 2 weeks

5-Fluorouracil: 500 mg/m² IV weekly for 2 weeks

Leucovorin: 20 mg/m² IV weekly for 2 weeks

Repeat cycle every 3 weeks (148).

Irinotecan + 5-Fluorouracil + Leucovorin (Douillard regimen)

Irinotecan: 180 mg/m² IV on day 1

5-Fluorouracil: 400 mg/m² IV bolus, followed by 600 mg/m² IV continuous infusion for 22 hours on days 1 and 2

Leucovorin: 200 mg/m² IV on days 1 and 2 as a 2-hour infusion prior to 5-fluorouracil

Repeat cycle every 2 weeks (149).

Irinotecan + 5-Fluorouracil + Leucovorin (FOLFIRI regimen)

Irinotecan: 180 mg/m² IV on day 1

5-Fluorouracil: 400 mg/m² IV bolus on day 1, followed by 2,400 mg/m² IV continuous infusion for 46 hours

Leucovorin: 200 mg/m² IV on day 1 as a 2-hour infusion prior to 5-fluorouracil

Repeat cycle every 2 weeks (150) .

Oxaliplatin + 5-Fluorouracil + Leucovorin (FOLFOX4)

Oxaliplatin:	85 mg/m^2 IV on day 1
5-Fluorouracil:	400 mg/m^2 IV bolus, followed by 600 mg/m^2 IV continuous infusion for 22 hours on days 1 and 2
Leucovorin:	200 mg/m^2 IV on days 1 and 2 as a 2-hour infusion before 5-fluorouracil
or	
L-Leucovorin	100 mg/m^2 IV on days 1 and 2 as a 2-hour infusion before 5-fluorouracil

Repeat cycle every 2 weeks (151) .

Oxaliplatin + 5-Fluorouracil + Leucovorin (FOLFOX6)

Oxaliplatin:	100 mg/m^2 IV on day 1
5-Fluorouracil:	400 mg/m^2 IV bolus on day 1, followed by 2,400 mg/m^2 IV continuous infusion for 46 hours
Leucovorin:	400 mg/m^2 IV on day 1 as a 2-hour infusion before 5-fluorouracil

Repeat cycle every 2 weeks (152) .

Oxaliplatin + 5-Fluorouracil + Leucovorin (FOLFOX7)

Oxaliplatin:	130 mg/m^2 IV on day 1
5-Fluorouracil:	2,400 mg/m^2 IV continuous infusion on days 1 and 2 for 46 hours
Leucovorin:	400 mg/m^2 IV on day 1 as a 2-hour infusion before 5-fluorouracil
or	
L-Leucovorin	200 mg/m^2 IV on days 1 and 2 as a 2-hour infusion before 5-fluorouracil

Repeat cycle every 2 weeks (153) .

Oxaliplatin + 5-Fluorouracil + Leucovorin (mFOLFOX7)

Oxaliplatin:	100 mg/m^2 IV on day 1
5-Fluorouracil:	3,000 mg/m^2 IV continuous infusion on days 1 and 2 for 46 hours
Leucovorin:	200 mg/m^2 IV on day 1 as a 2-hour infusion before 5-fluorouracil

Repeat cycle every 2 weeks (154) .

FOLFOXIRI Regimen

Irinotecan:	165 mg/m² IV on day 1
Oxaliplatin:	85 mg/m² IV on day 1
5-Fluorouracil:	3,200 mg/m² IV continuous infusion for 46 hours on days 1 and 2
Leucovorin:	200 mg/m² IV on day 1 as a 2-hour infusion prior to 5-fluorouracil

Repeat cycle every 2 weeks for a total of 12 cycles (155).

Cetuximab + Irinotecan

| Cetuximab: | 400 mg/m² IV loading dose, then 250 mg/m² IV weekly |
| Irinotecan: | 350 mg/m² IV on day 1 |

Repeat cycle every 21 days (156).

or

| Cetuximab: | 400 mg/m² IV loading dose, then 250 mg/m² IV weekly |
| Irinotecan: | 180 mg/m² IV on day 1 |

Repeat cycle every 14 days (156).

Capecitabine + Oxaliplatin (XELOX)

| Capecitabine: | 1,000 mg/m² PO bid on days 1–14 |
| Oxaliplatin: | 130 mg/m² IV on day 1 |

Repeat cycle every 21 days (157). May decrease dose of capecitabine to 850 mg/m² PO bid and dose of oxaliplatin to 100 mg/m² IV to reduce the risk of toxicity without compromising clinical efficacy.

or

| Capecitabine: | 1,750 mg/m² PO bid on days 1–7 |
| Oxaliplatin: | 85 mg/m² IV on day 1 |

Repeat cycle every 14 days (157). May decrease dose of capecitabine to 1,000–1,250 mg/m² PO bid to reduce the risk of toxicity without compromising clinical efficacy.

Capecitabine + Irinotecan (XELIRI)

| Capecitabine: | 1,000 mg/m² PO bid on days 1–14 |
| Irinotecan: | 250 mg/m² IV on day 1 |

Repeat cycle every 21 days (158). May decrease dose of capecitabine to 850 mg/m² PO bid and dose of irinotecan to 200 mg/m² IV to reduce the risk of toxicity without compromising clinical efficacy.

or

| Capecitabine: | 1,500 mg/m² PO bid on days 2–8 |
| Irinotecan: | 150 mg/m² IV on day 1 |

Repeat cycle every 14 days (159).

Oxaliplatin + Irinotecan (IROX regimen)
Oxaliplatin: 85 mg/m² IV on day 1
Irinotecan: 200 mg/m² IV on day 1
Repeat cycle every 3 weeks (160).

5-Fluorouracil + Leucovorin (Mayo Clinic schedule)
5-Fluorouracil: 425 mg/m² IV on days 1–5
Leucovorin: 20 mg/m² IV on days 1–5, administered before
                                5-fluorouracil
Repeat cycle every 4–5 weeks (161).

5-Fluorouracil + Leucovorin (Roswell Park schedule, high dose)
5-Fluorouracil: 500 mg/m² IV weekly for 6 weeks
Leucovorin: 500 mg/m² IV weekly for 6 weeks, adminis-
                                tered before 5-fluorouracil
Repeat cycle every 8 weeks (162).

5-Fluorouracil + Leucovorin + Bevacizumab
5-Fluorouracil: 500 mg/m² IV weekly for 6 weeks
Leucovorin: 500 mg/m² IV weekly for 6 weeks, adminis-
                                tered before 5-fluorouracil
Bevacizumab: 5 mg/kg IV every 2 weeks
Repeat cycle every 8 weeks (163).

5-Fluorouracil + Leucovorin (German schedule, low dose)
5-Fluorouracil: 600 mg/m² IV weekly for 6 weeks
Leucovorin: 20 mg/m² IV weekly for 6 weeks, administered
                                before 5-fluorouracil
Repeat cycle every 8 weeks (164).

5-Fluorouracil + Leucovorin (de Gramont regimen)
5-Fluorouracil: 400 mg/m² IV and then 600 mg/m² IV for 22
                                hours on days 1 and 2
Leucovorin: 200 mg/m² IV on days 1 and 2 as a 2-hour
                                infusion before 5-fluorouracil
Repeat cycle every 2 weeks (165).

FOLFOX4 + Bevacizumab
Oxaliplatin: 85 mg/m² IV on day 1
5-Fluorouracil: 400 mg/m² IV bolus, followed by 600 mg/m²
                                IV continuous infusion on days 1 and 2

| Leucovorin: | 200 mg/m² IV on days 1 and 2 as a 2-hour infusion before 5-fluorouracil |
| Bevacizumab: | 10 mg/kg IV every 2 weeks |

Repeat cycle every 2 weeks (166).

Capecitabine + Oxaliplatin (XELOX) + Bevacizumab

Capecitabine:	850 mg/m² PO bid on days 1–14
Oxaliplatin:	130 mg/m² IV on day 1
Bevacizumab:	7.5 mg/kg every 3 weeks

Repeat cycle every 21 days (167).

Cetuximab + Bevacizumab + Irinotecan

Cetuximab:	400 mg/m² IV loading dose, then 250 mg/m² IV weekly
Bevacizumab:	5 mg/kg IV every 2 weeks
Irinotecan:	180 mg/m² IV on day 1

Repeat cycle every 2 weeks (168).

Cetuximab + Bevacizumab

| Cetuximab: | 400 mg/m² IV loading dose, then 250 mg/m² IV weekly |
| Bevacizumab: | 5 mg/kg IV every 2 weeks |

Repeat cycle every 2 weeks (168).

Irinotecan + Cetuximab

| Irinotecan: | 125 mg/m² IV weekly for 4 weeks |
| Cetuximab: | 400 mg/m² IV loading dose, then 250 mg/m² IV weekly |

Repeat cycle every 6 weeks (169).
or
| Irinotecan: | 350 mg/m² IV on day 1 |
| Cetuximab: | 400 mg/m² IV loading dose, then 250 mg/m² IV weekly |

Repeat cycle every 3 weeks (170).

FOLFIRI + Cetuximab

Irinotecan:	180 mg/m² IV on day 1
5-Fluorouracil:	400 mg/m² IV bolus on day 1, followed by 2,400 mg/m² IV continuous infusion for 46 hours on days 1 and 2
Leucovorin:	400 mg/m² IV on day 1 as a 2-hour infusion prior to 5-fluorouracil

| Cetuximab: | 400 mg/m² IV loading dose, then 250 mg/m² IV weekly |

Repeat cycle every 2 weeks (171) .

FOLFOX4 + Cetuximab
Oxaliplatin:	85 mg/m² IV on day 1
5-Fluorouracil:	400 mg/m² IV bolus on day 1, followed by 600 mg/m² IV continuous infusion for 22 hours on days 1 and 2
Leucovorin:	400 mg/m² IV on days 1 and 2 as a 2-hour infusion prior to 5-fluorouracil
Cetuximab:	400 mg/m² IV loading dose, then 250 mg/m² IV weekly

Repeat cycle every 2 weeks (172) .

FOLFOX6 + Cetuximab
Oxaliplatin:	85 mg/m² IV on day 1
5-Fluorouracil:	2,400 mg/m² IV continuous infusion over 46 hours on days 1 and 2
Leucovorin:	200 mg/m² IV on day 1 as a 2-hour infusion prior to 5-fluorouracil
Cetuximab:	400 mg/m² IV loading dose and then 250 mg/m² IV weekly

Repeat cycle every 2 weeks (173) .

FOLFIRI + Bevacizumab
Irinotecan:	180 mg/m² IV on day 1
5-Fluorouracil:	400 mg/m² IV bolus on day 1, followed by 2,400 mg/m² IV continuous infusion for 46 hours on days 1 and 2
Leucovorin:	400 mg/m² IV on day 1 as a 2-hour infusion prior to 5-fluorouracil
Bevacizumab:	5 mg/kg IV every 2 weeks

Repeat cycle every 2 weeks (174) .

Hepatic Artery Infusion

Floxuridine
Floxuridine (FUDR):	0.3 mg/kg/day HAI on days 1–14
Dexamethasone:	20 mg HAI on days 1–14
Heparin:	50,000 U HAI on days 1–14

Repeat cycle every 14 days (175) .

Single-Agent Regimens

Capecitabine

Capecitabine: 1,250 mg/m^2 PO bid on days 1–14

Repeat cycle every 21 days (176) . Dose may be decreased to 850–1,000 mg/m^2 PO bid on days 1–14. This dose reduction may reduce the risk of toxicity without compromising clinical efficacy.

CPT-11 (weekly schedule)

CPT-11: 125 mg/m^2 IV over 90 minutes weekly for 4 weeks

Repeat cycle every 6 weeks (177) .

or

CPT-11: 125 mg/m^2 IV over 90 minutes weekly for 2 weeks

Repeat cycle every 3 weeks.

or

CPT-11: 175 mg/m^2 IV on days 1 and 10

Repeat cycle every 3 weeks (178) .

CPT-11 (monthly schedule)

CPT-11: 350 mg/m^2 IV on day 1

Repeat cycle every 3 weeks (179) .

Cetuximab

Cetuximab: 400 mg/m^2 IV loading dose, then 250 mg/m^2 IV weekly

Repeat cycle on a weekly basis (180) .

or

Cetuximab: 500 mg/m^2 IV every 2 weeks (no loading dose is necessary)

Repeat cycle every 2 weeks (181) .

Panitumumab

Panitumumab: 6 mg/kg every 2 weeks

Repeat cycle every 2 weeks (182) .

5-Fluorouracil (continuous infusion)

5-Fluorouracil: 2,600 mg/m^2 IV over 24 hours weekly

Repeat cycle weekly for 4 weeks (183) .

or

5-Fluorouracil: 1,000 mg/m^2/day IV continuous infusion on days 1–4

Repeat cycle every 21–28 days (184) .

or

5-Fluorouracil: 200 mg/m² /day IV continuous infusion on days 1–4

L-Leucovorin: 5 mg/m² /day IV on days 1-14

Repeat cycle every 28 days (185) .

ENDOMETRIAL CANCER

Combination Regimens

Paclitaxel + Carboplatin

Paclitaxel: 175 mg/m² IV over 3 hours on day 1

Carboplatin: AUC of 5–7, IV on day 1

Repeat cycle every 28 days (186) .

AC

Doxorubicin: 60 mg/m² IV on day 1

Cyclophosphamide: 500 mg/m² IV on day 1

Repeat cycle every 21 days (187) .

AP

Doxorubicin: 50 mg/m² IV on day 1

Cisplatin: 50 mg/m² IV on day 1

Repeat cycle every 21 days (188) .

Doxorubicin + Paclitaxel

Doxorubicin: 50 mg/m² IV on day 1

Paclitaxel: 150 mg/m² IV on day 1

Repeat cycle every 21 days (189) .

Cisplatin + Doxorubicin + Paclitaxel

Cisplatin: 50 mg/m² IV on day 1

Doxorubicin: 45 mg/m² IV on day 1

Paclitaxel: 160 mg/m² IV over 3 hours on day 2

Filgrastim: 5 µg/kg SC on days 3–12

Repeat cycle every 21 days (190) .

CAP

Cyclophosphamide: 500 mg/m² IV on day 1

Doxorubicin: 50 mg/m² IV on day 1

Cisplatin: 50 mg/m² IV on day 1
Repeat cycle every 21 days (191).

Carboplatin + Pegylated Liposomal Doxorubicin
Carboplatin: AUC of 5, IV on day 1
Pegylated Liposomal
Doxorubicin: 40 mg/m² IV on day 1
Repeat cycle every 28 days (192).

Paclitaxel + Ifosfamide (carcinosarcoma)
Paclitaxel: 135 mg/m² IV over 3 hours on day 1
Ifosfamide: 1,600 mg/m²/day IV on days 1–3
Repeat cycle every 21 days for up to 8 cycles (193). Mesna to be given as either IV or PO. G-CSF support at 5 µg/kg/day to be started on day 4.

Single-Agent Regimens
Doxorubicin
Doxorubicin: 60 mg/m² IV on day 1
Repeat cycle every 21 days (194).

Megestrol
Megestrol: 160 mg PO daily
Repeat on a daily basis (195).

Paclitaxel
Paclitaxel: 200 mg/m² IV over 3 hours on day 1
Repeat cycle every 21 days (196). Reduce dose to 175 mg/m² IV for patients with prior pelvic radiation therapy.

Topotecan
Topotecan: 1.0 mg/m²/day IV on days 1–5
Repeat cycle every 21 days (197). Reduce dose to 0.8 mg/m²/day IV on days 1–3 in patients with prior radiation therapy.

ESOPHAGEAL CANCER

Neoadjuvant Combined Modality Therapy

5-Fluorouracil + Cisplatin + Radiation Therapy (Herskovic regimen)

| 5-Fluorouracil: | 1,000 mg/m^2/day IV continuous infusion on days 1–4 |
| Cisplatin: | 75 mg/m^2 IV on day 1 |

Repeat on weeks 1, 5, 8, and 11 (198).

| Radiation therapy: | 200 cGy/day for 5 days per week (total dose, 3,000 cGy), followed by a boost to the field of 2,000 cGy. |

5-Fluorouracil + Cisplatin + Radiation Therapy (FFD French regimen)

5-Fluorouracil:	800 mg/m^2/day IV continuous infusion on days 1-5
Cisplatin:	15 mg/m^2 IV on days 1-5. Administer on days 1, 22, 43, 64, and 92
Radiation therapy:	200 cGy/day for 5 days per week to a total dose of 6,600 cGy over 6.5 weeks

Chemotherapy is given concurrently with radiation therapy, followed by surgical resection (199).

5-Fluorouracil + Cisplatin + Radiation Therapy (Hopkins/Yale regimen)

Preoperative Chemoradiation

5-Fluorouracil:	225 mg/m^2/day IV continuous infusion on days 1–30
Cisplatin:	20 mg/m^2/day IV on days 1–5 and 26–30
Radiation therapy:	200 cGy/day to a total dose of 4,400 cGy

Chemotherapy is given concurrently with radiation therapy. Followed by esophagectomy and then adjuvant chemotherapy in patients who had total gross removal of disease with negative margins.

Adjuvant Chemotherapy

| Paclitaxel: | 135 mg/m^2 IV for 24 hours on day 1 |
| Cisplatin: | 75 mg/m^2 IV on day 2 |

Adjuvant chemotherapy is given 8–12 weeks after esophagectomy, and each cycle is given every 21 days for a total of 3 cycles (200).

MAGIC Trial

Preoperative ECF Chemotherapy

Epirubicin:	50 mg/m² IV on day 1
Cisplatin:	60 mg/m² IV on day 1
5-Fluorouracil:	200 mg/m²/day IV continuous infusion on days 1–21

Repeat cycle every 21 days for 3 cycles (201).
Followed by esophagectomy and then adjuvant chemotherapy in patients who had total gross removal of disease with negative margins.

Adjuvant Chemotherapy

Epirubicin:	50 mg/m² IV on day 1
Cisplatin:	60 mg/m² IV on day 1
5-Fluorouracil:	200 mg/m²/day IV continuous infusion on days 1–21

Repeat cycle every 21 days for 3 cycles (201).

Metastatic Disease

Combination Regimens

5-Fluorouracil + Cisplatin

5-Fluorouracil:	1,000 mg/m²/day IV continuous infusion on days 1–5
Cisplatin:	100 mg/m² IV on day 1

Repeat cycle on weeks 1, 5, 8, and 11 (202).

Irinotecan + Cisplatin

Irinotecan:	65 mg/m² IV weekly for 4 weeks
Cisplatin:	30 mg/m² IV weekly for 4 weeks

Repeat cycle every 6 weeks (203).

Paclitaxel + Cisplatin

Paclitaxel:	200 mg/m² IV over 24 hours on day 1
Cisplatin:	75 mg/m² IV on day 2

Repeat cycle every 21 days (204). G-CSF support is recommended.

Capecitabine + Oxaliplatin

Capecitabine:	1,000 mg/m² PO bid on days 1–14

Oxaliplatin: 130 mg/m^2 IV on day 1
Repeat cycle every 21 days (205) .

ECF

Epirubicin: 50 mg/m^2 IV on day 1
Cisplatin: 60 mg/m^2 IV on day 1
5-Fluorouracil: 200 mg/m^2/day IV continuous infusion for 24 weeks
Repeat cycle every 21 days (206) .

EOF

Epirubicin: 50 mg/m^2 IV on day 1
Oxaliplatin: 130 mg/m^2 IV on day 1
5-Fluorouracil: 200 mg/m^2/day IV continuous infusion for 24 weeks
Repeat cycle every 21 days (206) .

ECX

Epirubicin: 50 mg/m^2 IV on day 1
Cisplatin: 60 mg/m^2 IV on day 1
Capecitabine: 625 mg/m^2 PO bid continuously
Repeat cycle every 21 days (206) .

EOX

Epirubicin: 50 mg/m^2 IV on day 1
Oxaliplatin: 130 mg/m^2 IV on day 1
Capecitabine: 625 mg/m^2 PO bid continuously
Repeat cycle every 21 days (206) .

Single-Agent Regimens

Paclitaxel

Paclitaxel: 250 mg/m^2 IV over 24 hours on day 1
Repeat cycle every 21 days (207) . G-CSF support is recommended.

GASTRIC CANCER

Adjuvant Therapy

One cycle of chemotherapy is administered as follows:

| 5-Fluorouracil: | 425 mg/m² IV on days 1–5 |
| Leucovorin: | 20 mg/m² IV on days 1–5 |

Chemoradiotherapy is then started 28 days after the start of the initial cycle of chemotherapy as follows:

Radiation therapy:	180 cGy/day to a total dose of 4,500 cGy, starting on day 28
5-Fluorouracil:	400 mg/m² IV on days 1–4 and days 23–25 of radiation therapy
Leucovorin:	20 mg/m² IV on days 1–4 and days 23–25 of radiation therapy

Chemoradiotherapy is followed by 2 cycles of chemotherapy that are given 1 month apart and include (208) :

| 5-Fluorouracil: | 425 mg/m² IV on days 1–5 |
| Leucovorin: | 20 mg/m² IV on days 1–5 |

Metastatic Disease

Combination Regimens

DCF

Docetaxel:	75 mg/m² IV on day 1
Cisplatin:	75 mg/m² IV over 1–3 hours on day 1
5-FU:	750 mg/m²/day IV continuous infusion on days 1–5

Repeat cycle every 21 days (209) .

CF

| Cisplatin: | 100 mg/m² IV over 1–3 hours on day 1 |
| 5-FU: | 1,000 mg/m²/day IV continuous infusion on days 1–5 |

Repeat cycle every 28 days (210) .

ECF

Epirubicin:	50 mg/m² IV on day 1
Cisplatin:	60 mg/m² IV on day 1
5-Fluorouracil:	200 mg/m²/day IV continuous infusion for 24 weeks

Repeat cycle every 21 days (206) .

EOF

| Epirubicin: | 50 mg/m² IV on day 1 |
| Oxaliplatin: | 130 mg/m² IV on day 1 |

| 5-Fluorouracil: | 200 mg/m^2/day IV continuous infusion for 24 weeks |

Repeat cycle every 21 days (206).

ECX

Epirubicin:	50 mg/m^2 IV on day 1
Cisplatin:	60 mg/m^2 IV on day 1
Capecitabine:	625 mg/m^2 PO bid continuously

Repeat cycle every 21 days (206).

EOX

Epirubicin:	50 mg/m^2 IV on day 1
Oxaliplatin:	130 mg/m^2 IV on day 1
Capecitabine:	625 mg/m^2 PO bid continuously

Repeat cycle every 21 days (206).

IP

| Irinotecan: | 70 mg/m^2 IV on days 1 and 15 |
| Cisplatin: | 80 mg/m^2 IV on day 1 |

Repeat cycle every 28 days (211).

IPB

Irinotecan:	65 mg/m^2 IV on days 1 and 8
Cisplatin:	30 mg/m^2 IV on days 1 and 8
Bevacizumab:	15 mg/kg IV on day 1

Repeat cycle every 21 days (212).

Docetaxel + Cisplatin

| Docetaxel: | 85 mg/m^2 IV on day 1 |
| Cisplatin: | 75 mg/m^2 IV on day 1 |

Repeat cycle every 21 days (213).

Capecitabine + Cisplatin

| Capecitabine: | 1,000 mg/m^2 PO bid on days 1–14 |
| Cisplatin: | 80 mg/m^2 IV on day 1 |

Repeat cycle every 21 days (214).

FLO

| 5-Fluorouracil: | 2,600 mg/m^2 IV on day 1 as a continuous infusion over 24 hours |
| Leucovorin: | 200 mg/m^2 IV on day 1 as a 2-hour infusion |

Oxaliplatin: 85 mg/m² IV on day 1
Repeat cycle every 14 days (215) .

Single-Agent Regimens

5-Fluorouracil
5-Fluorouracil: 500 mg/m² IV on days 1–5
Repeat cycle every 28 days (216) .

5-Fluorouracil + Leucovorin
5-Fluorouracil: 370 mg/m² IV on days 1–5
Leucovorin: 200 mg/m² IV on days 1–5
Repeat cycle every 21 days (217) .

Docetaxel
Docetaxel: 100 mg/m² IV on day 1
Repeat cycle every 21 days (218) .
or
Docetaxel: 36 mg/m² IV weekly for 6 weeks
Repeat cycle every 8 weeks
(219) .

GASTROINTESTINAL STROMAL TUMOR (GIST)

Adjuvant Therapy

Imatinib
Imatinib: 400 mg/day PO
Continue treatment for a total of one year (220) .

Metastatic Disease

Single-Agent Regimens

Imatinib
Imatinib: 400 mg/day PO
Continue treatment until disease progression (221) . May increase dose to
600 mg/day if no response is seen. In patients with exon 9 mutation, use
dose of 800 mg/day.

Nilotinib

Nilotinib: 400 mg PO bid

Continue treatment until disease progression (222).

Sunitinib

Sunitinib: 50 mg/day PO for 4 weeks

Repeat cycle every 6 weeks (223).

HEAD AND NECK CANCER

Combined Modality Therapy

Cetuximab + Radiation Therapy

Cetuximab: 400 mg/m^2 IV loading dose, 1 week before radiation therapy, then 250 mg/m^2 IV weekly

Radiation therapy: 200 cGy/day for 5 days per week (total dose, 7,000 cGy)

Cetuximab is given concurrently with radiation therapy (224).

TPF Induction Chemotherapy Followed by Carboplatin + Radiation Therapy

Docetaxel: 75 mg/m^2 IV on day 1

Cisplatin: 75–100 mg/m^2 IV on day 1

5-Fluorouracil: 1,000 mg/m^2/day IV continuous infusion on days 1–4

Repeat cycle every 3 weeks for 3 cycles followed by:

Carboplatin: AUC of 1.5, IV weekly for 7 weeks during radiation therapy

Radiation therapy: 200 cGy/day to a total dose of 7,400 cGy

At the completion of chemoradiotherapy, surgical resection as indicated (225).

Combination Regimens

TIP

Paclitaxel: 175 mg/m^2 IV over 3 hours on day 1

Ifosfamide: 1,000 mg/m^2 IV over 2 hours on days 1–3

Mesna: 400 mg/m^2 IV before ifosfamide and 200 mg/m^2 IV, 4 hours after ifosfamide

Cisplatin: 60 mg/m^2 IV on day 1

Repeat cycle every 21–28 days (226).

TPF

Docetaxel:	75 mg/m² IV on day 1
Cisplatin:	75–100 mg/m² IV over 24 hours on day 1
5-Fluorouracil:	1,000 mg/m² over 24 hours on days 1–4

Repeat cycle every 21 days (227) .

TIC

Paclitaxel:	175 mg/m² IV over 3 hours on day 1
Ifosfamide:	1,000 mg/m² IV over 2 hours on days 1–3
Mesna:	400 mg/m² IV before ifosfamide and 200 mg/m² IV, 4 hours after ifosfamide
Carboplatin:	AUC of 6, IV on day 1

Repeat cycle every 21–28 days (228) .

Paclitaxel + Carboplatin

Paclitaxel:	175 mg/m² IV over 3 hours on day 1
Carboplatin:	AUC of 6, IV on day 1

Repeat cycle every 21 days (229) .

Paclitaxel + Cisplatin

Paclitaxel:	175 mg/m² IV over 3 hours on day 1
Cisplatin:	75 mg/m² IV on day 2
G-CSF:	5 µg/kg/day SC on days 4–10

Repeat cycle every 21 days (230) .

PF

Cisplatin:	100 mg/m² IV on day 1
5-Fluorouracil:	1,000 mg/m²/day IV continuous infusion on days 1–5

Repeat cycle every 21–28 days (231) .

Carboplatin + 5-FU

Carboplatin:	AUC of 5, IV on day 1
5-Fluorouracil:	1,000 mg/m²/day IV continuous infusion on days 1–4

Repeat cycle every 21 days (232) .

PF + Cetuximab

Cisplatin:	100 mg/m² IV on day 1
5-Fluorouracil:	1,000 mg/m²/day IV continuous infusion on days 1–4

Cetuximab: 400 mg/m² IV loading dose, then 250 mg/m² IV weekly

Repeat cycle every 21 days for up to 6 cycles. If no evidence of disease progression at the end of 6 cycles, can continue with weekly cetuximab (233) .

Carboplatin + 5-FU + Cetuximab

Carboplatin: AUC of 5, IV on day 1

5-Fluorouracil: 1,000 mg/m²/day IV continuous infusion on days 1–4

Cetuximab: 400 mg/m² IV loading dose, then 250 mg/m² IV weekly

Repeat cycle every 21 days for up to 6 cycles. If no evidence of disease progression at the end of 6 cycles, can continue with weekly cetuximab (233) .

PF-Larynx Preservation

Cisplatin: 100 mg/m² IV on day 1

5-Fluorouracil: 1,000 mg/m²/day IV continuous infusion on days 1–5

Radiation therapy: 6,600–7,600 cGy in 180–200 cGy fractions

Repeat cycle every 21–28 days for 3 cycles (234) .

Concurrent Chemoradiation Therapy for Laryngeal Preservation

Cisplatin: 100 mg/m² IV on days 1, 22, and 43

Radiation therapy: 7,000 cGy in 200 cGy fractions

Administer cisplatin concurrently with radiation therapy (235) .

Chemoradiotherapy for Nasopharyngeal Cancer

Cisplatin: 100 mg/m² IV on days 1, 22, and 43 during radiotherapy

Radiation therapy: Total dose of 7,000 cGy in 180–200 cGy fractions

At the completion of chemoradiotherapy, chemotherapy is administered as follows:

Cisplatin: 80 mg/m² IV on day 1

5-Fluorouracil: 1,000 mg/m²/day IV continuous infusion on days 1–4

Repeat cycle every 28 days for a total of 3 cycles (236) .

VP

Vinorelbine: 25 mg/m² IV on days 1 and 8

Cisplatin: 80 mg/m² IV on day 1
Repeat cycle every 21 days (237) .

Single-Agent Regimens

Docetaxel
Docetaxel: 100 mg/m² IV on day 1
Repeat cycle every 21 days (238) .

Paclitaxel
Paclitaxel: 250 mg/m² IV over 24 hours on day 1
Repeat cycle every 21 days (239) .
or
Paclitaxel: 137–175 mg/m² IV over 3 hours on day 1
Repeat cycle every 21 days (239) .

Methotrexate
Methotrexate: 40 mg/m² IV or IM weekly
Repeat cycle every week (240) .

Vinorelbine
Vinorelbine: 30 mg/m² IV weekly
Repeat cycle every week (241) .

Cetuximab
Cetuximab: 400 mg/m² IV loading dose, then 250 mg/m²
                            IV weekly
Repeat cycle every week (242) .

HEPATOCELLULAR CANCER

Combination Regimens

GEMOX
Gemcitabine: 1,000 mg/m² IV on day 1
Oxaliplatin: 100 mg/m² IV on day 2
Repeat cycle every 2 weeks (243) .

Bevacizumab + Erlotinib
Bevacizumab: 10 mg/kg IV on days 1 and 14
Erlotinib: 150 mg PO daily

Repeat cycle every 28 days (244) .

Single-Agent Regimens

Sorafenib
Sorafenib: 400 mg PO bid

Continue until disease progression (245) . Dose may be reduced to 400 mg once daily or 400 mg every 2 days.

Doxorubicin
Doxorubicin: 20–30 mg/m^2 IV weekly

Repeat cycle every week (246) .

Cisplatin
Cisplatin: 80 mg/m^2 IV on day 1

Repeat cycle every week (247) .

Capecitabine
Capecitabine: 1,000 mg/m^2 PO bid on days 1–14

Repeat cycle every 21 days (248) . Dose may be reduced to 825–900 mg/m^2 PO bid on days 1–14. This dose reduction may decrease the risk of toxicity without compromising clinical efficacy.

Bevacizumab
Bevacizumab: 10 mg/kg IV on day 1

Repeat cycle every 14 days (249) .

KAPOSI'S SARCOMA

Combination Regimens

BV
Bleomycin: 10 U/m^2 IV on days 1 and 15
Vincristine: 1.4 mg/m^2 IV on days 1 and 15 (maximum, 2 mg)

Repeat cycle every 2 weeks (250) .

ABV
Doxorubicin: 40 mg/m^2 IV on day 1
Bleomycin: 15 U/m^2 IV on days 1 and 15
Vinblastine: 6 mg/m^2 IV on day 1

Repeat cycle every 28 days (251).

Single-Agent Regimens

Liposomal Daunorubicin
DaunoXome: 40 mg/m^2 IV on day 1
Repeat cycle every 14 days (252).

Pegylated Liposomal Doxorubicin
Doxil: 20 mg/m^2 IV on day 1
Repeat cycle every 21 days (253).

Paclitaxel
Paclitaxel: 135 mg/m^2 IV over 3 hours on day 1
Repeat cycle every 21 days (254).
or
Paclitaxel: 100 mg/m^2 IV over 3 hours on day 1
Repeat cycle every 2 weeks (255).

Docetaxel
Docetaxel: 25 mg/m^2 IV weekly for 8 weeks, then every other week
Continue until disease progression (256).

Etoposide
Etoposide: 50 mg PO daily on days 1–7
Repeat cycle every 2 weeks (257).

Vinorelbine
Vinorelbine: 30 mg/m^2 IV on day 1
Repeat cycle every 2 weeks (258).

Interferon-α
Interferon α-2a: 36 million IU/m^2 SC or IM, daily for 8–12 weeks (259).
Interferon α-2b: 30 million IU/m^2 SC or IM, 3 times weekly (260).

LEUKEMIA

Acute Lymphocytic Leukemia

Induction Therapy

Linker Regimen (261) (262)

Daunorubicin:	50 mg/m² IV every 24 hours on days 1–3
Vincristine:	2 mg IV on days 1, 8, 15, and 22
Prednisone:	60 mg/m² PO divided into 3 doses on days 1–28
L-Asparaginase:	6,000 U/m² IM on days 17–28

If bone marrow on day 14 is positive for residual leukemia,

Daunorubicin:	50 mg/m² IV on day 15

If bone marrow on day 28 is positive for residual leukemia,

Daunorubicin:	50 mg/m² IV on days 29 and 30
Vincristine:	2 mg IV on days 29 and 36
Prednisone:	60 mg/m² PO on days 29–42
L-Asparaginase:	6,000 U/m² IM on days 29–35

Consolidation Therapy

Linker Regimen (261) (262)

Treatment A (cycles 1, 3, 5, and 7)

Daunorubicin:	50 mg/m² IV on days 1 and 2
Vincristine:	2 mg IV on days 1 and 8
Prednisone:	60 mg/m² PO on days 1–14
L-Asparaginase:	12,000 U/m² on days 2, 4, 7, 9, 11, and 14

Treatment B (cycles 2, 4, 6, and 8)

Teniposide:	165 mg/m² IV on days 1, 4, 8, and 11
Cytarabine:	300 mg/m² IV on days 1, 4, 8, and 11

Treatment C (cycle 9)

Methotrexate:	690 mg/m² IV over 42 hours
Leucovorin:	15 mg/m² IV every 6 hours for 12 doses beginning at 42 hours

Maintenance Therapy

Linker Regimen (261) (262)

Methotrexate:	20 mg/m² PO weekly

6-Mercaptopurine: 75 mg/m² PO daily
Continue for a total of 30 months of complete response.

CNS Prophylaxis
Cranial irradiation: 1,800 rad in 10 fractions over 12–14 days
Methotrexate: 12 mg IT weekly for 6 weeks
Begin within 1 week of complete response.
In patients with documented CNS involvement at time of diagnosis,
intrathecal chemotherapy should begin during induction chemotherapy.
Methotrexate: 12 mg IT weekly for 10 doses
Cranial irradiation: 2,800 rad

Induction Therapy

Larson Regimen (263)
Induction (weeks 1–4)
Cyclophosphamide: 1,200 mg/m² IV on day 1
Daunorubicin: 45 mg/m² IV on days 1–3
Vincristine: 2 mg IV on days 1, 8, 15, and 22
Prednisone: 60 mg/m²/day PO on days 1–21
L-Asparaginase: 6,000 IU/m² SC on days 5, 8, 11, 15, 18, 22
Early Intensification (weeks 5–12)
Methotrexate: 15 mg IT on day 1
Cyclophosphamide: 1,000 mg/m² IV on day 1
6-Mercaptopurine: 60 mg/m²/day PO on days 1–14
Cytarabine: 75 mg/m² IV on days 1–4 and 8–11
Vincristine: 2 mg IV on days 15 and 22
L-Asparaginase: 6,000 IU/m² SC on days 15, 18, 22, and 25
Repeat the early intensification cycle once.

CNS Prophylaxis and Interim Maintenance (weeks 13–25)
Cranial irradiation: 2,400 cGy on days 1–12
Methotrexate: 15 mg IT on days 1, 8, 15, 22, and 29
6-Mercaptopurine: 60 mg/m²/day PO on days 1–70
Methotrexate: 20 mg/m² PO on days 36, 43, 50, 57, and 64
Late Intensification (weeks 26–33)
Doxorubicin: 30 mg/m² IV on days 1, 8, and 15
Vincristine: 2 mg IV on days 1, 8, and 15
Dexamethasone: 10 mg/m²/day PO on days 1–14
Cyclophosphamide: 1,000 mg/m² IV on day 29
6-Thioguanine: 60 mg/m²/day PO on days 29–42
Cytarabine: 75 mg/m² on days 29, 32, 36–39

Prolonged Maintenance (continue until 24 months after diagnosis)

Vincristine: 2 mg IV on day 1

Prednisone: 60 mg/m^2/day PO on days 1–5

Methotrexate: 20 mg/m^2 PO on days 1, 8, 15, and 22

6-Mercaptopurine: 80 mg/m^2/day PO on days 1–28

Repeat maintenance cycle every 28 days.

Hyper-CVAD Regimen

Cyclophosphamide: 300 mg/m^2 IV over 3 hours every 12 hours for 6 doses on days 1–3

Mesna: 600 mg/m^2 IV over 24 hours on days 1–3 ending 6 hours after the last dose of cyclophosphamide

Vincristine: 2 mg IV on days 4 and 11

Doxorubicin: 50 mg/m^2 IV on day 4

Dexamethasone: 40 mg PO or IV on days 1–4 and 11–14

Alternate cycles every 21 days with the following:

Methotrexate: 200 mg/m^2 IV over 2 hours, followed by 800 mg/m^2 IV over 24 hours on day 1

Leucovorin: 15 mg IV every 6 hours for 8 doses, starting 24 hours after the completion of methotrexate infusion

Cytarabine: 3,000 mg/m^2 IV over 2 hours every 12 hours for 4 doses on days 2–3

Methylprednisolone: 50 mg IV bid on days 1–3

Alternate 4 cycles of hyper-CVAD with 4 cycles of high-dose methotrexate and cytarabine therapy (264).

CNS Prophylaxis

Methorexate: 12 mg IT on day 2

Cytarabine: 100 mg IT on day 8

Repeat with each cycle of chemotherapy, depending on the risk of CNS disease.

Supportive Care

Ciprofloxacin: 500 mg PO bid

Fluconazole: 200 mg/day PO

Acyclovir: 200 mg PO bid

G-CSF: 10 µg/kg/day starting 24 hours after the end of chemotherapy (i.e., on day 5 of hyper-CVAD therapy and on day 4 of high-dose methotrexate and cytarabine therapy)

Single-Agent Regimens

Clofarabine
Clofarabine: 52 mg/m² IV for 5 days
Repeat cycle every 2–6 weeks (265).

Nelarabine
Nelarabine: 1.5 gm/m²/day IV on days 1, 3, and 5
Repeat cycle every 28 days up to a total of 4 cycles (266).

Imatinib
Imatinib: 600 mg PO daily
Continue until disease progression (267).

Dasatinib
Dasatinib: 70 mg PO bid
Continue until disease progression (268).

Nilotinib
Nilotinib: 400–600 mg PO bid
Continue until disease progression (269).

Acute Myelogenous Leukemia

Induction Regimens

Ara-C + Daunorubicin (7 + 3) (270)
Cytarabine: 100 mg/m²/day IV continuous infusion on days 1–7
Daunorubicin: 45 mg/m² IV on days 1–3

Ara-C + Idarubicin (271)
Cytarabine: 100 mg/m²/day IV continuous infusion on days 1–7
Idarubicin: 12 mg/m² IV on days 1–3

Ara-C + Doxorubicin (272)
Cytarabine: 100 mg/m²/day IV continuous infusion on days 1–7
Doxorubicin: 30 mg/m² IV on days 1–3

Ara-C + Clofarabine
Clofarabine: 40 mg/m^2 IV over 1 hour on days 2–6
Cytarabine: 1,000 mg/m^2 IV over 2 hours on days 1–5
Repeat cycles every 4–6 weeks for up to a total of 3 cycles (273) .

AIDA (acute promyelocytic leukemia only) (274)
ATRA: 45 mg/m^2 PO daily
Idarubicin: 12 mg/m^2 IV on days 2, 4, 6, and 8

ATRA + Arsenic Trioxide (acute promyelocytic leukemia only)
ATRA: 45 mg/m^2 PO daily
Arsenic trioxide: 0.15 mg/kg/day IV starting on day 10
Continue treatment until CR (275) . Once in CR, patients receive the following:
ATRA: 45 mg/m^2 PO daily on weeks 1-2, 5-6, 9-10, 13-14, 17-18, 21-22, and 25-26
Arsenic trioxide: 0.15 mg/kg/day IV on Monday-Friday on weeks 1-4, 9-12, 17-20, and 25-28
Therapy should be terminated 28 weeks after the CR date. If either ATRA or arsenic trioxide were discontinued, administer gemtuzumab at 9 gm/m^2 IV once monthly until 28 weeks had elapsed from the CR date.

Mitoxantrone + Etoposide (salvage regimen) (276)
Mitoxantrone: 10 mg/m^2/day IV on days 1–5
Etoposide: 100 mg/m^2/day IV on days 1–5

FLAG
Fludarabine: 30 mg/m^2 IV on days 1–5
Cytarabine: 2,000 mg/m^2/day IV over 4 hours on days 1–5 starting 3.5 hours after fludarabine
G-CSF: 5 µg/kg/day starting 24 hours before chemotherapy
An additional cycle may be given in the setting of a partial response (277) .

Consolidation Regimens

Ara-C + Daunorubicin (5 + 2) (278)
Cytarabine: 100 mg/m^2/day IV continuous infusion on days 1–5
Daunorubicin: 45 mg/m^2 IV on days 1 and 2

Ara-C + Idarubicin (279)

| Cytarabine: | 100 mg/m^2 IV continuous infusion on days 1–5 |
| Idarubicin: | 13 mg/m^2 IV on days 1 and 2 |

Repeat cycle every 21–28 days.

Single-Agent Regimens

Cladribine (280)
| Cladribine: | 0.1 mg/kg/day IV continuous infusion on days 1–7 |

High-Dose Cytarabine
| Cytarabine: | 3,000 mg/m^2 IV over 3 hours, every 12 hours on days 1, 3, and 5 |

Repeat cycle every 28 days (281) .

Clofarabine
| Clofarabine: | 40 mg/m^2 IV on days 1–5 |

Repeat cycle every 3–6 weeks (282) .

ATRA (acute promyelocytic leukemia only) (283)
| ATRA: | 45 mg/m^2 PO daily in 1–2 divided doses |

Arsenic Trioxide (acute promyelocytic leukemia only)
| Arsenic trioxide: | 0.15 mg/kg IV daily (284). |

Continue until bone marrow remission up to a maximum of 60 doses. Patients who meet the criteria for clinical CR can receive an additional course of arsenic trioxide as consolidation beginning 3-4 weeks after completion of induction therapy up to a cumulative total of 25 doses (284) .

Gemtuzumab
| Gemtuzumab: | 9 mg/m^2 IV as a 2-hour infusion |

Repeat with a second dose 14 days after administration of the first dose (285) . Premedicate with diphenhydramine 50 mg PO and acetaminophen 650–1,000 mg PO, 1 hour before drug infusion. Once the infusion is completed, give 2 additional doses of acetaminophen 650–1,000 mg PO every 4 hours.

Chronic Lymphocytic Leukemia

Combination Regimens

CVP

Cyclophosphamide: 400 mg/m² PO on days 1–5 (or 800 mg/m² IV on day 1)

Vincristine: 1.4 mg/m² IV on day 1 (maximum dose, 2 mg)

Prednisone: 100 mg/m² PO on days 1–5

Repeat cycle every 21 days (286) .

CF

Cyclophosphamide: 1,000 mg/m² IV on day 1

Fludarabine: 20 mg/m² IV on days 1–5

Bactrim DS: 1 tablet PO bid

Repeat cycle every 21–28 days (287) .

FP

Fludarabine: 30 mg/m² IV on days 1–5

Prednisone: 30 mg/m² IV on days 1–5

Repeat cycle every 28 days (288) .

CP

Chlorambucil: 30 mg/m² PO on day 1

Prednisone: 80 mg PO on days 1–5

Repeat cycle every 28 days (286) .

FR

Fludarabine: 25 mg/m² IV on days 1–5

Rituximab: 375 mg/m² IV on days 1 and 4 of cycle 1 and then on day 1 thereafter

Repeat cycle every 28 days for 6 cycles (289) .

FCR

Fludarabine: 25 mg/m² IV on days 1–3

Cyclophosphamide: 250 mg/m² IV on days 1–3

Rituximab: 375 mg/m² IV on day 1

Repeat cycle every 28 days for 6 cycles (290) . On cycles 2–6, rituximab is given at 500 mg/m².

PCR

Pentostatin: 2 mg/m² IV on day 1

Cyclophosphamide: 600 mg/m² IV on day 1

Rituximab: 375 mg/m² IV on day 1

Repeat cycle every 21 days (291) .

Single-Agent Regimens

Alemtuzumab

Alemtuzumab: 30 mg/day IV, 3 times per week

Repeat weekly for up to a maximum of 23 weeks (292) . Premedicate with diphenhydramine 50 mg PO and acetaminophen 625 mg PO 30 minutes before drug infusion. Patients should be placed on Bactrim DS PO bid and famciclovir 250 mg PO bid from day 8 through 2 months following completion of therapy.

Chlorambucil

Chlorambucil: 6–14 mg/day PO as induction therapy and then 0.7 mg/kg PO for 2–4 days

Repeat cycle every 21 days (293) .

Cladribine

Cladribine: 0.09 mg/kg/day IV continuous infusion on days 1–7

Repeat cycle every 28–35 days (294) .

Fludarabine

Fludarabine: 20–30 mg/m^2 IV on days 1–5

Repeat cycle every 28 days (295) .

Prednisone

Prednisone: 20–30 mg/m^2/day PO for 1–3 weeks (296) .

Rituximab

Rituximab: 375 mg/m^2 IV weekly for 4 weeks

Repeat cycle every 6 months for a total of 4 courses (297) .

Pentostatin

Pentostatin: 4 mg/m^2 IV on day 1

Repeat cycle every 14 days (298) .

Bendamustine

Bendamustine: 100 mg/m^2 IV on days 1 and 2

Repeat cycle every 28 days for up to 6 cycles (299) .

or

Bendamustine: 60 mg/m^2 IV on days 1–5

Repeat cycle every 28 days (300) . In patients >70 years, use dose of 50 mg/m^2 IV.

Lenalidomide

Lenalidomide: 10 mg PO daily on days 1-28
Increase dose by 5 mg every 28 days up to a maximum of 25 mg daily until disease progression or toxicity (301) .

Chronic Myelogenous Leukemia

Combination Regimens

Interferon + Cytarabine

Interferon α-2b: 5 million IU/m^2 SC daily
Cytarabine: 20 mg/m^2 SC daily for 10 days
Repeat cytarabine on a monthly basis (302) . The dose of interferon should be reduced by 50% when the neutrophil count drops below 1,500/mm^3, the platelet count drops below 100,000/m^3, or both. Interferon and cytarabine should both be discontinued when the neutrophil count drops below 1,000/mm^3, platelet count drops below 50,000/mm^3, or both.

Single-Agent Regimens

Imatinib

Imatinib: 400 mg/day PO (chronic phase); 600 mg/day PO (accelerated phase blast crisis) (303).

Dasatinib

Dasatinib: 70 mg PO bid (304).

Nilotinib

Nilotinib: 400 mg PO bid (305).

Busulfan

Busulfan: 1.8 mg/m^2/day PO (306).

Hydroxyurea

Hydroxyurea: 1–5 gm/day PO (307).

Interferon α-2a

Interferon α-2a: 9 million units/day SC (308).

Hairy Cell Leukemia

Cladribine
Cladribine: 0.09 mg/kg/day IV continuous infusion on
days 1–7
Administer one cycle (309).

Pentostatin
Pentostatin: 4 mg/m² IV on day 1
Repeat cycle every 14 days for 6 cycles (310).

Interferon α-2a
Interferon α-2a: 3 million IU SC or IM, 3 times per week
Continue treatment for up to 1 to 1.5 years (311).

LUNG CANCER

Non–Small Cell Lung Cancer

Combined Modality Therapy

Cisplatin + Etoposide + Radiation Therapy
Cisplatin: 50 mg/m² IV on days 1, 8, 29, and 36
Etoposide: 50 mg/m² IV on days 1-5 and 29-33
Radiation therapy: 180 cGy/day for a total dose of 4,500 cGy
Chemotherapy is given concurrently with radiation therapy (312).

Weekly Carboplatin + Paclitaxel + Radiation Therapy
Paclitaxel: 45 mg/m² IV weekly for 7 weeks
Carboplatin: AUC of 2, IV weekly for 7 weeks
Radiation therapy: 200 cGy/day for a total dose of 6,300 cGy over
7 weeks
Chemotherapy is given concurrently with radiation therapy (313). Three to
four weeks after the completion of chemoradiotherapy, 2 additional cycles
of the following chemotherapy are given:
Paclitaxel: 200 mg/m² IV on day 1
Carboplatin: AUC of 6, IV on day 1
Repeat cycle every 21 days for 2 cycles.

Adjuvant Therapy

Combination Regimens

Paclitaxel + Carboplatin
Paclitaxel: 175 mg/m^2 IV over 3 hours on day 1
Carboplatin: AUC of 6, IV on day 1
Repeat cycle every 21 days for 4 cycles (314) .

Vinorelbine + Cisplatin
Vinorelbine: 25 mg/m^2 IV weekly for 16 weeks
Cisplatin: 50 mg/m^2 IV on days 1 and 8
Repeat cycle every 28 days for 4 cycles (315) .

Metastatic Disease

Combination Regimens

Carboplatin + Paclitaxel (PC)
Carboplatin: AUC of 6, IV on day 1
Paclitaxel: 200 mg/m^2 IV over 3 hours on day 1
Repeat cycle every 21 days (316) .

Carboplatin + Paclitaxel (weekly regimen)
Carboplatin: AUC of 6, IV on day 1
Paclitaxel: 100 mg/m^2 IV weekly for 3 weeks
Repeat cycle every 4 weeks up to 4 cycles (317) . If response or stable disease, may then treat with maintenance chemotherapy of:
Paclitaxel: 70 mg/m^2 IV weekly for 3 weeks
Continue until disease progression.

Carboplatin + Paclitaxel + Bevacizumab (PCB)
Carboplatin: AUC of 6, IV on day 1
Paclitaxel: 200 mg/m^2 IV
Bevacizumab: 15 mg/kg IV on day 1
Repeat cycle every 21 days (316) .

Gemcitabine + Cisplatin + Bevacizumab (GCB)
Gemcitabine: 1,250 mg/m^2 IV on days 1 and 8
Cisplatin: 80 mg/m^2 IV on day 1
Bevacizumab: 7.5 or 15 mg/kg IV on day 1
Repeat cycle every 21 days for a total of 6 cycles (318) .

Cisplatin + Paclitaxel

Cisplatin: 80 mg/m² IV on day 1
Paclitaxel: 175 mg/m² IV over 3 hours on day 1
Repeat cycle every 21 days (319).

Docetaxel + Carboplatin

Docetaxel: 75 mg/m² IV on day 1
Carboplatin: AUC of 6, IV on day 1
Repeat cycle every 21 days (320).

Docetaxel + Cisplatin

Docetaxel: 75 mg/m² IV on day 1
Cisplatin: 75 mg/m² IV on day 1
Repeat cycle every 21 days (321).

Docetaxel + Gemcitabine

Docetaxel: 100 mg/m² IV on day 8
Gemcitabine: 1,100 mg/m² IV on days 1 and 8
Repeat cycle every 21 days (322). G-CSF support is required from day 9 to day 15.

Gemcitabine + Cisplatin

Gemcitabine: 1,250 mg/m² IV on days 1 and 8
Cisplatin: 100 mg/m² IV on day 1
Repeat cycle every 21 days (323).

Gemcitabine + Carboplatin

Gemcitabine: 1,000 mg/m² IV on days 1 and 8
Carboplatin: AUC of 5, IV on day 1
Repeat cycle every 21 days (324).

Gemcitabine + Vinorelbine

Gemcitabine: 1,200 mg/m² IV on days 1 and 8
Vinorelbine: 30 mg/m² IV on days 1 and 8
Repeat cycle every 21 days (325).

Vinorelbine + Cisplatin

Vinorelbine: 30 mg/m² IV on days 1, 8, and 15
Cisplatin: 120 mg/m² IV on day 1
Repeat cycle every 28 days (326).

Vinorelbine + Cisplatin + Cetuximab

Vinorelbine:	25 mg/m² IV on days 1 and 8
Cisplatin:	80 mg/m² IV on day 1
Cetuximab:	400 mg/m² IV loading dose, then 250 mg/m² IV weekly

Repeat cycle every 3 weeks up to 6 cycles (327).

Vinorelbine + Carboplatin

Vinorelbine:	25 mg/m² IV on days 1 and 8
Carboplatin:	AUC of 6, IV on day 1

Repeat cycle every 28 days (328).

Pemetrexed + Cisplatin

Pemetrexed:	500 mg/m² IV on day 1
Cisplatin:	75 mg/m² IV on day 1

Repeat cycle every 21 days up to 6 cycles (329). Folic acid at 350–1,000 µg PO q day beginning 1 week prior to therapy and vitamin B12 at 1,000 µg IM beginning 1–2 weeks prior to first dose of therapy and repeated every 9 weeks. Dexamethasone at 4 mg PO bid on the day before, the day of, and the day after pemetrexed.

Pemetrexed + Carboplatin

Pemetrexed:	500 mg/m² IV on day 1
Carboplatin:	AUC of 5, IV on day 1

Repeat cycle every 21 days up to 4 cycles (330). Folic acid at 350–1,000 µg PO q day beginning 1 week prior to therapy and vitamin B12 at 1,000 µg IM beginning 1–2 weeks prior to first dose of therapy and repeated every 9 weeks. Dexamethasone at 4 mg PO bid on the day before, the day of, and the day after pemetrexed.

EP

Etoposide:	120 mg/m² IV on days 1–3
Cisplatin:	60 mg/m² IV on day 1

Repeat cycle every 21–28 days (331).

EP and Docetaxel

Cisplatin:	50 mg/m² IV on days 1, 8, 29, and 36
Etoposide:	50 mg/m² IV on days 1–5 and 29–33

Administer concurrent thoracic radiotherapy, followed 4–6 weeks after the completion of combined modality therapy by

Docetaxel:	75 mg/m² IV on day 1

Repeat cycle every 21 days for 3 cycles (332). Dose of docetaxel can be escalated to 100 mg/m² IV on subsequent cycles in the absence of toxicity.

Docetaxel + Bevacizumab

Docetaxel: 75 mg/m^2 IV on day 1
Bevacizumab: 15 mg/kg IV on day 1
Repeat cycle every 21 days (333).

Pemetrexed + Carboplatin + Bevacizumab

Pemetrexed: 500 mg/m^2 IV on day 1
Carboplatin: AUC of 6, IV on day 1
Bevacizumab: 15 mg/kg IV on day 1
Repeat cycle every 21 days up to 6 cycles (334). Folic acid at 350-1,000 μg PO q day beginning 1 week prior to therapy and vitamin B12 at 1,000 μg IM beginnig 1-2 weeks prior to first dose of therapy and repeated every 9 weeks. Dexamethasone at 4 mg PO bid on the day before, the day of, and the day after pemetrexed.

Cisplatin + Vinorelbine + Cetuximab

Cisplatin: 80 mg/m^2 IV on day 1
Vinorelbine: 25 mg/m^2 IV continuous on days 1 and 8
Cetuximab: 400 mg/m^2 IV loading dose, then 250 mg/m^2 IV weekly
Repeat cycle every 21 days up to 6 cycles (335).

Platinum-Based Chemotherapy + Maintenance Pemetrexed (non-squamous histology)

Platinum-based chemotherapy x 4 cycles, followed by:
Pemetrexed: 500 mg/m^2 IV on day 1
Repeat cycle every 21 days up to 6 cycles (336). Folic acid at 350-1,000 μg PO q day beginning 1 week prior to therapy and vitamin B12 at 1,000 μg IM beginnig 1-2 weeks prior to first dose of therapy and repeated every 9 weeks. Dexamethasone at 4 mg PO bid on the day before, the day of, and the day after pemetrexed.

Single-Agent Regimens

Paclitaxel

Paclitaxel: 225 mg/m^2 IV over 3 hours on day 1
Repeat cycle every 21 days (337).
or
Paclitaxel: 80–100 mg/m^2 IV weekly for 3 weeks
Repeat cycle every 28 days after 1-week rest (338).

Docetaxel

Docetaxel: 75 mg/m^2 IV on day 1

Repeat cycle every 21 days (339).
or

Docetaxel: 36 mg/m² IV weekly for 6 weeks
Repeat cycle every 8 weeks after 2-week rest (340). Premedicate with
dexamethasone 8 mg PO at 12 hours and immediately before docetaxel
infusion and 12 hours after each dose.

Pemetrexed
Pemetrexed: 500 mg/m² IV on day 1
Repeat cycle every 21 days (341). Folic acid at 350–1,000 µg PO q day
beginning 1 week prior to therapy and vitamin B12 at 1,000 µg IM beginning 1–2 weeks prior to first dose of therapy and repeated every 3 cycles.

Gemcitabine
Gemcitabine: 1,000 mg/m² IV on days 1, 8, and 15
Repeat cycle every 28 days (342).

Vinorelbine
Vinorelbine: 25 mg/m² IV on day 1
Repeat cycle every 7 days (343).

Gefitinib
Gefitinib: 250 mg/day PO
Continue treatment until disease progression (344).

Erlotinib
Erlotinib: 150 mg/day PO
Continue treatment until disease progression (345).

Sunitinib
Sunitinib: 50 mg/day PO for 4 weeks
Repeat cycle every 6 weeks (346).

Cetuximab
Cetuximab: 400 mg/m² IV loading dose, then 250 mg/m²
                              IV weekly
Repeat cycle every week (347).

Small Cell Lung Cancer

Combination Regimens

EP
Etoposide:	80 mg/m² IV on days 1–3
Cisplatin:	80 mg/m² IV on day 1

Repeat cycle every 21 days (348) .

EC
Etoposide:	100 mg/m² IV on days 1–3
Carboplatin:	AUC of 6, IV on day 1

Repeat cycle every 28 days (349) .

Irinotecan + Cisplatin
Irinotecan:	60 mg/m² IV on days 1, 8, and 15
Cisplatin:	60 mg/m² IV on day 1

Repeat cycle every 28 days (350) .

Topotecan + Cisplatin
Topotecan:	1.7 mg/m²/day PO on days 1–5
Cisplatin:	60 mg/m² IV on day 5

Repeat cycle every 21 days up to 4 cycles or 2 cycles beyond best response (351) .

Carboplatin + Paclitaxel + Etoposide
Carboplatin:	AUC of 6, IV on day 1
Paclitaxel:	200 mg/m² IV over 1 hour on day 1
Etoposide:	50 mg alternating with 100 mg PO on days 1–10

Repeat cycle every 21 days (352) .

Carboplatin + Paclitaxel
Carboplatin:	AUC of 2, IV on day 1, 8, and 15
Paclitaxel:	80 mg/m² IV on days 1, 8, and 15

Repeat cycle every 28 days for 6 cycles (353) .

CAV
Cyclophosphamide:	1,000 mg/m² IV on day 1
Doxorubicin:	40 mg/m² IV on day 1
Vincristine:	1 mg/m² IV on day 1 (maximum, 2 mg)

Repeat cycle every 21 days (354) .

CAE

Cyclophosphamide:	1,000 mg/m^2 IV on day 1
Doxorubicin:	45 mg/m^2 IV on day 1
Etoposide:	50 mg/m^2 IV on days 1–5

Repeat cycle every 21 days (355).

Single-Agent Regimens

Etoposide

Etoposide:	160 mg/m^2 PO on days 1–5

Repeat cycle every 28 days (356).

or

Etoposide:	50 mg/m^2/day PO on days 1–21

Repeat cycle as tolerated (357).

Paclitaxel

Paclitaxel:	80–100 mg/m^2 IV weekly for 3 weeks

Repeat cycle every 28 days (358).

Topotecan

Topotecan:	1.5 mg/m^2 IV on days 1–5

Repeat cycle every 21 days (359).

LYMPHOMA

Hodgkin's Lymphoma

ABVD

Doxorubicin:	25 mg/m^2 IV on days 1 and 15
Bleomycin:	10 U/m^2 IV on days 1 and 15
Vinblastine:	6 mg/m^2 IV on days 1 and 15
Dacarbazine:	375 mg/m^2 IV on days 1 and 15

Repeat cycle every 28 days (360).

MOPP

Nitrogen mustard:	6 mg/m^2 IV on days 1 and 8
Vincristine:	1.4 mg/m^2 IV on days 1 and 8
Procarbazine:	100 mg/m^2 PO on days 1–14
Prednisone:	40 mg/m^2 PO on days 1–14

Repeat cycle every 28 days (361).

MOPP/ABVD Hybrid

Nitrogen mustard:	6 mg/m^2 IV on days 1 and 8
Vincristine:	1.4 mg/m^2 IV on day 1 (maximum dose, 2 mg)
Procarbazine:	100 mg/m^2 PO on days 1–14
Prednisone:	40 mg/m^2 PO on days 1–14
Doxorubicin:	35 mg/m^2 IV on day 8
Bleomycin:	10 U/m^2 IV on day 8
Hydrocortisone:	100 mg IV given before bleomycin
Vinblastine:	6 mg/m^2 IV on day 8

Repeat cycle every 28 days (362) .

MOPP Alternating with ABVD

See MOPP and ABVD regimens outlined above.

Stanford V

Nitrogen mustard:	6 mg/m^2 IV on day 1
Doxorubicin:	25 mg/m^2 IV on days 1 and 15
Vinblastine:	6 mg/m^2 IV on days 1 and 15
Vincristine:	1.4 mg/m^2 IV on days 8 and 22
Bleomycin:	5 U/m^2 IV on days 8 and 22
Etoposide:	60 mg/m^2 IV on days 15 and 16
Prednisone:	40 mg PO every other day

Repeat cycle every 28 days (363) . In patients >50 years of age, vinblastine dose reduced to 4 mg/m^2 and vincristine dose reduced to 1 mg/m^2 on weeks 9 and 12. Dose of prednisone tapered starting on week 10. Prophylactic Bactrim DS PO bid and acyclovir 200 mg PO tid.

EVA

Etoposide:	200 mg/m^2 IV on days 1–5
Vincristine:	2 mg/m^2 IV on day 1
Doxorubicin:	50 mg/m^2 IV on day 2

Repeat cycle every 28 days (364) .

EVAP

Etoposide:	120 mg/m^2 IV on days 1, 8, and 15
Vinblastine:	4 mg/m^2 IV on days 1, 8, and 15
Cytarabine:	30 mg/m^2 IV on days 1, 8, and 15
Cisplatin:	40 mg/m^2 IV on days 1, 8, and 15

Repeat cycle every 28 days (365) .

Mini-BEAM

BCNU:	60 mg/m^2 IV on day 1

Etoposide: 75 mg/m² IV on days 2–5
Ara-C: 100 mg/m² IV every 12 hours on days 2–5
Melphalan: 30 mg/m² IV on day 6
Repeat cycle every 4–6 weeks (366) .

BEACOPP

Bleomycin: 10 mg/m² IV on day 8
Etoposide: 100 mg/m² IV on days 1–3
Doxorubicin: 25 mg/m² IV on day 1
Cyclophosphamide: 650 mg/m² IV on day 1
Vincristine: 1.4 mg/m² IV on day 8 (maximum, 2 mg)
Procarbazine: 100 mg/m² PO on days 1–7
Prednisone: 40 mg/m² PO on days 1–14
Repeat cycle every 21 days (367) .

BEACOPP Escalated

Bleomycin: 10 mg/m² IV on day 8
Etoposide: 200 mg/m² IV on days 1–3
Doxorubicin: 35 mg/m² IV on day 1
Cyclophosphamide: 1,200 mg/m² IV on day 1
Vincristine: 1.4 mg/m² IV on day 8 (maximum dose, 2 mg)
Procarbazine: 100 mg/m² PO on days 1–7
Prednisone: 40 mg/m² PO on days 1–14
Repeat cycle every 21 days (368) . G-CSF support, at dose of 5 µg/kg/day
SC, starting on day 8 and continue until neutrophil recovery.

GVD

For transplant-naïve patients:
Gemcitabine: 1,000 mg/m² IV on days 1 and 8
Vinorelbine: 20 mg/m² IV on days 1 and 8
Doxil: 15 mg/m² IV on days 1 and 8
Repeat cycle every 21 days (369) .
or
For post-transplant patients:
Gemcitabine: 800 mg/m² IV on days 1 and 8
Vinorelbine: 15 mg/m² IV on days 1 and 8
Doxil: 10 mg/m² IV on days 1 and 8
Repeat cycle every 21 days (369) .

Gemcitabine

Gemcitabine: 1,250 mg/m² IV on days 1, 8, and 15
Repeat cycle every 28 days (370) .

Non-Hodgkin's Lymphoma

Low-Grade

Combination Regimens

CVP
Cyclophosphamide:	400 mg/m² PO on days 1–5 (or 800 mg/m² IV on day 1)
Vincristine:	1.4 mg/m² IV on day 1 (maximum, 2 mg)
Prednisone:	100 mg/m² PO on days 1–5

Repeat cycle every 21 days (371).

CHOP
Cyclophosphamide:	750 mg/m² IV on day 1
Doxorubicin:	50 mg/m² IV on day 1
Vincristine:	1.4 mg/m² IV on day 1 (maximum, 2 mg)
Prednisone:	100 mg/m² PO on days 1–5

Repeat cycle every 21 days (372).

CNOP
Cyclophosphamide:	750 mg/m² IV on day 1
Mitoxantrone:	10 mg/m² IV on day 1
Vincristine:	1.4 mg/m² IV on day 1 (maximum, 2 mg)
Prednisone:	50 mg/m² PO on days 1–5

Repeat cycle every 21 days (373).

FND
Fludarabine:	25 mg/m² IV on days 1–3
Mitoxantrone:	10 mg/m² IV on day 1
Dexamethasone:	20 mg PO on days 1–5
Bactrim DS:	1 tablet PO bid, 3 times per week

Repeat cycle every 21 days (374).

FC
Fludarabine:	20 mg/m² IV on days 1–5
Cyclophosphamide:	1,000 mg/m² IV on day 1
Bactrim DS:	1 tablet PO bid

Repeat cycle every 21–28 days (375).

FCR
Fludarabine:	25 mg/m² IV on days 1–3

Cyclophosphamide: 300 mg/m² IV on days 1–3
Rituximab: 375 mg/m² IV on day 1
Repeat cycle every 21 days for 4 cycles (376) .

R-CHOP

Cyclophosphamide: 750 mg/m² IV on day 1
Doxorubicin: 50 mg/m² IV on day 1
Vincristine: 1.4 mg/m² IV on day 1 (maximum, 2 mg)
Prednisone: 100 mg/day PO on days 1–5
Repeat cycle every 21 days up to 6 cycles (377) . Patients who experience a
response to therapy can then receive maintenance therapy with
Rituximab: 375 mg/m² IV on day 1
Repeat cycle every 3 months up to a maximum of 2 years.

R-FCM

Rituximab: 375 mg/m² IV on day 0
Fludarabine: 25 mg/m² IV on days 1–3
Cyclophosphamide: 200 mg/m² IV on days 1–3
Mitoxantrone: 8 mg/m² IV on day 1
Repeat cycle every 4 weeks for a total of 4 cycles (378) . Patients who experi-
ence a response can then receive maintenance therapy at 3 and 9 months
after completion of therapy with
Rituximab: 375 mg/m² IV weekly for 4 weeks

Bortezomib (mantle cell lymphoma)

Bortezomib: 1.3 mg/m² IV on days 1, 4, 8, and 11
Repeat cycle every 21 days for up to 17 cycles (379) .

Intermediate-Grade

CHOP

Cyclophosphamide: 750 mg/m² IV on day 1
Doxorubicin: 50 mg/m² IV on day 1
Vincristine: 1.4 mg/m² IV on day 1 (maximum, 2 mg)
Prednisone: 100 mg PO on days 1–5
Repeat cycle every 21 days (380) .

CHOP + Rituximab

Cyclophosphamide: 750 mg/m² IV on day 1
Doxorubicin: 50 mg/m² IV on day 1
Vincristine: 1.4 mg/m² IV on day 1 (maximum, 2 mg)

Prednisone: 40 mg/m² PO on days 1–5
Rituximab: 375 mg/m² IV on day 1
Repeat cycle every 21 days (381) . Rituximab is to be administered first
followed by cyclophosphamide, doxorubicin, and vincristine.
or

R-CHOP-14
Cyclophosphamide: 750 mg/m² IV on day 1
Doxorubicin: 50 mg/m² IV on day 1
Vincristine: 1.4 mg/m² IV on day 1 (maximum, 2 mg)
Prednisone: 100 mg/day PO on days 1–5
Rituximab: 375 mg/m² IV on day 1
Repeat cycle every 2 weeks up to 6 cycles (382) . G-CSF support to start on
day 4 of each cycle.

CNOP
Cyclophosphamide: 750 mg/m² IV on day 1
Mitoxantrone: 10 mg/m² IV on day 1
Vincristine: 1.4 mg/m² IV on day 1 (maximum, 2 mg)
Prednisone: 100 mg PO on days 1–5
Repeat cycle every 21 days (383) .

EPOCH
Etoposide: 50 mg/m²/day IV continuous infusion on days
                           1–4
Prednisone: 60 mg/m² PO on days 1–5
Vincristine: 0.4 mg/m²/day IV continuous infusion on days
                           1–4
Cyclophosphamide: 750 mg/m² IV on day 5, begin after infusion
Doxorubicin: 10 mg/m²/day IV continuous infusion on days
                           1–4
Bactrim DS: 1 tablet PO bid, 3 times per week
Repeat cycle every 21 days (384) .

EPOCH + Rituximab
Etoposide: 50 mg/m²/day IV continuous infusion on days
                           1–4
Prednisone: 60 mg/m² PO bid on days 1–5
Vincristine: 0.4 mg/m²/day IV continuous infusion on days
                           1–4
Cyclophosphamide: 750 mg/m² IV on day 5, begin after infusion

| Doxorubicin: | 10 mg/m²/day IV continuous infusion on days 1–4 |
| Rituximab: | 375 mg/m² IV on day 1 |

Repeat cycle every 21 days (385). Rituximab is to be administered first followed by infusions of etoposide, doxorubicin, and vincristine. Prophylaxis with Bactrim DS 1 tab PO bid, 3 times per week to reduce the risk of *Pneumocystis carinii* infection.

MACOP-B

Methotrexate:	400 mg/m² IV on weeks 2, 6, and 10
Leucovorin:	15 mg/m² PO every 6 hours for 6 doses, beginning 24 hours after methotrexate
Doxorubicin:	50 mg/m² IV on weeks 1, 3, 5, 7, 9, and 11
Cyclophosphamide:	350 mg/m² IV on weeks 1, 3, 5, 7, 9, and 11
Vincristine:	1.4 mg/m² IV on weeks 2, 4, 6, 8, 10, and 12
Prednisone:	75 mg/day PO for 12 weeks with taper over the last 2 weeks
Bleomycin:	10 U/m² IV on weeks 4, 8, and 12
Bactrim DS:	1 tablet PO bid
Ketoconazole:	200 mg/day PO

Administer one cycle (386).

m-BACOD

Methotrexate:	200 mg/m² IV on days 8 and 15
Leucovorin:	10 mg/m² PO every 6 hours for 8 doses, beginning 24 hours after methotrexate
Bleomycin:	4 U/m² IV on day 1
Doxorubicin:	45 mg/m² IV on day 1
Cyclophosphamide:	600 mg/m² IV on day 1
Vincristine:	1 mg/m² IV on day 1 (maximum, 2 mg)
Dexamethasone:	6 mg/m² PO on days 1–5

Repeat cycle every 21 days (387).

ProMACE/CytaBOM

Prednisone:	60 mg/m² PO on days 1–14
Doxorubicin:	25 mg/m² IV on day 1
Cyclophosphamide:	650 mg/m² IV on day 1
Etoposide:	120 mg/m² IV on day 1
Cytarabine:	300 mg/m² IV on day 8
Bleomycin:	5 U/m² IV on day 8
Vincristine:	1.4 mg/m² IV on day 8
Methotrexate:	120 mg/m² IV on day 8

| Leucovorin rescue: | 25 mg/m² PO every 6 hours for 6 doses, beginning 24 hours after methotrexate |
| Bactrim DS: | 1 tablet PO bid on days 1–21 |

Repeat cycle every 21 days (388) .

ESHAP (salvage regimen)
Etoposide:	40 mg/m² IV on days 1–4
Methylprednisolone:	500 mg IV on days 1–4
Cisplatin:	25 mg/m²/day IV continuous infusion on days 1–4
Cytarabine:	2,000 mg/m² IV on day 5 after completion of cisplatin and etoposide

Repeat cycle every 21 days (389) .

DHAP (salvage regimen)
Cisplatin:	100 mg/m² IV continuous infusion over 24 hours on day 1
Cytarabine:	2,000 mg/m² IV over 3 hours every 12 hours for 2 doses on day 2 after completion of cisplatin infusion
Dexamethasone:	40 mg PO or IV on days 1–4

Repeat cycle every 3–4 weeks (390) .

ICE (salvage regimen)
Ifosfamide:	5,000 mg/m² IV continuous infusion for 24 hours on day 2
Etoposide:	100 mg/m² IV on days 1–3
Carboplatin:	AUC of 5, IV on day 2
Mesna:	5,000 mg/m² IV in combination with ifosfamide dose

Repeat cycle every 14 days (391) . G-CSF support is administered at 5 µg/kg/day on days 5–12.

RICE (salvage regimen)
Rituximab	375 mg/m² IV on day 1
Ifosfamide:	5,000 mg/m² IV continuous infusion for 24 hours on day 4
Etoposide:	100 mg/m² IV on days 3–5
Carboplatin:	AUC of 5, IV on day 4
Mesna:	5,000 mg/m² IV in combination with ifosfamide dose

Repeat cycle every 14 days (392) . Rituximab is also given at 48 hours before the start of the first cycle. G-CSF is administered at 5 µg/kg/day on days 7–14 after the first 2 cycles and at 10 µg/kg/day after the 3rd cycle.

MINE (salvage regimen)

Mesna:	1,330 mg/m^2 IV administered at same time as ifosfamide on days 1–3, then 500 mg IV 4 hours after ifosfamide on days 1–3
Ifosfamide:	1,330 mg/m^2 IV on days 1–3
Mitoxantrone:	8 mg/m^2 IV on day 1
Etoposide:	65 mg/m^2 IV on days 1–3

Repeat cycle every 21 days (393) .

R-GemOx (salvage regimen)

Rituximab:	375 mg/m^2 IV on day 1
Gemcitabine:	1,000 mg/m^2 IV on day 2
Oxaliplatin:	50 mg/m^2 IV on day 2

Repeat cycle every 2 weeks for a total of 8 cycles (394) .

High-Grade

Magrath Protocol (Burkitt's lymphoma)

Cyclophosphamide:	1,200 mg/m^2 IV on day 1
Doxorubicin:	40 mg/m^2 IV on day 1
Vincristine:	1.4 mg/m^2 IV on day 1 (maximum, 2 mg)
Prednisone:	40 mg/m^2 PO on days 1–5
Methotrexate:	300 mg/m^2 IV on day 10, for 1 hour, then 60 mg/m^2 IV on days 10 and 11 for 41 hours
Leucovorin rescue:	15 mg/m^2 IV every 6 hours for 8 doses, starting 24 hours after methotrexate on day 12
Intrathecal Ara-C:	30 mg/m^2 IT on day 7, cycle 1 only
	45 mg/m^2 IT on day 7, all subsequent cycles
Intrathecal Methotrexate:	12.5 mg IT on day 10, all cycles

Repeat cycle every 28 days (395) .
or

Regimen A (CODOX-M) (396)

Cyclophosphamide:	800 mg/m^2 IV on day 1 and 200 mg/m^2 IV on days 2–5
Doxorubicin:	40 mg/m^2 IV on day 1
Vincristine:	1.5 mg/m^2 IV on days 1 and 8 in cycle 1 and on days 1, 8, and 15 in cycle 3

| Methotrexate: | 1,200 mg/m^2 IV over 1 hour, followed by 240 mg/m^2/hour for the next 23 hours on day 10 |
| Leucovorin: | 192 mg/m^2 IV starting at hour 36 after the start of the infusion and 12 mg/m^2 IV every 6 hours thereafter until serum MTX levels <50 nM |

CNS Prophylaxis
| Cytarabine: | 70 mg IT on days 1 and 3 |
| Methotrexate: | 12 mg IT on day 15 |

Regimen B (IVAC)
Ifosfamide:	1,500 mg/m^2 IV on days 1–5
Etoposide:	60 mg/m^2 IV on days 1–5
Cytarabine:	2 g/m^2 IV every 12 hours on days 1 and 2 for a total of 4 doses
Methotrexate:	12 mg IT on day 5

Stanford Regimen (small noncleaved cell and Burkitt's lymphoma)
Cyclophosphamide:	1,200 mg/m^2 IV on day 1
Doxorubicin:	40 mg/m^2 IV on day 1
Vincristine:	1.4 mg/m^2 IV on day 1 (maximum, 2 mg)
Prednisone:	40 mg/m^2 PO on days 1–5
Methotrexate:	3 g/m^2 IV over 6 hours on day 10
Leucovorin rescue:	25 mg/m^2 IV or PO every 6 hours for 12 doses, beginning 24 hours after methotrexate
Intrathecal Methotrexate:	12 mg IT on days 1 and 10

Repeat cycle every 21 days (397).

Hyper-CVAD/MTX-Ara-C
Cyclophosphamide:	300 mg/m^2 IV every 12 hours for 6 doses on days 1-3
Mesna:	600 mg/m^2/day continuous infusion on days 1-3 to start 1 hour before cyclophosphamide until 12 hours after completion of cyclophosphamide
Vincristine:	2 mg IV on days 4 and 11
Doxorubicin:	50 mg/m^2 IV over 24 hours on day 4
Dexamethasone:	40 mg PO or IV on days 1-4 and days 11-14

Administer every 3-4 weeks on cycles 1, 3, 5, and 7 (398).

| Methotrexate: | 200 mg/m^2 IV over 2 hours followed by 800 mg/m^2 continuous infusion over 22 hours on day 1 |

Cytarabine:	3 g/m^2 IV over 2 hours every 12 hours for 4 doses on days 2-3 (1 g/m^2 for patients over 60 years old)
Leucovorin:	50 mg IV every 6 hours starting 12 hours after completion of MTX until MTX level < 50 nM

Administer every 3-4 weeks on cycles 2, 4, 6, 8

Intrathecal Chemotherapy Prophylaxis:

Methotrexate:	12 mg IT on day 2 of each cycle for a total of 3-4 treatments
Cytarabine:	100 mg IT on day 8 of each cycle for a total of 3-4 treatments

Intrathecal Chemotherapy:

Administer intrathecal chemotherapy twice a week with methotrexate 12 mg and cytarabine 100 mg, respectively, until no more cancer cells in CSF, then decrease intrathecal chemotherapy to once a week for 4 weeks, followed by methotrexate 12 mg on day 2 and cytarabine 100 mg on day 8 for the remaining chemotherapy cycles.

Single-Agent Regimens

Rituximab

Rituximab:	375 mg/m^2 IV on days 1, 8, 15, and 22

Repeat one additional cycle (399) .

or

Rituximab (400)

Rituximab:	375 mg/m^2 IV on days 1, 8, 15, and 22 followed by 375 mg/m^2 IV at week 12 and at months 5, 7, and 9

Ibritumomab Tiuxetan Regimen

Rituximab:	250 mg/m^2 IV on days 1 and 8
^{111}In-Ibritumomab tiuxetan:	5 mCi of ^{111}In, 1.6 mg of ibritumomab tiuxetan IV on day 1
^{90}Y-Ibritumomab tiuxetan:	0.4 mCi/kg IV over 10 min on day 8 after the day 8 rituximab dose

The dose of ^{90}Y-ibritumomab tiuxetan is capped at 32 mCi (401) .

Fludarabine

Fludarabine:	25 mg/m^2 IV on days 1–5

Repeat cycle every 28 days (402) .

Cladribine

Cladribine: 0.5–0.7 mg/kg SC on days 1–5 or 0.1 mg/kg IV on days 1–7

Repeat cycle every 28 days (403).

Bendamustine
Bendamustine: 120 mg/m² IV on days 1 and 2

Repeat cycle every 21 days up to 8 cycles (404).

Primary CNS Lymphoma

Methotrexate:	3.5 g/m² IV over 2 hours every other week for 5 doses
Intrathecal Methotrexate:	12 mg IT weekly every other week after IV MTX
Leucovorin:	10 mg IV every 6 hours for 12 doses starting 24 hours after IV MTX; 10 mg IV every 12 hours for 8 doses starting 24 hours after IT MTX
Vincristine:	1.4 mg/m² IV every other week along with IV MTX
Procarbazine:	100 mg/m²/day PO for 7 days on 1st, 3rd, and 5th cycle of IV MTX

Once chemotherapy is completed, whole-brain radiation therapy is administered to a total dose of 45 cGy (405).

R-MPV + Radiation Therapy + Cytarabine

Rituximab:	500 mg/m² IV on day 1
Methotrexate:	3.5 g/m² IV on day 2
Leucovorin:	20-25 mg every 6 hours starting 24 hours after MTX infusion for 72 hours or until serum MTX level < 1 x 10⁻⁸ mg/dL. Increase leucovorin to 40 mg every 4 hour IV, if MTX level > 1 x 10⁻⁸ mg/dL at 48 hours or > 1 x 10⁻⁸ mg/dL at 72 hours
Vincristine:	1.4 mg/m² (max 2.8 mg) IV on day 2
Procarbazine:	100 mg/m² PO on days 1-7 of odd-numbered cycles only

If positive CSF cytology, administer 12 mg Methotrexate IT between days 5 and 12 of each cycle

Repeat cycle every 2 weeks for 5 cycles (406).

After 5 cycles of R-MPV:

If CR, whole-brain radiotherapy (WBRT) 180 cGy/day for 13 days to a total of 2340 cGy beginning 3-5 weeks after the completion of R-MPV.

If PR, administer 2 additional cycles of R-MPV. If CR is achieved after 7 cycles of R-MPV, administer WBRT 180 cGy/day x 13 days to a total of 2340 cGy beginning 3-5 weeks after completion of R-MPV.

If persistent disease exists after 7 cycles of R-MPV, administer WBRT 180 cGy/day x 25 days to a total of 4500 cGy beginning 3-5 weeks after the completion of R-MPV.

If stable or progressive disease after 5 cycles of R-MPV, administer WBRT 180 cGy/day for 25 days to a total of 4500 cGy beginning 3-5 weeks after the completion of R-MPV. Three weeks after the completion of WBRT, consolidation therapy is given with cytarabine 3 g/m²/day (max 6 g) IV over 3 hours for 2 days. A second cycle of cytarabine is given 1 month later.

High-Dose Methotrexate
Methotrexate: 8 g/m² IV on day 1
Repeat cycle every 2 weeks up to 8 cycles, followed by 8 gm/m² IV on day 1 every month up to 100 months (407).

Temozolomide
Temozolomide: 150 mg/m²/day PO on days 1–5
Repeat cycle every 4 weeks (408).

Topotecan
Topotecan: 1.5 mg/m² IV on days 1–5
Repeat cycle every 3 weeks (409).

MALIGNANT MELANOMA

Adjuvant Therapy

Interferon α-2b
Interferon α-2b: 20 million IU/m² IV, 5 times weekly for 4 weeks, then 10 million IU/m² SC, 3 times weekly for 48 weeks
Treat for a total of 1 year (410).

Metastatic Disease

Combination Regimens

DTIC + BCNU + Cisplatin
Dacarbazine: 220 mg/m² IV on days 1–3

| Carmustine: | 150 mg/m^2 IV on day 1 |
| Cisplatin: | 25 mg/m^2 IV on days 1–3 |

Repeat cycle with dacarbazine and cisplatin every 21 days and carmustine every 42 days (411) .

IFN + DTIC

Interferon α-2b:	15 million IU/m^2 IV on days 1–5, 8–12, and 15–19 as induction therapy
Interferon α-2b:	10 million IU/m^2 SC 3 times weekly after induction therapy
Dacarbazine:	200 mg/m^2 IV on days 22–26

Repeat cycle every 28 days (412) .

Temozolomide + Thalidomide

| Temozolomide: | 75 mg/m^2/day PO for 6 weeks |
| Thalidomide: | 200 mg/day PO for 6 weeks |

Repeat cycle every 8 weeks (413) . Consider dose escalation to 400 mg/day for patients >70 years and starting at a lower dose of 100 mg/day with dose escalation to 250 mg/day for patient ≥70 years.

Single-Agent Regimens

Dacarbazine

| Dacarbazine: | 250 mg/m^2 IV on days 1–5 |

Repeat cycle every 21 days (414) .

or

| Dacarbazine: | 850 mg/m^2 IV on day 1 |

Repeat cycle every 3–6 weeks (415) .

Interferon-α

| Interferon α-2b: | 20 million IU/m^2 IM, 3 times weekly for 12 weeks (416) . |

Aldesleukin

| Aldesleukin (IL-2): | 720,000 IU/kg IV every 8 hours on days 1–5 and 15–19 |

Repeat cycle in 6- to 12-week intervals (417) .

or

| Aldesleukin (IL-2): | 100,000 IU/kg IV every 4 hours on days 1–5 and 15–19 |

Repeat cycle in 12-week intervals up to a total of 3 cycles (418) .

or

Aldesleukin (IL-2):   720,000 IU/kg IV at 8 am and 6 pm on days 1–5 and 15–19

Treat up to a maximum of 8 total doses on days 1–5 and repeat on days 15–19. Repeat cycle in 8- to 12-week intervals (419).

Temozolomide
Temozolomide: 150 mg/m² PO on days 1–5

Repeat cycle every 28 days (420). If well tolerated, can increase dose to 200 mg/m² PO on days 1–5.

MALIGNANT MESOTHELIOMA

Combination Regimens

Doxorubicin + Cisplatin
Doxorubicin: 60 mg/m² IV on day 1
Cisplatin: 60 mg/m² IV on day 1

Repeat cycle every 21–28 days (421).

CAP
Cyclophosphamide: 500 mg/m² IV on day 1
Doxorubicin: 50 mg/m² IV on day 1
Cisplatin: 80 mg/m² IV on day 1

Repeat cycle every 21 days (422).

Gemcitabine + Cisplatin
Gemcitabine: 1,000 mg/m² IV on days 1, 8, and 15
Cisplatin: 100 mg/m² IV on day 1

Repeat cycle every 28 days (423).

Gemcitabine + Carboplatin
Gemcitabine: 1,000 mg/m² IV on days 1, 8, and 15
Carboplatin: AUC of 5, IV on day 1

Repeat cycle every 28 days (424).

Pemetrexed + Cisplatin
Pemetrexed: 500 mg/m² IV on day 1
Cisplatin: 75 mg/m² IV on day 1

Repeat cycle every 21 days (425). Folic acid at 350–1,000 µg PO q day beginning 1 week prior to therapy and vitamin B12 at 1,000 µg IM to start 1–2 weeks prior to first dose of therapy and repeated every 3 cycles.

Gemcitabine + Vinorelbine

Gemcitabine:	1,000 mg/m^2 IV on days 1 and 8
Vinorelbine:	25 mg/m^2 IV on days 1 and 8

Repeat cycle every 21 days (426).

Pemetrexed + Gemcitabine

Pemetrexed:	500 mg/m^2 IV on day 8
Gemcitabine:	1,250 mg/m^2 IV on days 1 and 8

Repeat cycle every 21 days (427). Folic acid at 350–1,000 µg PO q day beginning 1–2 weeks prior to therapy and vitamin B12 at 1,000 µg IM to start 1–2 weeks prior to first dose of therapy and repeated every 3 cycles.

Single-Agent Regimens

Pemetrexed

Pemetrexed:	500 mg/m^2 IV on day 1

Repeat cycle every 21 days (428). Folic acid at 350-1,000 µg PO q day beginning 1 week prior to therapy and vitamin B12 at 1,000 µg IM to start 1-2 weeks prior to first dose of therapy and repeated every 3 cycles. Dexamethasone 4 mg PO bid on the day before, day of, and day after each dose of pemetrexed.

Vinorelbine

Vinorelbine:	30 mg/m^2 IV weekly

One cycle consists of 6 weekly injections. Continue until disease progression (429).

MULTIPLE MYELOMA

Combination Regimens

MP

Melphalan:	8–10 mg/m^2 PO on days 1–4
Prednisone:	60 mg/m^2 on days 1–4

Repeat cycle every 42 days (430).

MPT

Melphalan:	0.25 mg/kg PO on days 1–4
Prednisone:	1.5 mg/kg PO on days 1–4
Thalidomide:	50–100 mg/day PO q day

Repeat cycle every 28 days (431).

or

Melphalan: 0.25 mg/kg/day PO on days 1–4
Prednisone: 2 mg/kg/day PO on days 1–4
Thalidomide: 100–400 mg PO q day
Repeat cycle every 42 days (432) .

MPL
Melphalan: 0.18 mg/kg PO on days 1–4
Prednisone: 2 mg/kg PO on days 1–4
Lenalidomide: 10 mg/day PO on days 1–21
Repeat cycle every 28 days (433) .

VAD
Vincristine: 0.4 mg/day IV continuous infusion on days 1–4

Doxorubicin: 9 mg/m^2/day IV continuous infusion on days 1–4
Dexamethasone: 40 mg PO on days 1–4, 9–12, and 17–20
Repeat cycle every 28 days (434) .

Thalidomide + Dexamethasone
Thalidomide: 200 mg/day PO
Dexamethasone: 40 mg/day PO on days 1–4, 9–12, and 17–20
                        for first 4 cycles and then 40 mg/day PO on
                        days 1–4
Repeat cycle every 28 days (435) .

Lenalidomide + Dexamethasone
Lenalidomide: 25 mg/day PO on days 1–21
Dexamethasone: 40 mg/day PO on days 1–4, 9–12, and 17–20
                        (first 4 cycles) and then 40 mg/day PO on days
                        1–4 with future cycles
Repeat cycles every 28 days (436) .
or
Lenalidomide: 25 mg/day PO on days 1–21
Dexamethasone: 40 mg/m^2/day PO on days 1, 8, 15, and 22
Repeat cycle every 28 days (437) .

DVD
Doxil: 40 mg/m^2 IV on day 1
Vincristine: 2 mg IV on day 1
Dexamethasone: 40 mg PO on days 1-4
Repeat cycles every 28 days (438) .

Bortezomib + Pegylated Liposomal Doxorubicin
Bortezomib: 1.3 mg/m² IV bolus on days 1, 4, 8, and 11
Doxil: 30 mg/m² IV infusion on day 4
Repeat cycle every 21 days (439).

Bortezomib + Melphalan
Bortezomib: 1.0 mg/m² IV on days 1, 4, 8, and 11
Melphalan: 0.10 mg/kg PO on days 1–4
Repeat cycle every 28 days up to 8 cycles (440).

BMP
Bortezomib: 1.3 mg/m² IV on days 1, 4, 8, 11, 22, 25, 29, and 32
Melphalan: 9 mg/m² PO on days 1–4
Prednisone: 60 mg/m² PO on days 1–4
Repeat cycle every 6 weeks for 4 cycles (441).
then
Bortezomib: 1.3 mg/m² IV on days 1, 8, 22, and 29
Melphalan: 9 mg/m² PO on days 1–4
Prednisone: 60 mg/m² PO on days 1–4
Repeat cycle every 6 weeks for 5 cycles.

BMPT
Bortezomib: 1–1.3 mg/m² IV on days 1, 4, 15, and 22
Melphalan: 6 mg/m² PO on days 1–5
Prednisone: 60 mg/m² PO on days 1–5
Thalidomide: 50 mg PO daily
Repeat cycle every 5 weeks for 6 cycles (442).

Single-Agent Regimens

Dexamethasone
Dexamethasone: 40 mg IV or PO on days 1–4, 9–12, and 17–20
Repeat cycle every 21 days (443).

Melphalan
Melphalan: 90–140 mg/m² IV on day 1
Repeat cycle every 28–42 days (444).

Thalidomide
Thalidomide: 200–800 mg PO daily
Continue treatment until disease progression or undue toxicity (445).

Lenalidomide

Lenalidomide: 30 mg PO daily on days 1–21
Repeat cycle every 28 days until disease progression or undue toxicity
(446).

Bortezomib

Bortezomib: 1.3 mg/m^2 IV on days 1, 4, 8, and 11
Repeat cycle every 21 days (447).

MYELODYSPLASTIC SYNDROME

Single-Agent Regimens

Azacitidine

Azacitidine: 75 mg/m^2 SC daily for 7 days
Repeat cycle every 4 weeks. Patients should be treated for at least 4 cycles
(448).

Decitabine

Decitabine: 15 mg/m^2 IV continuous infusion over 3 hours
                                every 8 hours for 3 days
Repeat cycle every 4 weeks. Patients should be treated for at least 4 cycles
(449).
or
Decitabine: 20 mg/m^2 IV continuous infusion over 1 hour
                                for 5 days
Repeat cycle every 4–6 weeks. Patients should be treated for at least 4 cycles
(450).

Lenalidomide

Lenalidomide: 10 mg PO daily
Continue until disease progression (451).
or
Lenalidomide: 10 mg PO daily for 21 days
Repeat cycle every 28 days (451).

Imatinib

Imatinib: 400 mg PO daily
Continue until disease progression (452).

OSTEOGENIC SARCOMA

Combination Regimens

Etoposide + Ifosfamide

Etoposide:	100 mg/m^2/day IV on days 1-5
Ifosfamide:	3,500 mg/m^2/day IV on days 1-5
Mesna:	700 mg/m^2 IV with first ifosfamide dose, then 3, 6, and 9 hours later on days 1-5

Repeat cycle every 21 days for 2 cycles (453). G-CSF support at 5 µg/kg/day to start on day 6. Followed by surgical resection of primary tumor and then intensive maintenance chemotherapy.

Methotrexate:	12 g/m^2 IV on weeks 1, 2, 6, 7, 11, 12, 16, 17, 30, 31
Leucovorin:	15 mg IV every 6 hours for 10 doses starting 24 hours after start of high-dose MTX

or

L-Leucovorin:	7.5 mg IV every 6 hours for 10 doses starting 24 hours after start of high-dose MTX
Doxorubicin:	37.5 mg/m^2/day IV on days 1–2 on weeks 3, 13, 21, 27, and 32
Cisplatin:	60 mg/m^2/day IV on days 1–2 on weeks 3, 13, 21, and 27
Ifosfamide:	2,400 mg/m^2/day IV on days 1–5 on weeks 8, 18, and 24

Administer G-CSF support at 5 µg/kg/day on weeks 8, 18, and 24.

Cisplatin + Doxorubicin + High-Dose Methotrexate

Doxorubicin:	25 mg/m^2/day IV on days 1-3 on weeks 0 and 5
Cisplatin:	120 mg/m^2 IV on day 1 on weeks 0 and 5
Methotrexate:	12 g/m^2 IV on day 1 on weeks 3, 4, 8, and 9
Leucovorin:	10 mg IV every 6 hours for 10 doses starting 24 hours after start of high-dose MTX

or

L-Leucovorin:	7.5 mg IV every 6 hours for 10 doses starting 24 hours after start of high-dose MTX

Induction chemotherapy is followed by surgical resection of primary tumor and then maintenance chemotherapy to begin on week 12 and continuing until week 31 (454).

Doxorubicin:	25 mg/m^2/day IV on days 1-3 on weeks 12, 17, 22, and 27
Cisplatin:	120 mg/m^2 IV on day 1 on weeks 12 and 17
Methotrexate:	12 g/m^2 IV on day 1 on weeks 15, 16, 20, 21, 25, 26, 30, and 31
Leucovorin:	10 mg IV every 6 hours for 10 doses starting 24 hours after start of high-dose MTX
or	
L-Leucovorin:	7.5 mg IV every 6 hours for 10 doses starting 24 hours after start of high-dose MTX

OVARIAN CANCER (Epithelial)

Combination Regimens

CC
| Carboplatin: | 300 mg/m^2 IV on day 1 |
| Cyclophosphamide: | 600 mg/m^2 IV on day 1 |

Repeat cycle every 28 days (455) .

CP
| Cisplatin: | 100 mg/m^2 IV on day 1 |
| Cyclophosphamide: | 600 mg/m^2 IV on day 1 |

Repeat cycle every 28 days (456) .

CT
| Cisplatin: | 75 mg/m^2 IV on day 2 |
| Paclitaxel: | 135 mg/m^2 IV over 24 hours on day 1 |

Repeat cycle every 21 days (457) .

Carboplatin + Paclitaxel
| Carboplatin: | AUC of 6-7.5, IV on day 1 |
| Paclitaxel: | 175 mg/m^2 IV over 3 hours on day 1 |

Repeat cycle every 21 days (458) .
or
| Carboplatin: | AUC of 2, IV on days 1, 8, and 15 |
| Paclitaxel: | 60 mg/m^2 IV on days 1, 8, and 15 |

Repeat cycle every 28 days (459) .

Carboplatin + Docetaxel
| Carboplatin: | AUC of 6, IV on day 1 |

Docetaxel: 60 mg/m² IV on day 1
Repeat cycle every 21 days (460).

Carboplatin + Pegylated Liposomal Doxorubicin
Carboplatin: AUC of 5, IV on day 1
Doxil: 30 mg/m² IV on day 1
Repeat cycle every 28 days (461).

Gemcitabine + Pegylated Liposomal Doxorubicin
Gemcitabine: 1,000 mg/m² IV on days 1 and 8
Doxil: 30 mg/m² IV on day 1
Repeat cycle every 21 days (462).

Gemcitabine + Cisplatin
Gemcitabine: 800–1,000 mg/m² IV on days 1 and 8
Cisplatin: 30 mg/m² IV on days 1 and 8
Repeat cycle every 21 days (463).

Gemcitabine + Carboplatin
Gemcitabine: 1,000 mg/m² IV on days 1 and 8
Carboplatin: AUC of 4, IV on day 1
Repeat cycle every 21 days (464).

Paclitaxel + IP Cisplatin + IP Paclitaxel
Paclitaxel: 135 mg/m² IV over 24 hours on day 1
Cisplatin: 100 mg/m² IP on day 2
Paclitaxel: 60 mg/m² IP on day 8
Repeat cycle every 21 days up to 6 cycles (465).

Pemetrexed + Carboplatin
Pemetrexed: 500 mg/m² IV on day 1
Carboplatin: AUC of 5, IV on day 1
Repeat cycle every 21 days (466). Folic acid at 350-1,000 µg PO q day
beginning 1-2 weeks prior to therapy and vitamin B12 at 1,000 µg IM to
start 1-2 weeks prior to first dose of therapy and repeated every 3 cycles.
Dexamethasone 4 mg PO bid on the day before, day of, and day after each
dose of pemetrexed.

Single-Agent Regimens

Altretamine

Altretamine: 260 mg/m² /day PO in 4 divided doses after
                                meals and at bedtime
Repeat cycle every 14–21 days (467) .

Pegylated Liposomal Doxorubicin
Pegylated Liposomal
Doxorubicin: 40-50 mg/m² IV over 1 hour on day 1
Repeat cycle every 28 days (468) .

Paclitaxel
Paclitaxel: 135 mg/m² IV over 3 hours on day 1
Repeat cycle every 21 days (469) .

Topotecan
Topotecan: 1.5 mg/m² IV on days 1–5
Repeat cycle every 21 days (470) .

Gemcitabine
Gemcitabine: 800 mg/m² IV weekly for 3 weeks
Repeat cycle every 4 weeks (471) .

Etoposide
Etoposide: 50 mg/m²/day PO on days 1–21
Repeat cycle every 28 days (472) .

Vinorelbine
Vinorelbine: 30 mg/m² IV on days 1 and 8
Repeat cycle every 21 days (473) .

Pemetrexed
Pemetrexed: 900 mg/m² IV on day 1
Repeat cycle every 21 days (474) . Folic acid at 350-1,000 µg PO q day
beginning 1 week prior to therapy and vitamin B12 at 1,000 µg IM to start
1-2 weeks prior to first dose of therapy and repeated every 3 cycles. Dexamethasone 4 mg PO bid on the day before, day of, and day after each dose of
pemetrexed.

Bevacizumab
Bevacizumab: 15 mg/kg IV on day 1
Repeat cycle every 21 days (475) .

OVARIAN CANCER (Germ Cell)

Combination Regimens

BEP

Bleomycin: 30 U IV on days 2, 9, and 16
Etoposide: 100 mg/m^2 IV on days 1–5
Cisplatin: 20 mg/m^2 IV on days 1–5
Repeat cycle every 21 days (476).

PANCREATIC CANCER

Adjuvant Therapy

Single-Agent Regimen

5-Fluorouracil + Leucovorin

5-Fluorouracil: 425 mg/m^2 IV on days 1-5
Leucovorin: 20 mg/m2 IV on days 1-5
Repeat cycle every 28 days for a total of 6 cycles (477).

Gemcitabine

Gemcitabine: 1,000 mg/m^2 IV on days 1, 8, and 15
Repeat cycle every 28 days for a total of 6 cycles (478).

Locally Advanced Disease

Combination Regimens

5-Fluorouracil + Radiation Therapy (GITSG regimen)

5-Fluorouracil: 500 mg/m^2/day IV on days 1–3 and 29–31, then weekly beginning on day 71
Radiation therapy: Total dose, 4,000 cGy
Chemotherapy and radiation therapy started on the same day and given concurrently (479).

RTOG Chemoradiation Regimen

Gemcitabine: 1,000 mg/m^2 IV on days 1, 8, and 15
Followed by concurrent chemoradiation:

5-Fluorouracil: 250 mg/m²/day IV continuous infusion during
radiation therapy
Radiation therapy: 180 cGy/day to a total dose of 5,040 cGy
Chemotherapy and radiation therapy started on the same day and given
concurrently.
After chemoradiation:
Gemcitabine: 1,000 mg/m² IV on days 1, 8, and 15
Repeat cycle every 4 weeks for a total of 3 cycles (480) .

Gemcitabine + Radiation Therapy (ECOG regimen)
Gemcitabine: 600 mg/m² IV weekly for 6 weeks
Radiation therapy: 180 cGy/day to a total dose of 5,040 cGy
Chemotherapy and radiation therapy started on the same day and given
concurrently.
Four weeks after the completion of chemoradiation:
Gemcitabine: 1,000 mg/m² IV on days 1, 8, and 15
Repeat cycle every 4 weeks for a total of 5 cycles (481) .

Metastatic Disease

Combination Regimens

5-Fluorouracil + Leucovorin
5-Fluorouracil: 425 mg/m² IV on days 1–5
Leucovorin: 20 mg/m² IV on days 1–5
Repeat cycle every 28 days (482) .

Gemcitabine + Capecitabine (GEM-CAP)
Gemcitabine: 1,000 mg/m² IV on days 1 and 8
Capecitabine: 650 mg/m² PO bid on days 1–14
Repeat cycle every 21 days (483) .
or
Gemcitabine: 1,000 mg/m² IV on days 1, 8, and 15
Capecitabine: 830 mg/m² PO bid on days 1–21
Repeat cycle every 28 days (484) .

Gemcitabine + Docetaxel + Capecitabine (GTX)
Gemcitabine: 750 mg/m² IV over 75 minutes on days 4 and
11
Docetaxel: 30 mg/m² IV on days 4 and 11
Capecitabine: 750 mg/m² PO bid on days 1–14
Repeat cycle every 3 weeks (485) .

Gemcitabine + Oxaliplatin

Gemcitabine:	1,000 mg/m^2 IV over 100 minutes on day 1
Oxaliplatin:	100 mg/m^2 over 2 hours on day 2

Repeat cycle every 2 weeks (486).
or

Gemcitabine:	1,000 mg/m^2 IV over 100 minutes on day 1
Oxaliplatin:	100 mg/m^2 over 2 hours on day 1

Repeat cycle every 2 weeks (487).

Gemcitabine + Erlotinib

Gemcitabine:	1,000 mg/m^2 IV weekly for 7 weeks, then 1 week rest; subsequent cycles 1,000 mg/m^2 IV weekly for 3 weeks with 1 week rest
Erlotinib:	100 mg PO daily

Repeat 3-week cycles every 28 days (488).

Capecitabine + Erlotinib

Capecitabine:	1,000 mg/m^2 PO bid on days 1–14
Erlotinib:	150 mg PO daily

Repeat cycle every 21 days (489).

Single-Agent Regimens

Gemcitabine

Gemcitabine:	1,000 mg/m^2 IV weekly for 7 weeks, then 1 week rest; subsequent cycles 1,000 mg/m^2 IV weekly for 3 weeks with 1 week rest

Repeat 3-week cycle every 28 days (490).
or

Gemcitabine:	1,000 mg/m^2 IV over 100 min at 10 mg/m^2/min on days 1, 8, and 15

Repeat cycle every 28 days (491).

Capecitabine

Capecitabine:	1,250 mg/m^2 PO bid on days 1–14

May decrease dose to 850–1,000 mg/m^2 PO bid on days 1–14 to reduce the risk of toxicity without compromising clinical efficacy. Repeat cycle every 21 days (492).

PROSTATE CANCER

Combination Regimens

Flutamide + Leuprolide (493)
Flutamide:	250 mg PO tid
Leuprolide:	7.5 mg IM every 28 days or 22.5 mg IM every 12 weeks

Flutamide + Goserelin (494)
Flutamide:	250 mg PO tid
Goserelin:	10.8 mg SC every 12 weeks

Estramustine + Etoposide
Estramustine:	15 mg/kg/day PO in 4 divided doses on days 1–21
Etoposide:	50 mg/m^2/day PO in 2 divided doses on days 1–21

Repeat cycle every 28 days (495) .

Estramustine + Vinblastine
Estramustine:	600 mg/m^2 PO daily on days 1–42
Vinblastine:	4 mg/m^2 IV weekly for 6 weeks

Repeat cycle every 8 weeks (496) .

Paclitaxel + Estramustine
Paclitaxel:	120 mg/m^2 IV continuous infusion on days 1–4
Estramustine:	600 mg/m^2 PO daily, starting 24 hours before paclitaxel

Repeat cycle every 21 days (497) .
or
Paclitaxel:	90 mg/m^2 IV weekly for 3 weeks
Estramustine:	140 mg PO tid, starting day before, day of, and day after paclitaxel

Repeat cycle every 28 days (498) .

Mitoxantrone + Prednisone
Mitoxantrone:	12 mg/m^2 IV on day 1
Prednisone:	5 mg PO bid daily

Repeat cycle every 21 days (499) .

Docetaxel + Estramustine

Docetaxel:	35 mg/m² IV on day 2 of weeks 1 and 2
Estramustine:	420 mg PO for the first 4 doses and 280 mg PO for the next 5 doses on days 1–3 of weeks 1 and 2

Repeat cycle every 21 days (500). Decadron is administered at 4 mg PO bid on days 1–3 of weeks 1 and 2.

or

Docetaxel:	60 mg/m² IV on day 2
Estramustine:	280 mg PO tid on days 1–5

Repeat cycle every 21 days (501).

Docetaxel + Prednisone

Docetaxel:	75 mg/m² IV on day 1
Prednisone:	5 mg PO bid

Repeat cycle every 21 days for up to a total of 10 cycles (502).

Single-Agent Regimens

Paclitaxel

Paclitaxel:	135–170 mg/m² IV as a 24-hour infusion on day 1

Repeat cycle every 3 weeks (503).

or

Paclitaxel:	150 mg/m² IV as a 1-hour infusion weekly for 6 weeks

Repeat cycle every 8 weeks (504).

Docetaxel

Docetaxel:	75 mg/m² IV on day 1

Repeat cycle every 21 days (505).

or

Docetaxel:	20–40 mg/m² weekly for 3 weeks

Repeat cycle every 4 weeks (506).

Estramustine

Estramustine:	14 mg/kg/day PO in 3–4 divided doses (507).

Goserelin

Goserelin:	3.6 mg SC on day 1

Repeat cycle every 28 days (508).

or

Goserelin: 10.8 mg SC on day 1
Repeat cycle every 12 weeks (508) .

Goserelin (Adjuvant Therapy)
Goserelin: 3.6 mg SC on day 1
Repeat cycle every 28 days for 24 months (509) .

Degarelix
Degarelix: 240 mg SC starting dose followed 28 days later
                              by the first maintenance dose of 80 mg SC
Repeat maintenance dose every 28 days (510) .

Leuprolide
Leuprolide: 7.5 mg IM on day 1
Repeat cycle every 28 days (511) .
or
Leuprolide: 22.5 mg IM on day 1
Repeat cycle every 12 weeks (512) .
or
Leuprolide: 30 mg IM on day 1
Repeat cycle every 16 weeks (513) .

Bicalutamide
Bicalutamide: 50 mg PO daily
In patients refractory to other antiandrogen agents, may start with a higher
dose of 150 mg PO daily (514) .

Flutamide
Flutamide: 250 mg PO tid (515).

Nilutamide
Nilutamide: 300 mg PO on days 1–30, then 150 mg PO daily
                              (516).

Prednisone
Prednisone: 5 mg PO bid (517).
or
Prednisone: 5 mg PO qid (518).

Ketoconazole
Ketoconazole: 1,200 mg PO daily (519).

Aminoglutethimide

Aminoglutethimide:	250 mg PO qid, if tolerated may increase to 500 mg PO qid (520).

RENAL CELL CANCER

Combination Regimens

Bevacizumab + Interferon-α

Bevacizumab:	10 mg/kg IV every 2 weeks
Interferon α-2a:	9 million units SC, 3 times per week, for 1 year

Continue until disease progression (521) .

Interferon-α + IL-2

Interferon α-2a:	9 million units SC on days 1–4, weeks 1–4
Interleukin-2:	12 million units SC on days 1–4, weeks 1–4

Repeat cycle every 6 weeks (522) .

Single-Agent Regimens

Bevacizumab

Bevacizumab:	10 mg/kg IV on day 1

Repeat cycle every 2 weeks (523) .

Sunitinib

Sunitinib:	50 mg PO daily for 4 weeks

Repeat cycle every 6 weeks (524) .

Sorafenib

Sorafenib:	400 mg PO bid

Continue until disease progression (525) .

Temsirolimus

Temsirolimus:	25 mg IV weekly

Continue until disease progression (526) .

Everolimus

Everolimus:	10 mg PO daily

Continue until disease progression (527) .

Aldesleukin

| IL-2: | 720,000 IU/kg IV every 8 hours on days 1–5 and 15–19 |

Repeat cycles in 6- to 12-week intervals up to a total of 3 cycles (528).
or

| IL-2: | 720,000 IU/kg IV at 8 am and 6 pm on days 1–5 and 15–19 |

Treat up to a maximum of 8 total doses on days 1–5 and repeat on days 15–19. Repeat cycles in 8- to 12-week intervals (419).

Interferon-α

| Interferon α-2a: | 5–15 million units SC daily or 3–5 times per week (529). |

SOFT TISSUE SARCOMAS

Combination Regimens

AD

| Doxorubicin: | 15 mg/m^2/day IV continuous infusion on days 1–4 |
| Dacarbazine: | 250 mg/m^2/day IV continuous infusion on days 1–4 |

Repeat cycle every 21 days (530).

AI

Doxorubicin:	20 mg/m^2/day IV continuous infusion on days 1–3
Ifosfamide:	1.5 g/m^2/day IV continuous infusion on days 1–4
Mesna:	225 mg/m^2 IV over 1 hr before ifosfamide and at 4 and 8 hours after ifosfamide

Repeat cycle every 21 days (531). G-CSF support at 5 µg/kg/day for 10 days starting on day 5.

MAID

Mesna:	2,500 mg/m^2/day IV continuous infusion on days 1–4
Doxorubicin:	20 mg/m^2/day IV continuous infusion on days 1–3
Ifosfamide:	2,500 mg/m^2/day IV continuous infusion on days 1–3

Dacarbazine: 300 mg/m² /day IV continuous infusion on
                             days 1–3
Repeat cycle every 21 days (532) .

CYVADIC
Cyclophosphamide: 500 mg/m² IV on day 1
Vincristine: 1.5 mg/m² IV on day 1 (maximum, 2 mg)
Doxorubicin: 50 mg/m² IV on day 1
Dacarbazine: 750 mg/m² IV on day 1
Repeat cycle every 21 days (533) .

Gemcitabine + Docetaxel
Gemcitabine: 900 mg/m² IV over 90 minutes on days 1 and
                             8
Docetaxel: 100 mg/m² IV on day 8
Repeat cycle every 21 days (534) .

Gemcitabine + Navelbine
Gemcitabine: 800 mg/m² IV over 90 minutes on days 1 and
                             8
Vinorelbine: 25 mg/m² IV on days 1 and 8
Repeat cycle every 21 days (535) .

CAV Alternating with IE (Ewing's sarcoma)
Cyclophosphamide: 1,200 mg/m² IV on day 1
Doxorubicin: 75 mg/m² IV on day 1
Vincristine: 2 mg IV on day 1
and
Ifosfamide: 1,800 mg/m² IV on days 1–5
Etoposide: 100 mg/m² IV on days 1–5
Alternate CAV with IE every 21 days for a total of 17 cycles (536) . When the
cumulative dose of doxorubicin reaches 375 mg/m², switch to dactinomycin
at 1.25 mg/m².

Single-Agent Regimens

Doxorubicin
Doxorubicin: 75 mg/m² IV on day 1
Repeat cycle every 21 days (533) .

Gemcitabine
Gemcitabine: 1,200 mg/m² IV on days 1 and 8

Repeat cycle every 21 days (534) .

Ifosfamide
Ifosfamide: 3 g/m²/day IV on days 1-3
Repeat cycle every 21 days (537) .

Liposomal Doxorubicin
Doxil: 50 mg/m² IV on day 1
Repeat cycle every 28 days (538) .

TESTICULAR CANCER

Adjuvant Therapy

PEB
Cisplatin: 20 mg/m² IV on days 1–5
Etoposide: 100 mg/m² IV on days 1–5
Bleomycin: 30 U IV on days 2, 9, and 16
Repeat cycle every 28 days for a total of 2 cycles (539) . Adjuvant therapy of stage II testicular cancer treated with orchiectomy and retroperitoneal lymph node dissection.

Carboplatin
Carboplatin: AUC of 7, IV on day 1
Administer one dose for adjuvant therapy of stage I seminoma (540) .

Advanced Disease

BEP
Bleomycin: 30 U IV on days 2, 9, and 16
Etoposide: 100 mg/m² IV on days 1–5
Cisplatin: 20 mg/m² IV on days 1–5
Repeat cycle every 21 days (541) .

EP
Etoposide: 100 mg/m² IV on days 1–5
Cisplatin: 20 mg/m² IV on days 1–5
Repeat cycle every 21 days (542) .

PVB

Cisplatin:	20 mg/m² IV on days 1–5
Vinblastine:	0.15 mg/kg IV on days 1 and 2
Bleomycin:	30 units IV on days 2, 9, and 16

Repeat cycle every 21 days (543) .

VAB-6

Vinblastine:	4 mg/m² IV on day 1
Dactinomycin:	1 mg/m² IV on day 1
Bleomycin:	30 U IV on day 1, then 20 U/m² continuous infusion on days 1–3
Cisplatin:	20 mg/m² IV on day 4
Cyclophosphamide:	600 mg/m² IV on day 1

Repeat cycle every 21 days (544) .

VeIP (salvage regimen)

Vinblastine:	0.11 mg/kg IV on days 1 and 2
Ifosfamide:	1,200 mg/m² IV on days 1–5
Cisplatin:	20 mg/m² IV on days 1–5
Mesna:	400 mg/m² IV, given 15 minutes before first ifosfamide dose, then 1,200 mg/m²/day IV continuous infusion for 5 days

Repeat cycle every 21 days (545) .

VIP (salvage regimen)

Etoposide (VP-16):	75 mg/m² IV on days 1–5
Ifosfamide:	1,200 mg/m² IV on days 1–5
Cisplatin:	20 mg/m² IV on days 1–5
Mesna:	400 mg/m² IV, given 15 minutes before first ifosfamide dose, then 1,200 mg/m²/day IV continuous infusion for 5 days

Repeat cycle every 21 days (545) .

TIP (salvage regimen)

Paclitaxel:	250 mg/m² IV over 24 hours on day 1
Ifosfamide:	1,500 mg/m² IV on days 2–5
Cisplatin:	25 mg/m² IV on days 1–5
Mesna:	500 mg/m² IV, given before ifosfamide dose, and at 4 and 8 hours after ifosfamide on days 2–5

Repeat cycle every 21 days for a total of 4 cycles (546) . G-CSF support at 5 µg/kg/day SC should be given on days 7–18.

Paclitaxel + Gemcitabine
Paclitaxel: 100 mg/m^2 IV on days 1, 8, and 15
Gemcitabine: 1,000 mg/m^2 IV on days 1, 8, and 15
Repeat cycle every 28 days for a total of 6 cycles (547) .

THYMOMA

CAP
Cyclophosphamide: 500 mg/m^2 IV on day 1
Doxorubicin: 50 mg/m^2 IV on day 1
Cisplatin: 50 mg/m^2 IV on day 1
Repeat cycle every 21 days (548) .

Cisplatin + Etoposide
Cisplatin: 60 mg/m^2 IV on day 1
Etoposide: 120 mg/m^2 IV on days 1–3
Repeat cycle every 21 days (549) .

ADOC
Cisplatin: 50 mg/m^2 IV on day 1
Doxorubicin: 40 mg/m^2 IV on day 1
Vincristine: 0.6 mg/m^2 IV on day 3
Cyclophosphamide: 700 mg/m^2 IV on day 4
Repeat cycle every 28 days (550) .

VIP
Etoposide (VP-16):   75 mg/m^2 IV on days 1–4
Ifosfamide: 1,200 mg/m^2 IV on days 1–4
Cisplatin: 20 mg/m^2 IV on days 1–4
Mesna: 240 mg/m^2 IV before first ifosfamide dose,
                          then 4 and 8 hours later on days 1–4
Repeat cycle every 21 days for a total of 4 cycles (551) . G-CSF support at 5 µg/kg/day on days 5–15.

THYROID CANCER

Combination Regimens

Doxorubicin + Cisplatin

| Doxorubicin: | 60 mg/m² IV on day 1 |
| Cisplatin: | 40 mg/m² IV on day 1 |

Repeat cycle every 21 days (552).

Single-Agent Regimens

Doxorubicin

| Doxorubicin: | 60 mg/m² IV on day 1 |

Repeat cycle every 21 days (552).

Sorafenib

| Sorafenib: | 400 mg PO bid |

Continue until disease progression (553).

References

1. Flam M, et al. *J Clin Oncol* 1996;14:2527–2539.
2. Bosset JF, et al. *Eur J Cancer* 2003;39:45–51.
3. Hung A, et al. *Cancer* 2003;97:1195–1202.
4. Eng C, et al. *J Clin Oncol* 2009;27:15S (abstract 4116).
5. Flam MS, et al. *J Clin Oncol* 1996;16:227–253.
6. Valle JW, et al. *J Clin Oncol* 2009; 27:15S (abstract 4503).
7. Thongprasert S, et al. *Ann Oncol* 2005;16:279-281.
8. Knox JJ, et al. *J Clin Oncol* 2005;23:2332–2338.
9. Andre T, et al. *Ann Oncol* 2004;15:1339–1343.
10. Taieb J, et al. *Ann Oncol* 2002;13:1192–1196.
11. Hong YS, et al. *Cancer Chemother Pharmacol* 2007;60:321–328.
12. Patt YZ, et al. *Cancer* 2004;101:578–586.
13. Papakostas P, et al. *Eur J Cancer* 2001;37:1833–1838.
14. Park JS, et al. *Jpn J Clin Oncol* 2005;35:68–73.
15. Bajorin DF, et al. *Cancer* 2000;88:1671–1678.
16. Kaufman D, et al. *J Clin Oncol* 2000;18:1921–1927.
17. Linardou H, et al. *Urology* 2004;64:479–484.
18. Meluch AA, et al. *J Clin Oncol* 2001;19:3018–3024.
19. Sternberg CN, et al. *Cancer* 2001;92:2993–2998.
20. Gitlitz BJ, et al. *Cancer* 2003;98:1863-1869.
21. Sternberg CN, et al. *Cancer* 1989;64:2448–2458.
22. Harker WG, et al. *J Clin Oncol* 1985;3:1463–1470.
23. Garcia del Muro X, et al. *Br J Cancer* 2002;86:326–330.
24. Vaughn D, et al. *Cancer* 2002;95:1022–1027.
25. Dreicer R, et al. *J Clin Oncol* 2000;18:1058–1061.

26. Moore MJ, et al. *J Clin Oncol* 1997;15:3441–3445.
27. Roth BJ, et al. *J Clin Oncol* 1994;12:2264–2270.
28. Vaughn D, et al. *J Clin Oncol* 2002;20:937–940.
29. Sweeney CJ, et al. *J Clin Oncol* 2006;24:3451–3457.
30. Stupp R, et al. *N Engl J Med* 2005;352:987–995.
31. Levin VA, et al. *Int J Radiat Oncol Biol Phys* 1990;18:321–324.
32. DeAngelis LM, et al. *Ann Neurol* 1998;44:691–695.
33. Buckner JC, et al. *J Clin Oncol* 2003;21:251–255.
34. Vredenburgh JJ, et al. *J Clin Oncol* 2007;25:4722–4729.
35. Nicholas MK, et al. *J Clin Oncol* 2009;27:15S (abstract 2016).
36. Yung A, et al. *Proc Am Soc Clin Oncol* 1999;18:139a.
37. Yung A, et al. *J Clin Oncol* 1999;17:2762–2771.
38. Raymond E, et al. *Ann Oncol* 2003;14:603–614.
39. Friedman H, et al. *J Clin Oncol* 1999;17:1516–1525.
40. Bear H, et al. *J Clin Oncol* 2003;21:4165–4174.
41. Fisher B, et al. *J Clin Oncol* 2000;8:1483–1496.
42. Hudis C, et al. *J Clin Oncol* 1999;17:93–100.
43. Sparano JA, et al. *N Engl J Med* 2008;358:1663–1671.
44. Sparano J, et al. *San Antonio Breast Cancer Symposium* 2005;abstract 48.
45. Jones S, et al. *J Clin Oncol* 2006;24:5381–5387.
46. Martin M, et al. *N Engl J Med* 2005;352:2302–2313.
47. Budman DR, et al. *J Natl Cancer Inst* 1998;90:1205–1211.
48. Weiss RB, et al. *Am J Med* 1987;83:455–463.
49. Poole CJ, et al. *N Engl J Med* 2006;355:1851–1862.
50. Coombes RC, et al. *J Clin Oncol* 1996;14:35–45.
51. Roche H, et al. *J Clin Oncol* 2006;24:5664–5671.
52. Burstein HJ, et al. *J Clin Oncol* 2005;23:8340–8347.
53. Citron M, et al. *J Clin Oncol* 2003;21:1431–1439.
54. Puhalla S, et al. *J Clin Oncol* 2008;26:1691–1697.
55. Romond E, et al. http://www.asco.org/ac/1.1003, fl12-002511-00fl18-0034-00fl19-005816-00fl21-001, 00 (accessed July 2005).
56. Dang C, et al. *J Clin Oncol* 2006;24:17S (abstract 582).
57. Slamon D, et al. *San Antonio Breast Cancer Symposium* 2006; abstract 52.
58. Joensuu H, et al. *N Engl J Med* 2006;354:809–820.
59. Fisher B, et al. *J Natl Cancer Inst* 1997;89:1673–1682.
60. Howell A, et al. *Lancet* 2005;365:60–62.
61. BIG I-98 Collaborative Group, et al. *N Engl J Med* 2009;361:766-776.
62. Goss PE, et al. *J Natl Cancer Inst* 2005;97:1262–1271.
63. Coombes RC, et al. *N Engl J Med* 2004;350:1081–1092.

64. Gnant M, et al. *N Engl J Med* 2009;360:679-691.
65. Sledge GE, et al. *J Clin Oncol* 2003;21:588–592.
66. Levine MN, et al. *J Clin Oncol* 1998;16:2651–2658.
67. O'Shaughnessy J, et al. *J Clin Oncol* 2002;20:2812–2823.
68. Biganzoli L, et al. *Oncologist* 2002;7 (Suppl):29–35.
69. Thomas ES, et al. *J Clin Oncol* 2007;25:5210–5217.
70. Dieras V. *Oncology* 1997;11:31–33.
71. Brufman G, et al. *Ann Oncol* 1997;8:155-162.
72. Sparano JA, et al. *J Clin Oncol* 2001;19:3117-3125 http://www.jco.org/cgi/reprint/19/12/3117.
73. The French Epirubicin Study Group. *J Clin Oncol* 1991;9:305–312.
74. O'Shaughnessy J, et al. *Proc Am Soc Clin Oncol* 2003;22:7 (abstract 25).
75. Perez EA, et al. *Cancer* 2000;88:124–131.
76. Fitch V, et al. *Proc Am Soc Clin Oncol* 2003;22:23 (abstract 90).
77. Miller K, et al. *N Engl J Med* 2007;35:2666–2676.
78. Slamon DJ, et al. *N Engl J Med* 2001;344:783–792.
79. Goldenberg MM, et al. *Clin Ther* 1999;21:309–318.
80. Francisco E, et al. *J Clin Oncol* 2002;20:1800–1808.
81. Pegram M, et al. *Proc Am Soc Clin Oncol* 2007;25:LBA1008.
82. Burstein HJ, et al. *J Clin Oncol* 2001;19:2722–2730.
83. O'Shaughnessy J, et al. *Clin Breast Cancer* 2004;5:142–147.
84. Schaller G, et al. *J Clin Oncol* 2007;25:3246–3250.
85. Bartsch R, et al. *J Clin Oncol* 2007;25:3853–3858.
86. O'Shaughnessy J, et al. *Proc Am Soc Clin Oncol* 2008;26:(abstract 1015).
87. Geyer CE, et al. *N Engl J Med* 2006;355:2733–2743.
88. Jaiyesimi IA, et al. *J Clin Oncol* 1995;13:513–529.
89. Hayes DF, et al. *J Clin Oncol* 1995;13:2556-2566.
90. Lonning PE, et al. *J Clin Oncol* 2000;18:2234–2244.
91. Buzdar A, et al. *J Clin Oncol* 1996;14:2000–2011.
92. Dombernowsky P, et al. *J Clin Oncol* 1998;16:453–461.
93. Howell A. *Clin Cancer Res* 2001;7 (Suppl 12):4402s–4410s.
94. Chia S, et al. *J Clin Oncol* 2008;26:1664–1670.
95. Kimmick GG, et al. *Cancer Treat Res* 1998;94:231–254.
96. Baselga J, et al. *Semin Oncol* 1999;26 (Suppl 12):78–83.
97. Baselga J, et al. *J Clin Oncol* 2005;23:2162–2171.
98. Blum JL, et al. *J Clin Oncol* 1999;17:485–493.
99. Chan S. *Oncology* 1997;11 (Suppl 8):19–24.
100. Baselga J, Tabernero JM. *Oncologist* 2001;6 (Suppl 3):26–29.
101. Holmes FA, et al. *J Natl Cancer Inst* 1991;83:1797–1805.
102. Perez EA. *Oncologist* 1998;3:373–389.

103. Perez EA et al. *J Clin Oncol* 2007;25:3407–3414.
104. Fumoleau P, et al. *Semin Oncol* 1995;22 (Suppl 5):22–28.
105. Torti FM, et al. *Ann Intern Med* 1983;99:745–749.
106. Carmichael J, et al. *Semin Oncol* 1996;23 (Suppl 10):77–81.
107. Al-Batran SE, *Oncol* 2006;70:141-146.
108. O'Shaughnessy J, et al. *Breast Cancer Res Treat* 2003;82:Suppl 1 (abstract 43).
109. O'Shaughnessy JA, et al. *Breast Cancer Res Treat* 2004;88:Suppl 1 (abstract 1070).
110. Hainsworth JD, et al. *J Clin Oncol* 1997;15:2385–2393.
111. Longeval E, et al. *Cancer* 1982;50:2751–2756.
112. Hainsworth JD, et al. *J Clin Oncol* 1992;10:912–922.
113. Greco FA, et al. *J Clin Oncol* 2002;20:1651–1656.
114. Hainsworth JD, et al. *J Clin Oncol* 2007;25:1747-1752.
115. Moertel CG, et al. *N Engl J Med* 1992;326:519–526.
116. Moertel CG, et al. *Cancer* 1991;68:227–232.
117. Saltz L, et al. *Cancer* 1993;72:244.
118. Kulke MH, et al. *J Clin Oncol* 2008;26:3403–3410.
119. Rose PG, et al. *N Engl J Med* 1995;15:1144.
120. Morris M, et al. *N Engl J Med* 1999;340:1137–1143.
121. Fiorica J, et al. *Gynecol Oncol* 2002;85:89–94.
122. Buxton EJ, et al. *J Natl Cancer Inst* 1989;81:359–361.
123. Murad AM, et al. *J Clin Oncol* 1994;12:55–59.
124. Whitney CW, et al. *J Clin Oncol* 1999;17:1339–1348.
125. Pignata S, et al. *J Clin Oncol* 1999;17:756–760.
126. Chitapanarux I, et al. *Gynecol Oncol* 2003;89:402–407.
127. Monk BJ, et al. *Proc Am Soc Clin Oncol* 2008;26:(LBA5504).
128. Nagao S, et al. *Gynecol Oncol* 2005;96:805–809.
129. Levy T, et al. *Proc Am Soc Clin Oncol* 1996;15:292a.
130. Thigpen T, et al. *Semin Oncol* 1997;24 (Suppl 2):41–46.
131. Verschraegen CF, et al. *J Clin Oncol* 1997;15:625–631.
132. Muderspach LI, et al. *Gynecol Oncol* 2001;81:213–215.
133. Sauer R, et al. *N Engl J Med* 2004;351:1731–1740.
134. Minsky BD. *Oncology* 1994;6:53–58.
135. Minsky BD. *Clin Colorectal Cancer* 2004;4 (Suppl 1):S29–36.
136. Ryan DP, et al. *J Clin Oncol* 2006;24:2557–2562.
137. Rodel C, et al. *J Clin Oncol* 2007;25:110–117.
138. O'Connell MJ, et al. *J Clin Oncol* 1997;15:246–250.
139. Wolmark N, et al. *J Clin Oncol* 1993;11:1879–1887.
140. Benson AB, et al. *Oncology* 2000;14:203–212.
141. Andre, T et al. *N Engl J Med* 2004;350:2343–2351.
142. Chung KY and Saltz LB. *Cancer J* 2007;13:192–197.

143. Kuebler JP, et al. *J Clin Oncol* 2007;25:2198–2204.
144. Schmoll HJ, et al. *J Clin Oncol* 2007;25:102–109.
145. Twelves C, et al. *N Engl J Med* 2005;352:2696–2704.
146. Saltz LB, et al. *N Engl J Med* 2000;343:905–914.
147. Hurwitz H, et al. *N Engl J Med* 2004;350: 2335–2342.
148. Hwang JJ, et al. *Am J Oncol Rev* 2003;2 (Suppl 5):15–25.
149. Douillard JY, et al. *Lancet* 2000;355:1041–1047.
150. Andre T, et al. *Eur J Cancer* 1999;35:1343–1347.
151. de Gramont A, et al. *J Clin Oncol* 2000;18:2938–2947.
152. Tournigand C, et al. *J Clin Oncol* 2004;22:229–237.
153. Andre T, et al. *Proc Am Soc Clin Oncol* 2003;22:253 (abstract 1016).
154. Maindrault-Goebel F, et al. *J Clin Oncol* 2006;24 (June 20 Supplement):3504.
155. Falcone A, et al. *J Clin Oncol* 2007;25:1670–1676.
156. Cunningham D, et al. *N Engl J Med* 2004;351:337–345.
157. Scheithauer W, et al. *J Clin Oncol* 2003;21:1307–1312.
158. Kerr D. *Oncology* 2002;16 (Suppl 14):12–15.
159. Borner MM, et al. *Ann Oncol* 2005;16:282–288.
160. Goldberg RM, et al. *J Clin Oncol* 2004;22:23–30.
161. Poon MA, et al. *J Clin Oncol* 1989;7:1407–1418.
162. Petrelli N, et al. *J Clin Oncol* 1989;7:1419–1426.
163. Kabbinavar F, et al. *J Clin Oncol* 2005;23:3697–3705.
164. Jager E, et al. *J Clin Oncol* 1996;14:2274–2279.
165. de Gramont A, et al. *J Clin Oncol* 1997;15:808–815.
166. Giantonio BJ, et al. *J Clin Oncol* 2007;25:1539–1544.
167. Hochster HS, et al. *J Clin Oncol* 2008;26;3523–3529.
168. Saltz L, et al. *J Clin Oncol* 2007;22:4557–4561.
169. Cunningham D, et al. *N Engl J Med* 2004;351:537–545.
170. Sobrero AF, et al. *J Clin Oncol* 2008;26:2311–2319.
171. Van Cutsem E, et al. *N Engl J Med* 2009; 360:1408-1417.
172. Bokemeyer C, et al. *J Clin Oncol* 2009;27:663-671.
173. Scott J, et al. *J Clin Oncol* 2005;23:16S (abstract 3705).
174. Kopetz S, et al. *J Clin Oncol* 2007;25:18S (abstract 4027).
175. Kemeny N, et al. *J Clin Oncol* 1994;12:2288–2295.
176. Hoff P, et al. *J Clin Oncol* 2001;15:2282–2292.
177. Pitot HC, et al. *J Clin Oncol* 1997;15:2910–2919.
178. Ulrich-Pur H, et al. *Ann Oncol* 2001;12:1269–1272.
179. Rougier P, et al. *J Clin Oncol* 1997;15:251–260.
180. Saltz LB, et al. *J Clin Oncol* 2004;22:1201–1208.
181. Tabernero J, et al. *J Clin Oncol* 2006;24:18S (abstract 3085).
182. Van Cutsem E, et al. *J Clin Oncol* 2007;25:1658–1664.
183. Leichman CG, et al. *J Clin Oncol* 1995;13:1303–1311.

184. Leichman CG, *Oncology* 1999;13 (Suppl 3):26-32.
185. Falcone A, et al. *Cancer Chemother Pharmacol* 1999;44:159-163.
186. Hoskins PJ, et al. *J Clin Oncol* 2001;19:4048–4053.
187. Thigpen JT, et al. *J Clin Oncol* 1994;12:1408–1414.
188. Deppe G, et al. *Eur J Gynecol Oncol* 1994;15:263–266.
189. Fiorica JV. *Oncologist* 2002;7 (Suppl 5):36–45.
190. Fleming GF, et al. *J Clin Oncol* 2004;22:2159–2165.
191. Burke TW, et al. *Gynecol Oncol* 1994;55:47–50.
192. Pignata S, et al. *Br J Cancer* 2007;96:1639–1643.
193. Homesley HD, et al. *J Clin Oncol* 2007;25:526–531.
194. Muss HB. *Semin Oncol* 1994;21:107–113.
195. Thigpen JT, et al. *J Clin Oncol* 1999;17:1736–1744.
196. Ball H, et al. *Gynecol Oncol* 1996;62:278–282.
197. Wadler S, et al. *J Clin Oncol* 2003;21:2110–2114.
198. Herskovic A, et al. *N Engl J Med* 1992;326:1593–1598.
199. Bedenne L, et al. *J Clin Oncol* 2007;25:1160-1168.
200. Heath EI, et al. *J Clin Oncol* 2000;18:868–876.
201. Cunningham D, et al. *N Engl J Med* 2006;355:11–20.
202. Kies MS, et al. *Cancer* 1987;60:2156–2160.
203. Ilson DH, et al. *J Clin Oncol* 1999;17:3270–3275.
204. Ilson DH, et al. *J Clin Oncol* 1998;16:1826–1834.
205. Van Meerten E, et al. *Br J Cancer* 2007;96:1348–1352.
206. Cunningham D, et al. *N Engl J Med* 2008;358:36-46.
207. Ajani JA, et al. *Semin Oncol* 1995;22 (Suppl 6):35–40.
208. MacDonald JS, et al. *N Engl J Med* 2001;345:725–730.
209. Ajani JA, et al. *J Clin Oncol* 2007;25:3205–3209.
210. Wilke M, et al. *J Clin Oncol* 1989;7:1318–1326.
211. Shirao K, et al. *J Clin Oncol* 1997;15:921–927.
212. Shah MA, et al. *J Clin Oncol* 2006;24:5201–5206.
213. Ajani JA, et al. *Proc Am Soc Clin Oncol* 2000;20:165a (abstract 657).
214. Kang Y, et al. *J Clin Oncol* 2006;24:18S, LBA4018.
215. Al-Batran SE, et al. *J Clin Oncol* 2008;26:1435–1442.
216. Cullinan SA, et al. *J Clin Oncol* 1994;12:412–416.
217. Cascinu S, et al. *J Chemother* 1992;4:185–188.
218. O'Connell MJ. *J Clin Oncol* 1985;3:1032–1039.
219. Ajani JA, *Oncology* 2002;16 (suppl 6):89-96.
220. DeMatteo RP, et al. *Lancet* 2009;373:1097-1104.
221. Demetri GD, et al. *N Engl J Med* 2002;347:472–480.
222. Montemurro M, et al. *Eur J Cancer* 2009;May 19 (Epub ahead of print).
223. Demetri GD, et al. *Proc GI ASCO* 2006,Abstract 8.
224. Bonner JA, et al. *N Engl J Med* 2006;354:567–578.

225. Posner MR, et al. *N Engl J Med* 2007;357:1705-1715.
226. Shin DS, et al. *J Clin Oncol* 1998;16:1325–1330.
227. Posner M, et al. *J Clin Oncol* 2001;19:1096–1104.
228. Shin DM, et al. *Cancer* 1999;91:1316–1323.
229. Fountzilas G, et al. *Semin Oncol* 1997;24 (Suppl 2):65–67.
230. Hitt R, et al. *Semin Oncol* 1995;22 (Suppl 15):50–54.
231. Kish JA, et al. *Cancer* 1984;53:1819–1824.
232. Vokes EE, et al. *Cancer* 1989;63 (Suppl 6):1048–1053.
233. Vermorken JB, et al. *N Engl J Med* 2008;359:1116-1127.
234. Veterans Affairs Laryngeal Cancer Study Group. *N Engl J Med* 1991;324:1685–1690.
235. Forastiere AA, et al. *N Engl J Med* 2003;349:2091–2098.
236. Al-Sarraf M, et al. *J Clin Oncol* 1998;16:1310–1317.
237. Gebbia V, et al. *Am J Clin Oncol* 1995;18:293–296.
238. Dreyfuss A, et al. *Proc Am Soc Clin Oncol* 1995;14:875a.
239. Forastiere AA. *Ann Oncol* 1994;5 (Suppl 6):51–54.
240. Hong WK, et al. *N Engl J Med* 1983;308:75–79.
241. Degardin M, et al. *Ann Oncol* 1998;9:1103–1107.
242. Vermorken JB, et al. *J Clin Oncol* 2007;25:2171-2177.
243. Taieb J, et al. *Cancer* 2003;98:2664–2670.
244. Thomas MB, et al. *J Clin Oncol* 2009;27:843-850.
245. Llovet J, et al. *N Engl J Med* 2008;359:378–390.
246. Venook AP. *J Clin Oncol* 1994;12:1323–1334.
247. Okada S, et al. *Oncology* 1993;50:22–26.
248. Patt YZ, et al. *Cancer* 2004;101:578–586.
249. Siegel AB, et al. *J Clin Oncol* 2008;26:2992-2998.
250. Ireland-Gill A, et al. *Semin Oncol* 1992;19 (Suppl 5):32–37.
251. Laubenstein LL, et al. *J Clin Oncol* 1984;2:1115–1120.
252. Gill PS, et al. *J Clin Oncol* 1996;14:2353–2364.
253. Northfelt DW, et al. *J Clin Oncol* 1997;15:653–659.
254. Gill PS, et al. *J Clin Oncol* 1999;17:1876–1880.
255. Gill PS, et al. *Cancer* 2002;95:147–154.
256. Lim ST, et al. *Cancer* 2005;103:417–421.
257. Evans SR, et al. *J Clin Oncol* 2002;20:3236–3241.
258. Nasti G, et al. *J Clin Oncol* 2000;18:1550–1557.
259. Real FX, et al. *J Clin Oncol* 1986;4:544–551.
260. Groopman JE, et al. *Ann Intern Med* 1984;100:671–676.
261. Linker CA, et al. *Blood* 1987;69:1242–1248.
262. Linker CA, et al. *Blood* 1991;78:2814–2822.
263. Larson R, et al. *Blood* 1995;85:2025–2037.
264. Kantarjian H, et al. *J Clin Oncol* 2000;18:547–561.
265. Faderl S, et al. *Cancer* 2005;103:1985–1995.

266. DeAngelo DJ, et al. *Blood* 2007;109:5136-5142.
267. Ottman OG, et al. *Blood* 2002;100:1965–1971.
268. Talpaz M, et al. *N Engl J Med* 2006;354:2531–2541.
269. Kantarjian H, et al. *N Engl J Med* 2006;354:2542–2551.
270. Yates JW, et al. *Cancer Chemother Rep* 1973;57:485–488.
271. Preisler H, et al. *Blood* 1987;69:1441–1449.
272. Preisler H, et al. *Cancer Treat Rep* 1977;61:89–92.
273. Faderi S, et al. *Blood* 2006;108:45–51.
274. Mandelli F, et al. *Blood* 1997;90:1014–1021.
275. Estey E. et al. *Blood* 2006;107:3469-3473.
276. Ho AD, et al. *J Clin Oncol* 1988;6:213–217.
277. Montillo M, et al. *Am J Hematol* 1998;58:105–109.
278. Wiernik PH, et al. *Blood* 1992;79:313–319.
279. Tallman MS, et al. *Blood* 2005;106:1154–1163.
280. Santana VM, et al. *J Clin Oncol* 1992;10:364–369.
281. Mayer RJ, et al. *N Engl J Med* 1994;331:896–903.
282. Kantarjian H, et al. *Blood* 2003;102:2379–2386.
283. Degos L, et al. *Blood* 1995;85:2643–2653.
284. Soignet SL, et al. *J Clin Oncol* 2001;19:3852-3860.
285. Sievers EL, et al. *Blood* 1999;11:3678–3684.
286. Raphael B, et al. *J Clin Oncol* 1991;9:770–776.
287. Keating MJ, et al. *Blood* 1998;92:1165–1171.
288. O'Brien S, et al. *Blood* 1993;82:1695–1700.
289. Byrd JC, et al. *Blood* 2003;101:6–14.
290. Keating M, et al. *J Clin Oncol* 2005;22:4079–4088.
291. Kay NE, et al. *Blood* 2004;104:Abstract 339.
292. Osterborg A, et al. *J Clin Oncol* 1997;15:1567–1574.
293. Dighiero G, et al. *N Engl J Med* 1998;338:1506–1514.
294. Saven A, et al. *J Clin Oncol* 1995;13:570–574.
295. Keating MJ, et al. *Blood* 1988;92:1165–1171.
296. Sawitsky A, et al. *Blood* 1977;50:1049.
297. Hainsworth JD, et al. *J Clin Oncol* 2003;21:1746–1751.
298. Grever MR, et al. *J Clin Oncol* 1985;3:1196–1201.
299. Alvado M, et al. *Semin Oncol* 2002;29(4 Suppl 13):19–22.
300. Kath R, et al. *J Cancer Res Clin Oncol* 2001;127:48–54.
301. Ferrajoli A, et al. *Blood* 2008;111:5291-5297.
302. Guilhot F, et al. *N Engl J Med* 1997;337:223–229.
303. Druker BJ, et al. *N Engl J Med* 2001;344:1031–1037.
304. Kantarjian HM, et al. *Blood* 2007;110:3540–3546.
305. Kantarjian HM, et al. *Blood* 2007;109:5143–5150.
306. Hehlmann R, et al. *Blood* 1993;82:398–407.
307. Hehlmann R, et al. *Blood* 1994;84:4064–4077.

308. The Italian Cooperative Study Group on Chronic Myelogenous Leukemia. *N Engl J Med* 1994;330:820–825.
309. Saven A, et al. *Blood* 1992;79:111–1120.
310. Cassileth PA, et al. *J Clin Oncol* 1991;9:243–246.
311. Ratain MJ, et al. *Blood* 1985;65:644–648.
312. Gandara DR, et al. *J Clin Oncol* 2003;21:2004-2010.
313. Belani CP, et al. *J Clin Oncol* 2005;23:5883-5891.
314. Strauss GM, et al. *J Clin Oncol* 2004;621S (abstract 7019).
315. Winton T, et al. *N Engl J Med* 2005;352:2589–2597.
316. Sandler AB, et al. *N Engl J Med* 2006;355:2542–2560.
317. Belani CP, et al. *J Clin Oncol* 2008;26:468–473.
318. Manegold C, et al. *Proc Am Soc Clin Oncol* 2007;25:LBA7514.
319. Giaccone G, et al. *J Clin Oncol* 1998;16:2133–2141.
320. Fossella F, et al. *J Clin Oncol* 2003;21:3016–3024.
321. Belani CP, et al. *Clin Lung Cancer* 1999;1:144–150.
322. Georgoulias V, et al. *Lancet* 2001;357:1478–1484.
323. Abratt RP, et al. *J Clin Oncol* 1997;15:744–749.
324. Langer CJ, et al. *Semin Oncol* 1999;26 (Suppl 4):12–18.
325. Frasci G, et al. *J Clin Oncol* 2000;18:2529–2536.
326. Smith TJ, et al. *J Clin Oncol* 1995;13:2166–2173.
327. Pirker R, et al. *Proc Am Soc Clin Oncol* 2008;26 (abstract 3).
328. Cremonesi M, et al. *Oncology* 2003;64:97–101.
329. Scagliotti GV, et al. *J Clin Oncol* 2008;21:3543–3551.
330. Scagliotti GV. *Semin Oncol* 2005;32 (2 Suppl 2):S5–8.
331. Longeval E, et al. *Cancer* 1982;50:2751–2756.
332. Gandara D, et al. *J Clin Oncol* 2003;21:2004–2010.
333. Herbst RS, et al. *J Clin Oncol* 2007;25:4734–4750.
334. Patel JD, et al. *J Clin Oncol* 2009;27:3284-3289.
335. Pirker R, et al. *Lancet* 2009;373:1525-1531.
336. Belani CP, et al. *J Clin Oncol* 2009;27:18S (abstract CRA8000).
337. Lilenbaum RC, et al. *J Clin Oncol* 2005;23:190–196.
338. Tester WJ, et al. *Cancer* 1997;79:724–729.
339. Miller VA, et al. *Semin Oncol* 2000;27 (Suppl 3):3–10.
340. Hainsworth JD, et al. *Cancer* 2000;89:328–333.
341. Hanna N, et al. *J Clin Oncol* 2004;22:1589–1597.
342. Manegold C, et al. *Ann Oncol* 1997;8:525–529.
343. Furuse K, et al. *Ann Oncol* 1996;7:815–820.
344. Herbst RS. *Semin Oncol* 2003;30 (Suppl 1):30–38.
345. Shepherd FA, et al. *J Clin Oncol* 2004;22 (Suppl 1):14S (abstract 7022).
346. Socinski MA, et al. *J Clin Oncol* 2008;26:650–656.
347. Hanna N, et al. *J Clin Oncol* 2006;24:5253-5258.

348. Ihde DC, et al. *J Clin Oncol* 1994;12:2022–2034.
349. Viren M, et al. *Acta Oncol* 1994;33:921–924.
350. Noda K, et al. *N Engl J Med* 2002;346:85–91.
351. Eckardt JR, et al. *J Clin Oncol* 2006;24:2044–2051.
352. Hainsworth JD, et al. *J Clin Oncol* 1997;15:3464–3470.
353. Neubauer M, et al. *J Clin Oncol* 2004;22:1872-1877.
354. Roth BJ, et al. *J Clin Oncol* 1992;10:282–291.
355. Aisner J, et al. *Semin Oncol* 1986;(Suppl 3):54–62.
356. Johnson DH. *Semin Oncol* 1993;20:315–325.
357. Johnson DH, et al. *J Clin Oncol* 1990;8:1013–1017.
358. Hainsworth JD, et al. *Semin Oncol* 1999;26 (Suppl 2):60–66.
359. Ardizzoni A, et al. *J Clin Oncol* 1997;15:2090–2096.
360. Bonadonna G, et al. *Cancer* 1975;36:252–259.
361. DeVita VT Jr, et al. *Ann Intern Med* 1970;73:881–895.
362. Klimo P, et al. *J Clin Oncol* 1985;3:1174–1182.
363. Bartlett NL, et al. *J Clin Oncol* 1995;13:1080–1088.
364. Radford JA, et al. *J Clin Oncol* 1995;13:2379–2385.
365. Longo DL. *Semin Oncol* 1990;17:716–735.
366. Colwill R, et al. *J Clin Oncol* 1995;13:396–402.
367. Diehl V, et al. *J Clin Oncol* 1998;16:3810–3821.
368. Tesch H, et al. *Blood* 1998;15:4560–4567.
369. Bartlett NL, et al. *Ann Oncol* 2007;18:1071–1079.
370. Santoro A, et al. *J Clin Oncol* 2000;18:2615–2619.
371. Bagley CM Jr, et al. *Ann Intern Med* 1972;76:227–234.
372. Urba WJ, et al. *J Natl Cancer Ins Monogr* 1990;10:29-37.
373. Sonnevald P, et al. *J Clin Oncol* 1995;13:2530–2539.
374. McLaughlin P, et al. *J Clin Oncol* 1996;14:1262–1268.
375. Hochster H, et al. *Blood* 1994;84 (Suppl 1):383a.
376. Sacchi S, et al. *Cancer* 2007;110:121–128.
377. van Oers MHJ, et al. *Blood* 2006;108:3295–3301.
378. Forstpointer R, et al. *Blood* 2006;108:4033–4008.
379. Fisher RI, et al. *J Clin Oncol* 2006;24:4867–4874.
380. Klimo P, et al. *J Clin Oncol* 1985;3:1174-1182.
381. Coiffier B, et al. *N Engl J Med* 2002;346:235–242.
382. Pfreundschuh M, et al. *Lancet Oncol* 2008;9:105-116.
383. Vose JM, et al. *Leuk Lymphoma* 2002;43:799–804.
384. Wilson WH, et al. *J Clin Oncol* 1993;11:1573–1582.
385. Wilson WH. *Semin Oncol* 2000;27 (Suppl 12):30–36.
386. Klimo P, et al. *Ann Intern Med* 1985;102:596–602.
387. Shipp MA, et al. *Ann Intern Med* 1986;104:757–765.
388. Longo DL, et al. *J Clin Oncol* 1991;9:25–38.
389. Velasquez WS, et al. *J Clin Oncol* 1994;12:1169–1176.

390. Velasquez WS, et al. *Blood* 1988;71:117–122.
391. Moskowitz C, et al. *J Clin Oncol* 1999;17:3776–3785.
392. Kewairamani T, et al. *Blood* 2004;103;3684–3688.
393. Rodriguez MA, et al. *Ann Oncol* 1995;6: 609–611.
394. El Gnaoui T, et al. *Ann Oncol* 2007;18:1363–1368.
395. Magrath I, et al. *Blood* 1984;63:1102–1111.
396. Magrath I, et al. *J Clin Oncol* 1996;14:925.
397. Berstein JI, et al. *J Clin Oncol* 1986;4:847–858.
398. Thomas DA, et al. *Blood* 2004;104:1624-1630.
399. McLaughlin P, et al. *J Clin Oncol* 1998;16:2825–2833.
400. Ghielmini M, et al. *Blood* 2004;103:4416-4423.
401. Witzig TE, et al. *J Clin Oncol* 2002;20:2453–2463.
402. Falkson CI. *Am J Clin Oncol* 1996;19:268–270.
403. Betticher DC, et al. *J Clin Oncol* 1998;16:850–858.
404. Friedberg JW, et al. *J Clin Oncol* 2008;26:204–210.
405. Abrey LE, et al. *J Clin Oncol* 2002;18:3144–3150.
406. Shah GD, et al. *J Clin Oncol* 2007;25:4730-4735.
407. Batchelor T, et al. *J Clin Oncol* 2003;21:1044–1049.
408. Reni M, et al. *Br J Cancer* 2007;96:864–867.
409. Fischer L, et al. *Ann Oncol* 2006;17:1141–1145.
410. Kirkwood JM, et al. *J Clin Oncol* 1996;14:7–17.
411. Creagen ET, et al. *J Clin Oncol* 1999;17:1884–1890.
412. Falkson CI, et al. *J Clin Oncol* 1998;16:1743–1751.
413. Hwu WJ, et al. *J Clin Oncol* 2003;21:3351–3356.
414. Luce JK, et al. *Cancer Chemother Rep* 1970;54:119–124.
415. Pritchard KI, et al. *Cancer Treat Rep* 1980;64:1123–1126.
416. Kirkwood JM, et al. *Semin Oncol* 1997;24 (Suppl 4):1–48.
417. Atkins MB, et al. *J Clin Oncol* 1999;17:2105–2116.
418. Parkinson DR, et al. *J Clin Oncol* 1990;8:1650–1656.
419. Acquavella N, et al. *J Immunother* 2008;31:569–576.
420. Middleton MR, et al. *J Clin Oncol* 2000;18:158–166.
421. Ardizzoni A, et al. *Cancer* 1991;67:2984–2987.
422. Shin DM, et al. *Cancer* 1995;76:2230–2236.
423. Nowak AK, et al. *Br J Cancer* 2002;87:491–496.
424. Favaretto AG, et al. *Cancer* 2003;97:2791–2797.
425. Vogelzang NJ, et al. *J Clin Oncol* 2003;21:2636–2644.
426. Zucali PA, et al. *Cancer* 2008;112:1555–1561.
427. Simon GR, et al. *J Clin Oncol* 2008;21:3567–3572.
428. Jassem J, et al. *J Clin Oncol* 2008;26:1698-1704.
429. Steele JPC, et al. *J Clin Oncol* 2000;18:3912–3917.
430. Southwest Oncology Group Study. *Arch Intern Med* 1975;135:147–152.
431. Palumbo A, et al. *Lancet* 2006;367:835.

432. Facon T, et al. *Proc Am Soc Clin Oncol* 2006;24 (abstract 1).
433. Palumbo A, et al. *J Clin Oncol* 2007;25:4459–4465.
434. Barlogie B, et al. *N Engl J Med* 1984;310:1353–1356.
435. Rajkumar SV, et al. *J Clin Oncol* 2002;20:4319–4323.
436. Richardson PG, et al. *Blood* 2006;108:3458-3464.
437. Rajkumar SV, et al. *Proc Am Soc Clin Oncol* 2007;25:LBA8025.
438. Hussein MA, et al. *Cancer* 2002;95:2160-2168.
439. Orlowski RZ, et al. *Proc Am Soc Hematol* 2006 (abstract 404).
440. Berenson JR, et al. *J Clin Oncol* 2006;24:937–944.
441. San Miguel JF, et al. *N Engl J Med* 2008;359:906–917.
442. Palumbo A et al *Blood* 2007;109:2757-2762.
443. Alexanian R, et al. *Ann Intern Med* 1986;105:8–11.
444. Cunningham D, et al. *J Clin Oncol* 1994;12:764–768.
445. Singhal S, et al. *N Engl J Med* 1999;341:1565–1571.
446. Richardson PG, et al. *Blood* 2006;108:3458–3464.
447. Richardson P, et al. *N Engl J Med* 2003;348:2609–2617.
448. Silverman LR, et al. *J Clin Oncol* 2006;24:3895–3903.
449. Kantarjian H, et al. *Cancer* 2006;106:1794–1780.
450. Kantarjian H, et al. *Semin Hematology* 2005;32 (Suppl 2):S17–S22.
451. Galili N, et al. *Expert Opin Investig Drugs* 2006;15:805–813.
452. David M, et al. *Blood* 2007;109:61-64.
453. Goorin A, et al. *Med Pediatr Oncol* 1995;24:362-367.
454. Meyers PA, et al. *J Clin Oncol* 2005;23:2004-2011.
455. Swenerton K, et al. *J Clin Oncol* 1992;10:718–726.
456. Alberts D, et al. *J Clin Oncol* 1992;10:706–717.
457. McGuire WP, et al. *N Engl J Med* 1996;334:1–6.
458. Ozols RE. *Semin Oncol* 1995;22 (Suppl 15):1-6.
459. Pignata S, et al. *Crit Rev Oncol Hematol* 2008;66:229-236.
460. Markman M, et al. *J Clin Oncol* 2001;19:1901–1905.
461. Pignant S, et al. *J Clin Oncol* 2009;27:18S (LBA5509).
462. D'Agostino G, et al. *Br J Cancer* 2003;89:1180–1184.
463. Nagourney RA, et al. *Gynecol Oncol* 2003;88:35–39.
464. Thigpen T. *Semin Oncol* 2006;33 (Suppl 6):S26–32.
465. Armstrong DK, et al. *N Engl J Med* 2006;354:34–43.
466. Matulonis UA, et al. *J Clin Oncol* 2008;26:5761-5766.
467. Markman M. *Gynecol Oncol* 1998;69:226–229.
468. Rose PG, et al. *Gynecol Oncol* 2001;82:323-328.
469. McGuire WP, et al. *Ann Intern Med* 1989;111:273–279.
470. Kudelka AP, et al. *J Clin Oncol* 1996;14:1552–1557.
471. Lund B, et al. *J Natl Cancer Inst* 1994;86:1530–1533.
472. Ozols RF. *Drugs* 1999;58 (Suppl 3):43–49.
473. Sorensen P, et al. *Gynecol Oncol* 2001;81:58–62.

474. Miller DS, et al. *J Clin Oncol* 2009;27:2686-2691.

475. Burger RA, et al. *J Clin Oncol* 2007; 25:5165-5171.

476. Dimopoulos MA, et al. *Gynecol Oncol* 2004;95:695–700.

477. Neoptolemos J, et al. *J Clin Oncol* 2009;27:18S (abstract LBA4505).

478. Oettle H, et al. *JAMA* 2007;297:267–277.

479. Gastrointestinal Tumor Study Group. *Int J Radiat Oncol Biol Phys* 1979;5:1643–1647.

480. Regine WF, et al. *Proc Am Soc Clin Oncol* 2006;25 (abstract 4007).

481. Loehrer PJ, et al. *Proc Am Soc Clin Oncol* 2008;26 (abstract 4506).

482. DeCaprio JA, et al. *J Clin Oncol* 1991;9:2128–2133.

483. Hess V, et al. *J Clin Oncol* 2003;21:66–68.

484. Cunningham D, et al. *Proc. ECCO* 2005;13 (abstract 11).

485. Fine RL, et al. *Cancer Chemother Pharmacol* 2008;61:167–175.

486. Louvet C, et al. *J Clin Oncol* 2002;20:1512–1518.

487. Louvet C, et al. *Proc Am Soc Clin Oncol* 2007;25:18S (abstract 4592).

488. Moore MJ, et al. *J Clin Oncol* 2005;23:16S (abstract 1).

489. Kulke MH, et al. *J Clin Oncol* 2007;25:4787–4792.

490. Burris HA, et al. *J Clin Oncol* 1997;15:2403–2413.

491. Brand R, et al. *Invest New Drugs* 1997;15:331–341.

492. Cartwright TH, et al. *J Clin Oncol* 2002;20:160–164.

493. Eisenberger MA, et al. *Semin Oncol* 1994;21:613–619.

494. Jurincic CD, et al. *Semin Oncol* 1991;18 (Suppl 6):21–25.

495. Pienta KJ, et al. *J Clin Oncol* 1994;12:2005–2012.

496. Hudes GR, et al. *J Clin Oncol* 1992;11:1754–1761.

497. Hudes GR, et al. *J Clin Oncol* 1997;15:3156–3163.

498. Vaughn DJ, et al. *Cancer* 2004;100:746–750.

499. Tannock IF, et al. *J Clin Oncol* 1996;14:1756–1764.

500. Copur MS, et al. *Semin Oncol* 2001;28:16–21.

501. Petrylak DP, et al. *N Engl J Med* 2004;351:1513–1520.

502. Tannock IF, et al. *N Engl J Med* 2004;351:1502–1512.

503. Roth BJ, et al. *Cancer* 1993;72:2457–2260.

504. Ahmed S, et al. *Proc Am Soc Clin Oncol* 1998;17:325a.

505. Petrylak DP. *Semin Oncol* 2000;27 (Suppl 3):24–29.

506. Dreicer R. *Hematol Oncol Clin North Am* 2006;20:935–946.

507. Murphy GP, et al. *Urology* 1984;23:54–63.

508. Dijkman GA, et al. *Eur Urol* 1995;27:43–46.

509. Hanks GE, et al. *J Clin Oncol* 2003;21:3972–3978.

510. Klotz L, et al. *BJU Int* 2008;10:1531-1538.

511. The Leuprolide Study Group. *N Engl J Med* 1984;311:1281–1286.

512. Sharifi R, et al. *Clin Ther* 1996;18:647–657.

513. *Please see package insert for Lupron Depot-4 month 30 mg and go to http://rx.lupron.com/landing/prostate/ (accessed Sept. 2008).*

514. Schellhammer PF, et al. *Urology* 1997;50:330-336.
515. McLeod DG, et al. *Cancer* 1993;72:3870–3873.
516. Janknegt RA, et al. *J Urol* 1993;149:77–82.
517. Tannock IF, et al. *J Clin Oncol* 1989;7:590-597.
518. Fossa SD, et al. *J Clin Oncol* 2001;19:62-71.
519. Johnson DE, et al. *Urology* 1988;31:132–134.
520. Havlin KA, et al. *Cancer Treat Res* 1988;39:83–96.
521. Escudier B, et al. *Lancet* 2007;370:2103-2111.
522. Atzpodien J, et al. *Semin Oncol* 1993;20 (Suppl 9):22.
523. Yang JC, et al. *N Engl J Med* 2003;349:427–434.
524. Motzer RJ, et al. *J Clin Oncol* 2006;24:16–24.
525. Ratain MJ, et al. *J Clin Oncol* 2006;24:2505–2512.
526. Hudes G, et al. *N Engl J Med* 2007;356:2271–2281.
527. Motzer RJ, et al. *Lancet* 2008;372:449-456.
528. Fyfe G, et al. *J Clin Oncol* 1995;13:688–696.
529. Minasian LM, et al. *J Clin Oncol* 1993;11:1368–1375.
530. Antman K, et al. *J Clin Oncol* 1993;11:1276–1285.
531. Worden FP, et al. *J Clin Oncol* 2005;23:105–112.
532. Elias A, et al. *J Clin Oncol* 1989;7:1208–1216.
533. Santoro A, et al. *J Clin Oncol* 1995;13:1537–1545.
534. Maki RG, et al. *J Clin Oncol* 2007;25:2755–2763.
535. Dileo P, et al. *Cancer* 2007;109:1863–1869.
536. Holcombe E, et al. *N Engl J Med* 2003;348:694–701.
537. Van Oosterom AT, et al. *Eur J Cancer* 2002;38:2397-2406.
538. Judson I, et al. *Eur J Cancer* 2001;37:870-877.
539. Einhorn LH, et al. *J Clin Oncol* 1989;7:387–391.
540. Oliver RT, et al. *Lancet* 2005;366:293-300.
541. Williams SD, et al. *N Engl J Med* 1987;316:1435–1440.
542. Bosl G, et al. *J Clin Oncol* 1988;6:1231–1238.
543. Einhorn LH, et al. *Ann Intern Med* 1977;87:293–298.
544. Vugrin D, et al. *Ann Intern Med* 1981;95:59–61.
545. Loehrer PJ, et al. *Ann Intern Med* 1988;109:540–546.
546. Kondagunat GV, et al. *J Clin Oncol* 2005;23:6549–6555.
547. Einhorn LH, et al. *J Clin Oncol* 2007;25:513–516.
548. Loehrer PJ, et al. *J Clin Oncol* 1994;12:1164–1168.
549. Giaccone G, et al. *J Clin Oncol* 1996;14:814–820.
550. Fornasiero A, et al. *Cancer* 1991;68:30–33.
551. Loehrer PJ, et al. *Cancer* 2001;91:2010–2015.
552. Shimaoka K, et al. *Cancer* 1985;56:2155–2160.
553. Gupta-Abramson V, et al. *J Clin Oncol* 2008;26:2010–2015.

5

Antiemetic Agents for the Treatment of Chemotherapy-Induced Nausea and Vomiting

Hari Deshpande, M. Sitki Copur, Laurie J. Harrold,
Edward Chu, and Arthur L. Levy

This chapter presents an overview of the common antiemetic agents as well as selected regimens for the treatment of chemotherapy-induced nausea and vomiting. The specific agents are organized alphabetically, and the various regimens selected are used in clinical practice in the medical oncology community. It should be emphasized that not all of the drugs and dosages in the regimens have been officially approved by the Food and Drug Administration (FDA). This chapter should serve as a quick reference for physicians and healthcare professionals, and it provides several options for treating both acute and delayed nausea and vomiting. It is not intended to be an all-inclusive review of antiemetic agents and treatment regimens, nor is it intended to endorse and/or prioritize any particular drug or regimen.

A

Aprepitant

Trade Name

Emend

Classification

Substance P/NK1 receptor antagonist

Category

Antiemetic agent

Drug Manufacturer

Merck

Mechanism of Action

- Selective high-affinity antagonist of substance P/neurokinin 1 (NK1) receptors.
- Inhibits the acute and delayed phases of chemotherapy-induced emesis.
- Little to no affinity for 5-HT3, dopamine, or corticosteroid receptors.

Absorption

Well absorbed by the gastrointestinal (GI) tract, and oral bioavailability is on the order of 60%–65%. Peak plasma levels reached in 4 hours. Ingestion of food does not alter the extent of absorption.

Distribution

Crosses the blood-brain barrier and enters the central nervous system (CNS). Greater than 95% of drug is bound to plasma proteins.

Metabolism

Undergoes extensive metabolism in the liver, principally by the CYP3A4 liver microsomal system. The main route of elimination of parent drug is via liver metabolism. The parent drug and its metabolites are not renally excreted. The elimination half-life ranges from 9–13 hours.

Indications

1. Prevention of acute and delayed nausea and vomiting associated with highly emetogenic cancer chemotherapy, including high-dose cisplatin.

2. Prevention of nausea and vomiting associated with moderately emetogenic cancer chemotherapy.

3. Prevention of postoperative nausea and vomiting (PONV).

Dosage Range

1. Oral: Recommended dose is 125 mg PO given 1 hour before chemotherapy and 80 mg PO on days 2 and 3 after chemotherapy.

2. Intravenous: Recommended dose is 115 mg IV 30 minutes before chemotherapy on day 1 only.

3. PONV: 40 mg PO within 3 hours prior to induction of anesthesia.

Special Considerations

1. Use with caution in patients on chronic warfarin anticoagulation. Coagulation parameters, PT/INR, should be closely monitored in the 2-week period, especially at days 7 and 10, following aprepitant therapy.

2. Patients should be advised to report to their physician the use of any non-prescription or herbal medications, as significant drug interactions can occur with aprepitant and other drugs.

3. Well tolerated in patients with mild to moderate liver dysfunction. Caution should be exercised in patients with severe hepatic insufficiency (Child-Pugh score >9).

4. No dose adjustment is required for patients with renal insufficiency and/or those undergoing hemodialysis.

5. Pregnancy category B. Breast-feeding should be avoided.

Toxicity 1

Fatigue is most common side effect. CNS effects include headache and insomnia.

Toxicity 2

GI side effects include constipation and/or diarrhea.

Toxicity 3

Hiccups observed in 10% of patients.

Toxicity 4

Anorexia.

Dexamethasone

Trade Name

Decadron

Classification

Glucocorticoid steroid

Category

Antiemetic agent

Drug Manufacturer

Merck

Mechanism of Action

- Precise mechanism of action in preventing and/or treating chemotherapy-induced nausea and vomiting is not known.
- Suppresses prostaglandin release from hypothalamus, which may then inhibit the subsequent process of nausea and vomiting.
- Possesses anti-inflammatory and immunosuppressive effects with minimal mineralocorticoid properties.

Absorption

Well absorbed by the GI tract, and oral bioavailability is on the order of 60%–70%. Peak plasma levels are observed in 1–2 hours after doses of 0.5–3.0 mg and are independent of the route of administration.

Distribution

Dexamethasone binds corticosteroid-binding globulin and corticosteroid-binding albumin to significantly less extent than does hydrocortisone.

Metabolism

Metabolism occurs primarily in the liver, and about 20% of the drug is conjugated via glucuronidation. The main route of elimination is through renal excretion with biliary excretion playing a minor role. The elimination half-life is 3–4 hours.

Indications

Treatment of nausea and vomiting associated with cancer chemotherapy in combination with other antiemetics, including serotonin (5-HT3) receptor antagonists, metoclopramide, and lorazepam.

Dosage Range

1. The optimal dose of dexamethasone for the prevention and/or treatment of cancer chemotherapy-induced nausea and vomiting has not been established.

2. Oral: Recommended dose is 4 mg PO every 4–6 hours for four doses with first dose given 1–6 hours before chemotherapy.

3. Intravenous (IV): Recommended dose is 10–20 mg IV before chemotherapy and then 10–20 mg IV every 4–6 hours.

Special Considerations

1. Contraindicated in patients with an underlying psychiatric disorder, including psychosis and depression.

2. Efficacy of dexamethasone may be decreased when used in the presence of drugs that induce the liver microsomal P450 system, including phenytoin, phenobarbital, and carbamazepine. In this setting, the dose of drug may need to be increased.

3. Use with caution in patients with liver impairment and/or hypothyroidism as increased drug effects may be observed.

4. Patients should be cautioned about possible neuropsychiatric side effects, including mood changes, euphoria, depression, insomnia, and in extreme cases, psychosis.

Toxicity 1

Electrolyte abnormalities with hypokalemia and hyperglycemia.

Toxicity 2

Fluid retention, leg edema, hypertension, and rarely, exacerbation of congestive heart failure (CHF).

Toxicity 3

Neuropsychiatric effects, including mood changes, euphoria, headache, insomnia, depression, and psychosis.

Toxicity 4

Increased white blood count (WBC) secondary to demargination.

Diphenhydramine

Name

Benadryl

Classification

Antihistamine

Category

Antiemetic agent

Drug Manufacturer

Parke-Davis

Mechanism of Action

- Antihistamine with anticholinergic and sedative effects. Competes with histamine for receptor sites on effector cells.
- Blocks the chemoreceptor trigger zone and decreases vestibular stimulation.

Absorption

Well absorbed by the GI tract, and oral bioavailability is on the order of 40%–60%. Peak plasma levels reached in 1–4 hours.

Distribution

Widely distributed throughout the body, including the CNS. Crosses the placenta and is excreted in breast milk. About 80%–85% of drug is bound to plasma proteins.

Metabolism

Metabolism occurs in the liver, principally to diphenylmetoxyacetic, which may then undergo conjugation. The main route of elimination of parent drug and its metabolites is through renal excretion. The elimination half-life ranges from 2.5–9 hours.

Indications

1. Prevention of nausea and vomiting associated with cancer chemotherapy in combination with other antiemetics, including 5-HT3 receptor antagonists, metoclopramide, and lorazepam.
2. Active treatment of motion sickness.
3. Prevention and/or treatment of allergic, hypersensitivity reactions.
4. Temporary relief of cough caused by minor irritation of upper airways.
5. Treatment of Parkinsonism.

Dosage Range

1. Oral: Recommended dose is 25–50 mg PO before chemotherapy and then every 4–6 hours thereafter.
2. IV: Recommended dose is 25–50 mg IV before chemotherapy.

Special Considerations

1. Use with caution in patients with a history of increased intraocular pressure, narrow-angle glaucoma, bladder-neck obstruction, bronchial asthma, cardiovascular disease, and/or hypertension.
2. Use with caution in elderly patients as they are more likely to exhibit altered sensorium with drowsiness and confusion.
3. Patients should be advised against performing activities that require mental alertness, including operating heavy machinery and driving.
4. Useful to treat and/or prevent extrapyramidal side effects related to antiemetic therapy.
5. Pregnancy category B. Breast-feeding should be avoided.

Toxicity 1

CNS effects are most commonly observed with sedation, drowsiness, dizziness, and confusion. Alterations in coordination, irritability, and insomnia.

Toxicity 2

Dryness of mucous membranes, including mouth, nose, and throat.

Toxicity 3

Hypotension, palpitations, and tachycardia.

Toxicity 4

Anorexia.

Dolasetron

Trade Name
Anzemet

Classification
5-HT3 receptor antagonist

Category
Antiemetic agent

Drug Manufacturer
Aventis

Mechanism of Action
- Competitive, highly selective antagonist of type 3, 5-HT3 receptors.
- 5-HT3 receptors are present centrally, in the chemoreceptor trigger zone of the area postrema of brain, and peripherally, on vagal nerve terminals. Antiemetic action of dolasetron may be mediated centrally, peripherally, or at both sites.
- Does not have direct dopamine-receptor antagonist activity.
- Effective in acute nausea and vomiting but plays only a limited role in delayed emesis.

Absorption
Well absorbed by the GI tract. Oral bioavailability is approximately 75%. Food does not affect oral absorption.

Distribution
Widely distributed in the body. Approximately 70%–80% of drug is bound to plasma proteins.

Metabolism
Parent drug is rarely detected in plasma due to rapid and complete metabolism to hydrodolasetron, which is further metabolized by the liver

P450 microsomal system. Main routes of metabolism include hydroxylation and glucuronidation. Hydrodolasetron is eliminated by both renal and hepatic excretion, with about 60% of an administered dose recovered in the urine and 30% in the feces. The mean elimination half-life in adult cancer patients is approximately 8 hours.

Indications

1. Prevention of nausea and vomiting associated with initial and repeat courses of moderately emetogenic cancer chemotherapy.

2. Prevention of postoperative nausea and vomiting.

Dosage Range

1. Oral: Recommended dose is 100 mg PO once daily given 1 hour before chemotherapy.

2. Prevention of postoperative nausea and vomiting: 100 mg PO within 2 hours before surgery.

3. IV: Recommended dose is 1.8 mg/kg IV as a single dose administered 30 minutes before chemotherapy. As an alternative, a fixed dose of 100 mg IV can be administered 30 minutes before chemotherapy.

Special Considerations

1. No dose adjustment is required in elderly patients or in those with hepatic and/or renal impairment.

2. Use with caution in patients who have or may develop cardiac conduction abnormalities, including those with prolonged PR and QT intervals. Baseline electrocardiograms should be performed before administration of dolasetron and chemotherapy.

3. Use with caution in patients who are receiving antiarrhythmic agents or other drugs that can prolong the PR, QRS, and QT intervals.

4. Careful monitoring of electrolytes, including potassium and magnesium, is required to reduce the occurrence of arrhythmias.

5. Pregnancy category B. Breast-feeding should be avoided.

Toxicity 1

Headache is most common side effect (18%–25%).

Toxicity 2

Diarrhea and/or abdominal pain.

Toxicity 3

Fever, fatigue, and dizziness.

Toxicity 4

Hypotension, chest pain, orthostatic hypotension, syncope, bradycardia and Mobitz I atrioventricular (AV) block, and atrial arrhythmias, including atrial flutter and atrial fibrillation.

Toxicity 5

Agitation, sleep disorder, confusion, depersonalization, anxiety, and abnormal dreams.

Toxicity 6

Transient elevations in liver function tests (LFTs). Usually clinically asymptomatic.

Toxicity 7

Hypersensitivity reactions with dyspnea, skin rash, urticaria, bronchospasm, and hypotension have been reported in rare instances.

Dronabinol

Name

Marinol

Classification

Cannabinoid

Category

Antiemetic agent

Drug Manufacturer

Roxane and Unimed

Mechanism of Action

- Precise mechanism of action in preventing and/or treating cancer chemotherapy-induced nausea and vomiting is not known.
- Complex effects on the CNS with central sympathomimetic activity.
- Binding to cannabinoid receptors in CNS may contribute to its antiemetic effect.
- Inhibition of vomiting control mechanism in the medulla oblongata.

Absorption

Nearly completely absorbed (90%–95%) by the GI tract. Onset of action occurs within 0.5–1 hour after ingestion. Peak plasma levels are observed in 2–4 hours with 3–6 hours duration of action.

Distribution

Because of extensive first-pass metabolism in the liver, only 10% of an administered dose reaches the systemic circulation. Highly bound to plasma proteins (97%).

Metabolism

Undergoes extensive first-pass metabolism in the liver microsomal system. Both active and inactive metabolites are formed. The main active metabolite is 11-hydroxy-delta tetrahydrocannabinol (THC). Dronabinol and the 11-hydroxy metabolite are present in nearly equal concentrations in plasma. The main route of elimination is via biliary excretion. The elimination half-life of the parent drug is 25–36 hours, while that of the 11-hydroxy metabolite is 15–18 hours.

Indications

1. Treatment of nausea and vomiting associated with cancer chemotherapy in patients who have failed to respond to conventional antiemetic agents.

2. Stimulates appetite and prevents weight loss in patients with AIDS.

Dosage Range

Recommended dose is 5–15 mg/m^2 PO 1–3 hours before chemotherapy and then every 4–6 hours PO thereafter.

Special Considerations

1. Use with caution in elderly patients due to an increased risk of neuropsychoactive effects.

2. Use with caution in patients with a history of alcohol and/or substance abuse.

3. Prescriptions should be limited to only one course of chemotherapy.

4. Use with caution in patients with underlying psychiatric disorders, including mania, depression, or schizophrenia.

5. Patients should be cautioned about possible neuropsychiatric side effects, including mood changes, euphoria, depression, insomnia, and, in extreme cases, psychosis.

6. Pregnancy category C.

Toxicity 1

Mood changes, drowsiness, confusion, and dizziness. Impairment in perception, coordination, and sensory function. Visual distortions, nightmares, hallucinations, and depersonalization are also observed.

Toxicity 2

Orthostatic hypotension, tachycardia, facial flush, conjunctival injection, and palpitations.

Toxicity 3

Dry mouth, abdominal pain, and diarrhea occur in less than 10% of patients.

Granisetron

Trade Name

Kytril

Classification

5-HT3 receptor antagonist

Category

Antiemetic agent

Drug Manufacturer

Roche

Mechanism of Action

- Highly selective antagonist of type 3, 5-HT receptors.
- 5-HT3 receptors are present centrally, in the chemoreceptor trigger zone of the area postrema of brain, and peripherally, on vagal nerve terminals. Antiemetic action of granisetron may be mediated centrally, peripherally, or at both sites.
- Does not have direct dopamine-receptor antagonist activity.
- Effective in preventing acute chemotherapy-induced nausea and vomiting.

Absorption

Well absorbed by the GI tract. Bioavailability is 60%. Absorption is decreased in the presence of food (AUC decreased by 5%; Cmax increased by 30%).

Distribution

Distributes freely between plasma and red blood cells. Approximately 65% of drug is bound by plasma proteins.

Metabolism

Undergoes extensive metabolism in the liver by the cytochrome P450 microsomal system. Main routes of metabolism include N-demethylation and oxidation followed by conjugation. Some of the metabolites may have 5-HT3 antagonist activity. About 11% of an administered dose is recovered as the parent compound in the urine. The mean elimination half-life in adult cancer patients ranges from 2.9 to 6.2 hours.

Indications

1. Prevention of nausea and vomiting associated with initial and repeat courses of emetogenic cancer chemotherapy, including high-dose cisplatin.

2. Prevention of nausea and vomiting associated with radiation, including total body irradiation and fractionated abdominal radiation (oral solution and tablets only).

3. Prevention of postoperative nausea and vomiting (PONV) (injection only).

Dosage Range

1. Oral: Recommended dose is 2 mg PO once daily given 1 hour before chemotherapy. An alternative regimen is 1 mg PO bid with the first 1 mg dose given 1 hour before chemotherapy and the second dose given 12 hours after the first dose.

2. For the prevention of radiotherapy-induced nausea and vomiting: 2 mg PO once daily (oral) to be taken within 1 hour of radiation therapy.

3. IV: Recommended dose is 10 µg/kg IV administered 30 minutes before chemotherapy, only on days of chemotherapy.

4. IV: Recommended dose for prevention of PONV is 1 mg IV, administered before induction of anesthesia or immediately before reversal of anesthesia.

Special Considerations

1. No dose adjustment is required in elderly patients or in those with hepatic and/or renal impairment.

2. There appears to be little difference in clinical efficacy between oral dosing of 1 mg bid or a single daily dose of 2 mg.

3. Granisetron is especially effective when combined with dexamethasone in treating cisplatin-associated nausea and vomiting.

4. Granisetron does not induce or inhibit the liver microsomal P450 system.

5. Granisetron can be administered by IV in pediatric patients ages 2–16.

6. Pregnancy category B. It is not known whether granisetron is excreted in human milk. Caution should be exercised when granisetron is administered to a nursing woman.

Toxicity 1

Headache is the most common side effect (15%–20%).

Toxicity 2

Constipation, diarrhea, and/or abdominal pain.

Toxicity 3

Asthenia.

Toxicity 4

Transient elevations in LFTs. Usually clinically asymptomatic.

Toxicity 5

Hypersensitivity reactions with dyspnea, skin rash, urticaria, bronchospasm, and hypotension have been reported in rare instances.

Lorazepam

Name
Ativan

Classification
Benzodiazepine

Category
Antiemetic agent

Drug Manufacturer
Elkins-Sinn and Watson

Mechanism of Action

- Interacts with the γ-aminobutyric acid (GABA)-benzodiazepine receptor complex, which is widely expressed in the brain.
- Exhibits relatively high affinity for GABA recognition site and enhances the binding affinity of GABA for its receptor site on the same receptor complex.
- Intensity of action, including antianxiety effects, sedation, and reduction of seizure activity, appears to be directly related to the occupancy status of the receptor.

Absorption

Well absorbed by the GI tract with an oral bioavailability of nearly 90%. Peak concentrations in plasma occur approximately 2 hours following oral or intramuscular (IM) administration. Absorption after IM injection is rapid and complete.

Distribution

Widely distributed in body tissues and crosses the blood-brain barrier. Lorazepam and its metabolites cross the placenta and are distributed into milk. Approximately 90% of parent drug and its metabolites are bound to plasma proteins.

Metabolism

Undergoes extensive conjugation in the liver to the glucuronide metabolite, which is then excreted mainly into the urine. The mean half-lives of unconjugated lorazepam and its major metabolite, lorazepam glucuronide, are 12 and 18 hours, respectively.

Indications

1. Management of nausea and vomiting associated with emetogenic cancer chemotherapy either alone or in combination with other drugs, such as 5-HT3 receptor antagonists and/or corticosteroids.
2. Management of anxiety disorders and acute relief of symptoms of anxiety and/or anxiety associated with depressive symptoms.
3. Management of preoperative anxiety.
4. Management of status epilepticus.

Dosage Range

1. Dosage of lorazepam must be individualized, and the smallest effective dose should be used, especially in those with low serum albumin.
2. Recommended oral dose as an antiemetic agent is 2.5 mg of lorazepam PO on the evening before and just after initiation of chemotherapy.
3. Recommended IV dose is 1.5 mg/m^2 (maximum, 3 mg) IV administered 45 minutes before the initiation of chemotherapy.

Special Considerations

1. Contraindicated in patients with known hypersensitivity to benzodiazapines or any ingredients in the formulation.
2. Contraindicated in patients with acute angle-closure glaucoma.
3. Use with caution in geriatric patients, debilitated patients, and patients with underlying pulmonary disease.
4. Use with caution in patients with liver impairment.
5. Patients should be warned about the possibility of impaired ability to perform activities that require mental alertness or physical coordination, including operating machinery and driving.
6. Pregnancy category D.

Toxicity 1

Sedation, depression, headache, sleep disturbance, dizziness, weakness, and unsteadiness are most commonly observed.

Toxicity 2

Changes in appetite, nausea, and GI symptoms may occur infrequently.

Toxicity 3

Reduction in blood pressure without clinical significance.

Toxicity 4

Transient amnesia or memory impairment.

Metoclopramide

$$Cl \diagdown \underset{H_2N \diagup \qquad \diagdown OCH_3}{\bigcirc}^{CONHCH_2CH_2N(C_2H_5)_2}$$

Trade Name
Reglan

Classification
Substituted benzamide

Category
Antiemetic agent

Drug Manufacturer
Baxter and Geneva

Mechanism of Action
- Precise mechanism of antiemetic action is unclear.
- Acts centrally by directly blocking the dopamine receptors in the chemoreceptor trigger zone of the area postrema of brain.
- Acts peripherally to enhance the action of acetylcholine at muscarinic synapses.
- Stimulates GI motility through increasing gastric emptying via cholinergic excitatory processes.
- Inhibits 5-HT3 receptors at high doses.

Absorption
Rapidly and completely absorbed by the GI tract. Peak plasma levels occur 1–2 hours after an oral dose.

Distribution
Extensively distributed to body tissues and crosses the blood-brain barrier. Distributes into the placenta and found in breast milk. Approximately 30% of drug is bound by plasma proteins.

Metabolism
Precise metabolism of drug has not been clearly established. Main routes of metabolism involve conjugation with glucuronic acid and sulfuric acid. Primary route of elimination is through the kidneys. About 85% of an administered dose is recovered as the parent compound and metabolites in the urine. Only 5% is eliminated via biliary excretion. The mean elimination half-life in adult cancer patients is approximately 5–6 hours.

Indications

1. Prevention and/or treatment of nausea and vomiting associated with cancer chemotherapy.
2. Prevention of postoperative nausea and vomiting.
3. Treatment of GI motility disorders, diabetic gastroparesis, and/or gastroesophageal reflux.

Dosage Range

1. Oral: Recommended dose is 20–40 mg PO every 4–6 hours as needed.
2. IV: Recommended dose is 1–2 mg/kg IV administered 30 minutes before chemotherapy and repeated every 4–6 hours as needed.

Special Considerations

1. Contraindicated in patients with pheochromocytoma as it may induce a hypertensive crisis.
2. Contraindicated in patients with seizure disorders because the frequency and severity of seizures may be increased.
3. Use with caution in patients with renal impairment. Dose adjustment is required in patients with decreased renal function.
4. Use with caution in patients with Parkinson's disease as symptoms may be worsened with metoclopramide.
5. Extrapyramidal symptoms typically occur within 24–48 hours of metoclopramide treatment. Most commonly seen with high-dose therapy and in pediatric patients and young adults. Diphenhydramine 50 mg IV or IM can provide immediate relief.
6. Use with caution in patients with a history of mental depression and/or suicidal tendencies as exacerbation or worsening of underlying depression may occur.
7. Pregnancy category B. Breast-feeding should be avoided.

Toxicity 1

Headache, fatigue, drowsiness, restlessness, and insomnia are the most common side effects (10%–15%).

Toxicity 2

Diarrhea and/or abdominal pain.

Toxicity 3

Dry mouth.

Toxicity 4

Hypersensitivity reactions with dyspnea, skin rash, urticaria, bronchospasm, and hypotension.

Toxicity 5

Extrapyramidal reactions with motor restlessness, tremor, akasthesia, dystonia, and tardive dyskinesia.

Nabilone

N

Name

Cesamet

Classification

Cannabinoid

Category

Antiemetic agent

Drug Manufacturer

Valeant Pharmaceuticals

Mechanism of Action

- Precise mechanism of action in preventing and/or treating cancer chemotherapy-induced nausea and vomiting is not known.
- Complex effects on the CNS with central sympathomimetic activity.
- Binding to cannabinoid receptors in CNS may contribute to its antiemetic effect.

Absorption

Nearly completely absorbed by the GI tract. Peak plasma levels are observed within 2 hours of ingestion. Food does not affect the rate or extent of absorption.

Distribution

Highly bound to plasma proteins (97%).

Metabolism

Undergoes extensive metabolism in the liver microsomal system. Precise information relating to the relative activities of the metabolites and parent drug has not been established. The main route of elimination is via biliary excretion, with approximately 60% of nabilone and its metabolites being recovered in stool and approximately 24% being recovered in urine. The elimination half-life of the parent drug is 2 hours, whereas that of the metabolites is up to 35 hours.

Indications

1. Treatment of nausea and vomiting associated with cancer chemotherapy in patients who have failed to respond to conventional antiemetic agents.
2. Should not be used as the initial antiemetic agent for a patient.

Dosage Range

Recommended dose is 1–2 mg PO given daily 1–3 hours before chemotherapy. The maximal daily dose is 6 mg given in divided doses 2 to 3 times a day during the entire course of chemotherapy.

Special Considerations

1. Use with caution in older patients and in those with hypertension or heart disease, as there is an increased risk of postural hypotension.

2. Use with caution in patients with a history of alcohol and/or substance abuse.

3. Use with caution in patients with underlying hepatic and/or renal dysfunction, as the safety aspects of this agent have not been investigated in these patient populations.

4. Use with caution in patients with underlying psychiatric disorders, including mania, depression, or schizophrenia.

5. Patients should be cautioned about possible neuropsychiatric side effects, including mood changes, euphoria, depression, insomnia, and in extreme cases, psychosis.

6. Patients should be warned not to drive, operate machinery, or engage in any type of hazardous activity while on treatment.

7. Pregnancy category C.

Toxicity 1

Mood changes, drowsiness, confusion, and vertigo. Impairment in perception, coordination, and sensory function. Visual distortions, nightmares, hallucinations, and depersonalization are also observed.

Toxicity 2

Orthostatic hypotension, tachycardia, facial flush, and palpitations.

Toxicity 3

Dry mouth, anorexia, and nausea/vomiting.

Ondansetron

Name
Zofran

Classification
5-HT3 receptor antagonist

Category
Antiemetic agent

Drug Manufacturer
GlaxoSmithKline

Mechanism of Action
- Competitive, highly selective antagonist of type 3, 5-HT3 receptors.
- 5-HT3 receptors are present centrally, in the chemoreceptor trigger zone of the area postrema of brain, and peripherally, on vagal nerve terminals. Antiemetic action of ondansetron may be mediated centrally, peripherally, or at both sites.
- Does not have direct dopamine-receptor antagonist activity.
- Effective in acute nausea and vomiting but plays only a limited role in delayed emesis.

Absorption
Well absorbed by the GI tract. Mean bioavailability in healthy subjects from 48% to 75%.

Distribution
Nearly 40% of circulating drug is distributed in red blood cells.

Metabolism
Undergoes extensive metabolism in the liver by the cytochrome P450 microsomal system. The main metabolic pathway is hydroxylation followed by glucuronide or sulfate conjugation. Less than 5% of an administered dose is recovered as the parent compound in the urine. The mean elimination half-life in adult cancer patients is 4 hours.

Indications

1. Treatment of nausea and vomiting associated with moderately or highly emetogenic cancer chemotherapy.
2. Prevention and/or management of postoperative nausea and vomiting.
3. Prevention of nausea and vomiting associated with radiotherapy in patients receiving total body irradiation or single high-dose fraction or daily fractions to the abdomen.

Dosage Range

1. Oral: Recommended dose is 8 mg PO bid with the first dose given 30 minutes before chemotherapy. Continue for 1–2 days after chemotherapy is completed.
2. For the prevention of radiotherapy-induced nausea and vomiting, 8 mg PO to be taken 1–2 hours before radiotherapy and then 8 mg PO every 8 hours post radiotherapy.
3. IV: Recommended dose is a single 32 mg IV dose administered 30 minutes before chemotherapy or 0.15 mg/kg IV every 4 hours for three doses given 30 minutes before chemotherapy.

Special Considerations

1. Use with caution in patients with severe hepatic impairment as the clearance of ondansetron is decreased, resulting in an increased plasma half-life. Dose modification is warranted in such patients, and the total daily dose should not exceed 8 mg.
2. Ondansetron may, on rare occasions, cause hypersensitivity reactions. Patients should be warned of this possibility and be advised to contact their physician at the first sign of a skin rash or any other sign of hypersensitivity.
3. Use with caution in elderly patients, especially patients older than 75 years of age, as the plasma clearance may be decreased, resulting in increased drug levels.
4. Patients with phenylketonuria should be informed that oral tablets of ondansetron contain aspartame, which is metabolized in the GI tract to phenylalanine.
5. Pregnancy category B. Breast-feeding should be avoided.

Toxicity 1

Fever, headache, malaise, and fatigue occur in 10% of patients.

Toxicity 2

Constipation, diarrhea, and/or abdominal pain.

Toxicity 3

Transient elevations in LFTs. Usually clinically asymptomatic.

Toxicity 4

Local reaction at site of injection with pain, redness, and burning.

Toxicity 5

Hypersensitivity reactions with dyspnea, skin rash, urticaria, bronchospasm, and hypotension have been reported in rare instances.

Palonosetron

·HCl

Trade Name
Aloxi

Classification
5-HT3 receptor antagonist

Category
Antiemetic agent

Drug Manufacturer
MGI Pharma

Mechanism of Action
- Competitive, highly selective antagonist of type 3, 5-HT3 receptors.
- 5-HT3 receptors are present centrally, in the chemoreceptor trigger zone of the area postrema of brain, and peripherally, on vagal nerve terminals. Antiemetic action of palonosetron may be mediated centrally, peripherally, or at both sites.
- Does not have direct dopamine-receptor antagonist activity.
- Effective in both acute and delayed nausea and vomiting.

Absorption
Not available for oral use and is administered only via the parenteral route.

Distribution
Nearly 60% of circulating drug is bound to plasma proteins.

Metabolism
Undergoes metabolism by multiple routes with about 50% of parent drug metabolized to two main metabolites, N-oxide-palonosetron and 6-S-hydroxy-palonosetron. Each of these metabolites has less than 1% of the 5-HT3 receptor antagonist activity of the parent compound. In vitro studies show that CYP2D6 is the main liver microsomal enzyme involved in palonosetron

metabolism. The mean elimination half-life in adult cancer patients is 40 hours.

Indications

1. Prevention of acute nausea and vomiting associated with initial and repeat courses of moderately or highly emetogenic cancer chemotherapy.
2. Prevention of delayed nausea and vomiting associated with initial and repeat courses of moderately emetogenic cancer chemotherapy.

Dosage Range

IV: Recommended dose is a single 0.25 mg IV dose administered 30 minutes before chemotherapy. Repeat dosing of drug within a 7 day interval is not recommended as the safety and efficacy of consecutive and/or alternate dosing in patients has not been evaluated.

Special Considerations

1. Use with caution in patients who have or may develop prolongation of cardiac conduction intervals, especially QTc. These include patients with hypokalemia or hypomagnesemia, patients taking diuretics with potential for inducing electrolyte abnormalities, patients with QT syndrome, patients taking antiarrhythmic drugs or other drugs that lead to QT prolongation, and cumulative high dose anthracycline therapy.
2. Palonosetron may cause hypersensitivity reactions as have been observed with other 5-HT3 receptor antagonists. Patients should be warned of this possibility and be advised to contact their physician at the first sign of a skin rash or any other sign of hypersensitivity.
3. Dose reduction is not required in patients with impaired liver and/or renal dysfunction.
4. Pregnancy category B. Breast-feeding should be avoided.

Toxicity 1

Headache occurs in 10% of patients.

Toxicity 2

Constipation, diarrhea, and/or abdominal pain.

Toxicity 3

Transient elevations in LFTs. Usually clinically asymptomatic.

Toxicity 4

Somnolence, dizziness, insomnia, and fatigue. Anxiety and euphoria have also been observed.

Toxicity 5

Hypersensitivity reactions have been reported in rare instances.

Prochlorperazine

Trade Name
Compazine

Classification
Phenothiazine

Category
Antiemetic agent

Drug Manufacturer
GlaxoSmithKline

Mechanism of Action
- Precise mechanism of antiemetic action is unclear.
- Blocks dopamine receptors in the chemoreceptor trigger zone.
- Inhibits vagal stimulation of the vomiting center by peripheral afferents.

Absorption
Following oral administration of tablet form, onset of action is 30–40 minutes with 3–4 hours duration of action. Oral extended-release formulation prolongs duration of action up to 10–12 hours. Rectal suppository form has a 60-minute onset of action with 3–4 hours of duration. IM route has a 10–20 minutes onset of action and lasts for up to 12 hours.

Distribution
Large volume of distribution. Drug crosses the placenta and is excreted in breast milk.

Metabolism
Metabolism occurs in the liver with excretion mainly in the kidneys. Terminal elimination half-life is 7–8 hours.

Indications

1. Control of nausea and vomiting of various etiologies.
2. Management of the manifestations of psychotic disorders.
3. Acute treatment of generalized nonpsychotic anxiety.

Dosage Range

1. Oral: Recommended dose is 10 mg PO every 4–6 hours. For the slow-release form, dose ranges from 10 to 30 mg PO every 12 hours.
2. Rectal: Recommended dose is 25 mg per rectum (PR) every 12 hours.
3. IM: Recommended dose is 10–25 mg IM every 4–6 hours.
4. IV: Recommended dose is 10–25 mg IV every 4–6 hours.

Special Considerations

1. Contraindicated in patients with known hypersensitivity to phenothiazines.
2. Use with caution in patients who are receiving CNS depressants.
3. Use with caution in elderly patients.
4. Use with caution in patients with glaucoma.
5. Patients should be advised to avoid heat exposure as prochlorperazine may interfere with thermoregulatory mechanisms.
6. Use with caution in patients under the age of 35 years as there is an increased risk of dystonic reactions.
7. Patients should be advised to avoid sun exposure to prevent photosensitivity reactions.

Toxicity 1

Drowsiness, sedation, insomnia, dizziness, and blurred vision.

Toxicity 2

Extrapyramidal reactions in the form of motor restlessness, tremor, akathisia, dystonia, pseudoparkinsonism, and tardive dyskinesia.

Toxicity 3

Dry mouth, constipation.

Toxicity 4

Orthostatic hypotension.

Toxicity 5

Mild photosensitivity, skin rash, and urticaria.

COMMON ANTIEMETIC REGIMENS FOR CHEMOTHERAPY-INDUCED NAUSEA AND VOMITING:

Mildly Emetogenic Chemotherapy (Levels 1 and 2):

1. Prochlorperazine 10–25 mg PO, 5–25 mg IV, or 25 mg PR before chemotherapy and then 10–25 mg PO every 4–6 hours as needed.
2. Thiethylperazine 10 mg PO, 10 mg IM, or 10 mg PR every 4–6 hours as needed.
3. Ondansetron 8 mg PO bid with the first dose 30 minutes before the start of chemotherapy and a subsequent dose 8 hours after the first dose or 32 mg IV.
4. Dexamethasone 4–8 mg PO or 10–20 mg IV before chemotherapy and every 4-6 hours as needed.
5. Prochlorperazine 10–25 mg PO, 5–25 mg IV, or 25 mg PR before chemotherapy and then 10–25 mg PO every 6 hours as needed; dexamethasone 4 mg PO or 10–20 mg IV before chemotherapy and continue with 4 mg PO every 6 hours up to a total of 4 doses as needed.
6. Prochlorperazine 10–25 mg PO, 5–25 mg IV, or 25 mg PR before chemotherapy and then 10–25 mg PO every 6 hours as needed; dexamethasone 4 mg PO or 10–20 mg IV before chemotherapy and continue with 4 mg PO every 6 hours up to a total of 4 doses as needed; and lorazepam 1.5 mg/m^2 IV administered 45 minutes before chemotherapy.
7. Metoclopramide 20–40 mg PO and diphenhydramine 25–50 mg PO every 4–6 hours as needed.
8. Metoclopramide 1–2 mg/kg IV and diphenhydramine 25–50 mg IV every 4–6 hours as needed.

Moderately Emetogenic Chemotherapy (Level 3):

1. Ondansetron 32 mg IV and dexamethasone 4–8 mg PO or 10–20 mg IV given 30 minutes before chemotherapy. In the next 1–2 mornings, give ondansetron 16 mg PO and dexamethasone 8 mg PO along with prochlorperazine 10 mg PO every 6 hours as needed.
2. Dolasetron 100 mg PO or IV and dexamethasone 8 mg IV 30 minutes before chemotherapy. In the next 1–2 mornings, give dolasetron 100 mg PO and dexamethasone 8 mg PO along with prochlorperazine 10 mg PO every 6 hours as needed.
3. Granisetron 1–2 mg PO 1 hour before chemotherapy or 1 mg or 10 μg/kg IV and dexamethasone 8 mg IV 30 minutes before chemotherapy. In the next 1–2 mornings, give granisetron 1 mg PO and dexamethasone 8 mg PO along with prochlorperazine 10 mg PO every 6 hours as needed.

4. Aprepitant 125 mg PO taken 60 minutes before chemotherapy; dexamethasone 12 mg PO and ondansetron 32 mg IV given 30 minutes before chemotherapy.

5. Aprepitant 125 mg PO taken 60 minutes before chemotherapy; dexamethasone 12 mg PO and granisetron 1–2 mg PO or 10 µg/kg IV given 30 minutes before chemotherapy.

6. Aprepitant 115 mg IV taken 30 minutes before chemotherapy; dexamethasone 12 mg PO and granisetron 1–2 mg PO or 10 µg/kg IV given 30 minutes before chemotherapy.

7. Dexamethasone 4–8 mg PO or 10–20 mg IV for one dose before chemotherapy; lorazepam 1.5 µg/m² IV before chemotherapy; and prochlorperazine 5–25 mg PO or IV before chemotherapy.

8. Palonosetron 0.25 mg IV given 30 minutes before chemotherapy.

9. Palonosetron 0.25 mg IV given 30 minutes before chemotherapy; aprepitant 125 mg PO taken 60 minutes before chemotherapy on day 1, and 80 mg PO on days 2–3; dexamethasone 12 mg PO taken 30 minutes before chemotherapy on day 1, and 8 mg PO on days 2–3.

Highly Emetogenic Chemotherapy (Levels 4 and 5):

1. Ondansetron 32 mg IV and dexamethasone 10–20 mg IV plus lorazepam 1 mg PO or IV given 30 minutes before chemotherapy and then every 6 hours as needed. Ondansetron 16 mg PO and dexamethasone 8 mg PO in the next 2–3 mornings along with prochlorperazine 10 mg PO every 6 hours as needed.

2. Dolasetron 100 mg IV and dexamethasone 10–20 mg IV 30 minutes before chemotherapy or the same doses given orally 1 hour before chemotherapy. Dolasetron 100 mg PO and dexamethasone 8 mg PO in the next 2–3 mornings along with prochlorperazine 10 mg PO every 6 hours as needed.

3. Dolasetron 200 mg PO and dexamethasone 20 mg PO 30 minutes before chemotherapy.

4. Granisetron 1 mg or 10 µg/kg IV and dexamethasone 10–20 mg IV 30 minutes before chemotherapy. Granisetron 1 mg PO and dexamethasone 8 mg PO in the next 2–3 mornings along with prochlorperazine 10 mg PO every 6 hours as needed.

5. Aprepitant 125 mg PO taken 60 minutes before chemotherapy on day 1 and 80 mg PO on days 2–3; dexamethasone 12 mg PO and ondansetron 32 mg IV given 30 minutes before chemotherapy.

6. Aprepitant 125 mg PO taken 60 minutes before chemotherapy on day 1 and 80 mg PO on days 2–3; dexamethasone 12 mg PO and granisetron 1–2 mg PO or 10 µg/kg IV given 30 minutes before chemotherapy.

7. Aprepitant 115 mg IV taken 30 minutes before chemotherapy on day 1 and 80 mg PO on days 2–3; dexamethasone 12 mg PO and

granisetron 1–2 mg PO or 10 μg/kg IV given 30 minutes before chemotherapy.

8. Metoclopramide 2–3 mg/kg IV, dexamethasone 10–20 mg IV; and diphenhydramine 25–50 mg IV to be given 1 hour before chemotherapy or orally at the same doses 30 minutes before chemotherapy. Metoclopramide 20–40 mg PO, dexmethasone 8 mg PO in the next 2–3 mornings along with prochlorperazine 10 mg PO every 6 hours as needed.

9. Metoclopramide 2–3 mg/kg IV before chemotherapy and then 2 hours post chemotherapy; dexamethasone 10–20 mg IV; diphenhydramine 25–50 mg IV; and lorazepam 1–2 mg IV.

10. Palonosetron 0.25 mg IV given 30 minutes before chemotherapy.

11. Palonosetron 0.25 mg IV given 30 minutes before chemotherapy; aprepitant 125 mg PO taken 60 minutes before chemotherapy on day 1, and 80 mg PO on days 2–3; dexamethasone 12 mg PO taken 30 minutes before chemotherapy on day 1, and 8 mg PO on days 2–3.

COMMON REGIMENS FOR DELAYED AND/OR BREAKTHROUGH NAUSEA AND VOMITING:

1. Metoclopramide 40 mg PO every 4–6 hours and dexamethasone 4–8 mg PO every 4–6 hours for 4 days.

2. Metoclopramide 40 mg PO every 4–6 hours; dexamethasone 4–8 mg PO every 4–6 hours; and prochlorperazine 10–25 mg PO every 4–6 hours.

3. Aprepitant 80 mg PO and dexamethasone 8–12 mg PO once daily on days 2 and 3.

4. Aprepitant 80 mg PO daily, dexamethasone 8–12 mg PO daily, and ondansetron 8 mg PO bid on days 2 and 3.

5. Aprepitant 80 mg PO daily, dexamethasone 8–12 mg PO daily, and granisetron 1 mg PO bid on days 2 and 3.

6. Aprepitant 80 mg PO daily, dexamethasone 8–12 mg PO daily, and dolasetron 100 mg PO daily on days 2 and 3.

7. Ondansetron 8 mg PO bid for up to 2–3 days after chemotherapy.

8. Ondansetron (orally dissolving tablets) 8 mg sublingual every 8 hours as needed.

9. Metoclopramide 20–40 mg PO and diphenhydramine 50 mg PO every 3–4 hours.

10. Prochlorperazine suppository 25 mg PR every 12 hours.

11. Dolasetron 100 mg PO daily.

12. Nabilone 1–2 mg PO bid.

13. Dronabinol 5–10 mg PO every 4–6 hours.

Table 1. Emetogenic Potential of Chemotherapy Agents

Level	Frequency of Emesis (%)	Agent
5	>90	AC regimen (doxorubicin plus cyclophosphamide)
		Actinomycin-D
		Altretamine
		Carmustine >250 mg/m^2
		Cisplatin ≥50 mg/m^2
		Cyclophosphamide >1,500 mg/m^2
		Dacarbazine >500 mg/m^2
		Mechlorethamine
		Pentostatin
		Procarbazine
		Streptozocin
4	60–90	Carboplatin
		Carmustine 250 mg/m^2
		Cisplatin <50 mg/m^2
		Cyclophosphamide 750–1,500 mg/m^2
		Cytarabine >1 g/m^2
		Doxorubicin >60 mg/m^2
		Irinotecan
		Melphalan (IV)
		Methotrexate >1,000 mg/m^2
3	30–60	Aldesleukin
		Arsenic trioxide
		Cyclophosphamide ≤750 mg/m^2
		Cyclophosphamide (oral)
		Cytarabine (conventional doses)
		Doxorubicin 20–60 mg/m^2
		Epirubicin ≤90 mg/m^2
		5-Fluorouracil >1,000 mg/m^2
		Idarubicin
		Ifosfamide
		Imatinib

Level	Frequency of Emesis (%)	Agent
3	30–60	Methotrexate 250–1,000 mg/m^2
		Mitoxantrone <15 mg/m^2
		Temozolomide
2	10–30	Albumin-bound paclitaxel
		Asparaginase
		Bexarotene
		Capecitabine
		Cetuximab
		Cytarabine 100-200 mg/m^2
		Daunorubicin
		Docetaxel
		Doxorubicin <20 mg/m^2
		Etoposide
		5-Fluorouracil <1,000 mg/m^2
		Gemcitabine
		Liposomal doxorubicin
		Lomustine
		Methotrexate 50–250 mg/m^2
		Mitomycin-C
		Paclitaxel
		Pemetrexed
		Thiotepa
		Topotecan
		Vorinostat
1	<10	Alemtuzumab
		Asparaginase
		Bevacizumab
		Bleomycin
		Bortezomib
		Busulfan
		Cetuximab
		Chlorambucil (oral)
		Cladribine
		Dasatinib
		Decitabine
		Denileukin diftitox
		Erlotinib
		Fludarabine

Level	Frequency of Emesis (%)	Agent
I	<10	Gefitinib
		Gemtuzumab
		Hydroxyurea
		Interferon-α
		Lapatinib
		Lenalidomide
		Melphalan (oral)
		6-Mercaptopurine
		Methotrexate $\leq$50 mg/m^2
		Nelarabine
		Nilotinib
		Panitumumab
		Pentostatin
		Rituximab
		Sorafenib
		Sunitinib
		Temsirolimus
		Thalidomide
		6-Thioguanine (oral)
		Trastuzumab
		Tretinoin
		Vinblastine
		Vincristine
		Vinorelbine

Adapted and taken from: Hesketh et al. *J Clin Oncol* 1997;15:103–109; Gralla et al. *J Clin Oncol* 1998;17:2971–2994; Grunberg et al. *Support Care Cancer* 2005;13:80–84; and NCCN Clinical Practice Guidelines in Oncology, V.3.2009. Antiemesis. NCCN 2009.

Single agents are divided into five different levels of emetogenic potential. They are as follows:

1. Level 1: <10% of patients experience acute (<24 hours after chemotherapy) emesis without antiemetic prophylaxis.
2. Level 2: 10%–30% of patients experience acute emesis without antiemetic prophylaxis.
3. Level 3: 30%–60% of patients experience acute emesis without antiemetic prophylaxis.
4. Level 4: 60%–90% of patients experience acute emesis without antiemetic prophylaxis.
5. Level 5: >90% of patients experience acute emesis without antiemetic prophylaxis.

With regard to combination regimens, the emetogenic levels are determined by identifying the most emetogenic agent in the combination and then assessing the relative contribution of the other agents based on the following:

1. Level 1 agents do not contribute to the emetogenic potential of the combination.
2. The presence of one or more level 2 agents increases the emetogenic potential of the combination by one level greater than the most emetogenic agent in the combination.
3. The presence of level 3 or level 4 agents increases the emetogenic potential of the combination by one level per given agent.

Index